Health effects of environmental pollutants

Health effects of environmental pollutants

GEORGE L. WALDBOTT, M.D.

With 117 illustrations

THE C. V. MOSBY COMPANY

Saint Louis   1973

VH/M/M   9   8   7   6   5   4   3

PREFACE

During the past two decades an abundance of technical, biological, and legal information dealing with air pollution has accumulated; however, there is an extraordinary paucity of data on how pollutants affect human health. Indeed, a survey of the air pollution literature conveys the impression that animals, plants, and materials are adversely affected by polluted air but that, at levels in which pollutants are present in the atmosphere, little if any serious damage to human health ensues. The question arises whether humans are really not subject to adverse effects from polluted air or whether damage to health actually occurs but is not being recognized by the scientific community. A number of circumstances render damage caused by polluted ambient air difficult to identify with its sources.

In the past, environmental health has been largely the domain of physicians associated with industry and with public health. The practicing clinician has had relatively little exposure to environmental diseases.

Furthermore, diseases resulting from air pollutants develop slowly and inconspicuously. They are, therefore, difficult to relate to their cause. When pathologists find at autopsy a chronic condition within the kidney, liver, or bone disease, their mission is regarded accomplished. Only in exceptional cases can they pinpoint the original source of a chronic illness, a task as difficult as detection of the cause or causes of cancer.

Those of us who have been engaged in the specialty of allergy frequently encounter patients in whom air pollution either precipitated or aggravated respiratory illness or an allergic skin disease. To document such cases in a scientifically convincing manner is almost insurmountable. Most clinicians lack the tools to relate an illness to a specific pollutant. Laboratory facilities to analyze blood, urine, and organ tissue for a suspected poison are not readily available. Furthermore, the interpretation of findings gleaned from laboratory tests is difficult. Relatively few physicians have been alerted to the manner in which a specific air pollutant interferes with human health. In small communities where the populace relies upon an industry for its livelihood, even the patients themselves are reluctant to cooperate because they fear unpleasant repercussions.

The statistical approach for documenting illness resulting from air pollution is effective only in rare instances. Because of the numerous variables, which are difficult to control, sampling must cover many thousands or even millions of individuals. Furthermore, the interaction between airborne agents alters the effects of an individual pollutant.

Because of the above-mentioned sparsity of data on how ambient air affects humans, I was obliged to resort to data gleaned from animal experiments and from occupational exposures in which the concentrations are much higher than those associated with ambient air. Attempts have been made throughout the book to distinguish between such effects and those of low-grade, long-term exposures.

In selection of the bibliography emphasis has been placed on the clinical aspect of the problem.

To facilitate assessment of a disease caused by a specific agent, pollutants have been classified according to their health effects. Since most pollutants exhibit diverse effects to multiple organs, some overlapping in the various categories was inevitable.

The Environmental Protection Agency in Durham, North Carolina, particularly through Wave Elaine Culver; the librarians Helene Norris, Barbara Johnson, and Ann Vander at Hutzel and Harper Hospitals of Detroit; and the personnel of the Shiffman Medical Library have given me valuable assistance.

Others who have given me helpful advice in the preparation of this book are Dr. Carole B. Boyd, Wayne State University, School of Medicine, Department of Pathol-ogy, Detroit; Prof. Albert W. Burgstahler, University of Kansas, Department of Chemistry; Dr. Harold Chen, Children's Hospital of Michigan, Bio-statistic Department, Detroit; Dr. Basil Considine, Jr., Hutzel Hospital, Department of Radiology, Detroit; Dr. Harriet L. Hardy, Massachusetts General Hospital, Boston; Mr. James P. Lodge, National Center for Atmospheric Research, Boulder, Colorado; Dr. F. A. Prantl, Atomic Energy of Canada Limited, Environmental Research Branch, Chalk River, Ontario; Dr. Irving J. Selikoff, Mount Sinai School of Medicine, Environmental Sciences Laboratory, New York; Dr. William G. Van de Riet, Wayne State University, Department of Radiology and Medicine, Detroit. I am particularly grateful to members of the Hutzel Hospital staff, especially Drs. Boris K. Silberberg and Kenneth M. Nowicki, to Jim Hanna and John Shay, the hospital's photographer. My secretary Linda Pasco has displayed unremitting interest in completing the book, and this book could not have been written without the invaluable assistance of my wife, Edith M. Waldbott.

To them, as well as to many others who have cooperated and encouraged me in collecting the material, I wish to express my appreciation.

George L. Waldbott
28411 Hoover Road
Warren, Michigan 48093

CONTENTS

Health effects of environmental pollutants

1
DISASTERS

FROM BELGIUM TO NEW JERSEY

Meuse Valley disaster. On December 3 to 5, 1930, the densely populated Meuse River Valley west of Liège, Belgium, was the scene of the first significant, and one of the worst, industrial air pollution disasters. Several thousand persons became violently ill and sixty persons died during the three-day period.

During the three fatal days, the mist that covered the entire country of Belgium was particularly concentrated along the narrow valley of the River Meuse from the town of Huy to Liège in a strip 20 km (12 miles) long, about 1 to 2 km (0.6 to 1.2 miles) wide, and 60 to 80 meters deep (Fig. 1-1). The barometric pressure was high. Temperatures during the day were at or below freezing. Except for a slight easterly breeze, there was no wind. The smoke from the factories, combined with fog, had turned into a familiar "soupy" mixture that settled on the ground.

People became ill simultaneously throughout the entire valley on December 3, when the mist reached its maximum density. The victims became hoarse and short of breath. A persistent cough yielded a frothy phlegm succeeded by a puslike mass. Many became nauseated and vomited. The sixty deaths were the result of acute heart failure. No new cases occurred after December 5, when the fog cleared.

The majority of the affected individuals were elderly people whose lungs or hearts were already weakened by other causes. However, young and perfectly healthy persons also became seriously ill. Curiously, cattle contracted the same illness, marked by fast, shallow breathing and acute emphysema. Some eventually died. Rats and birds in the area were also affected.

Donora. Because of the general lack of interest in air pollution, which prevailed at that time, the Belgian disaster failed to arouse sufficient interest for significant preventive measures to be instituted elsewhere. Had precautions been taken, the greatest air pollution disaster in the United States, which occurred 18 years later on the last few days of October, 1948, in Donora, Pennsylvania, could have been averted.

The circumstances surrounding the Donora disaster resembled remarkably those of the Meuse Valley. Large zinc smelters, plants producing wire, steel, and sulfuric acid, as well as many other factories, lined the river front solidly for 3 miles in the horseshoe-shaped Monongahela Valley. Freight trains, operating day and night on both sides of the river and propelled by steam locomotives burning high-volatile soft coal, emitted clouds of smoke that were trapped by hills surrounding the river, some of which rise abruptly as high as 350 feet (Fig. 1-2).

A high-pressure condition had moved into western Pennsylvania, eastern Ohio, parts of Virginia, West Virginia, and Maryland. Rainfall had added fog and moisture

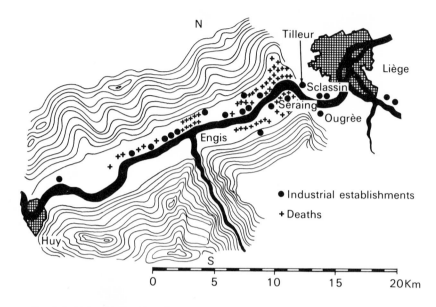

Fig. 1-1. Meuse Valley. Distribution of deaths in relation to location of factories.

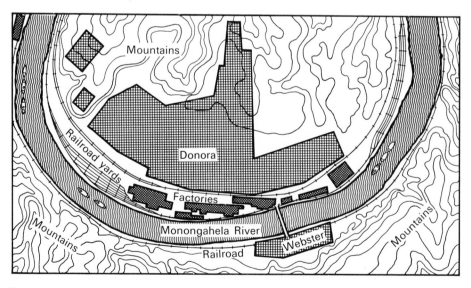

Fig. 1-2. The environs of Donora. The horseshoe curve of the Monongahela River is surrounded by mountains. Railroad tracks are located on both sides of the river. The low-lying stretch of the Monongahela Valley between railroad and river is a natural trap for pollutants.

to the valley's air. On October 26, the first day of the inversion (Fig. 1-3), the weather was cold and wind velocity was near zero. A constant smog blanket produced a virtually airtight chamber, day and night, for more than 5 days, during which time the air was permeated by an odor of sulfur.

Twenty persons, seventeen in Donora and three in nearby Webster, died during the fateful days and 5910 persons, representing 42% of the people of that area, were stricken with irritation in eyes, nose, and throat, pains and constriction in the chest, cough, labored breathing, severe headaches, and nausea and vomiting.

At a football game between Donora and Monongahela High Schools, players were obliged to drop out of the game because of chest pains, cough, and shortness of breath. Patients improved temporarily when they stayed in their homes and closed their doors. According to health authorities the older the Donorian, the more likely he was to become ill from the polluted air. Some of those exposed to it were perma-

nently injured and subsequent deaths were attributed by Public Health Service physicians to the air contamination. A veterinarian sent in by the Public Health Service reported that two dogs, seven chickens, three cats, two canaries, and two rabbits died from the smoke. According to a follow-up study 10 years later,[1] Donorians who became acutely ill at the time of the smog episode showed a higher mortality and illness prevalence than others who were residing in the town at that time. The highest illness rates following the disaster were among smokers who had become ill during the episode; the lowest rates were in nonsmokers who were not ill during the inversion.

London. A different picture unfolded in London, England, on December 4, 1952. A high pressure mass of cold air was moving from Europe across the English Channel toward the Thames Valley. Unlike the deep valleys in the Monongahela and Meuse topography, the broad stretch of the relatively low Thames Valley extends over many square miles. Because of cold

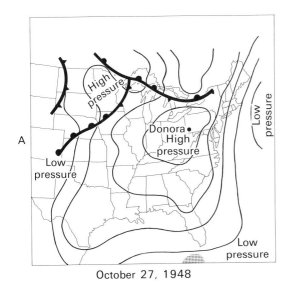

October 27, 1948

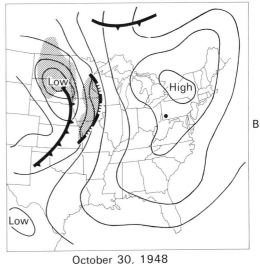

October 30, 1948

Fig. 1-3. Surface weather charts for October 27 and 30, 1948, during the Donora, Pennsylvania, air pollution episode.

temperature and moist air, Londoners' fireplaces were working overtime.

There was practically a complete cessation of air movement. For 5 days the city was engulfed in a heavy cloud of smoke that had condensed in the moisture of London's fog. Within a radius of 20 miles the smoke had rendered the atmosphere so opaque that there were collisions of automobiles and trains on land. A steam ferry collided with a vessel at anchor on the Thames. At Earls' Court, where a show of prize cattle had been in progress, some 160 animals developed fast, labored breathing and fever. Among the dozen animals that were autopsied, inflammatory changes in the bronchial tree, pneumonia, and emphysema were found.

When the fog lifted after 5 days, most Londoners had not as yet realized the seriousness of the disaster in terms of sickness and deaths in the population. During the week ending December 13, *2851 persons above the usual death rate had lost their lives. During the following weeks, another 1224 deaths were attributed to the fog.* Even today it is impossible to assess adequately the death toll caused by respiratory and heart diseases in the wake of this disaster.

In 1956 London was again the scene of a fog disaster. This time there were *about 1000 deaths above the usual death rate*, although the fog lasted only 18 hours.

Los Angeles. In the Meuse Valley and in Donora, industrial complexes emitted their poisonous fumes; in London, the smoke originated from fireplaces and became mixed with the moisture of the British fog. In Los Angeles, California, however, a combination of automobile exhaust and the California sunshine produced a special brand of pollution called "smog." The conditions that produce smog are being duplicated in other large United States and foreign metropolitan areas where sunshine and heavy automobile traffic prevail and in cities like New York, where high buildings interfere with the dispersion of toxic pollutants.

In Los Angeles, pollution is at its worst during the day, when traffic is heavy and the sun is shining[2]; in London, pollution is most severe at night, when fireplaces and coal furnaces are working at their peak and when fog blankets the city. In Los Angeles, the highly oxidizing type of "smog" contains a mixture of ozone, oxides of nitrogen, and peroxidized organic compounds, especially peroxyacetyl nitrate (PAN), which are formed in the air under the influence of the sun's ultraviolet rays.

Hydrocarbons and nitric acid reach their peak concentrations with the early morning traffic; whereas the maximum concentrations of oxidants is not reached until the sunlight is sufficiently intense for the photochemical reactions to gather speed.

Since 1943, residents of Los Angeles have been concerned about this greatest nuisance of their city. According to a California State Health Department Survey[3] about three fourths of the population of metropolitan areas in southern California experience a peculiar burning and annoying irritation of their eyes at peak periods of smog. Health officials have assured the people that they need not worry about any permanent eye damage; but, in spite of an impressive body of valuable research, no adequate *clinical* assessment of the potential hazard to the general health of the community is available.

In Los Angeles as in London, Donora, and the Meuse Valley, the constant outpouring of pollutants led to several acute episodes, namely in 1942, 1954, and in late August and early September of 1955. At the time of the last-mentioned incident a severe heat wave with temperatures above 100° had engulfed Los Angeles for over a week. The clouds of automobile exhaust in the streets, triggered by the intense ultraviolet radiation of sunshine, led to formation of the irritating chemicals, particularly ozone and peroxyacetyl nitrates.

Asthma and bronchitis appeared in epidemic proportions and raised the local mortality among persons of 65 and over from an average of about 70 to 317 a day.[4] Persons with heart and lung disease were particularly hard hit.

Numerous minor episodes of air pollution have occurred in the United States and in other countries, the impact of which is rarely recognized. Only when damage occurs in startling proportions, do health authorities become cognizant of the seriousness of the pollution with respect to human health.

Piscataway. On September 16, 1971, Quibbletown Junior High School in Piscataway, a New Jersey town 20 miles south of the Newark Airport and 30 miles southwest of New York, was the focal point of a serious inversion (Fig. 1-4).[5] By early afternoon the temperature was 86°, humidity 68%, and winds a feeble 2 knots per hour. Seven major state and federal highways, which are linked together by busy boulevards, pass within 8 miles of the school. Dozens of factories including many chemical plants are located close to the railroads and expressways.

The 8 A.M. count of oxidants at a Newark parking lot, as registered by pollution gauges, was .022 ppm (parts per million), a level higher than usual but not considered cause for alarm. However, by 3 P.M. the oxidant count was abnormally high, namely .080 ppm in Newark and .096 ppm at another monitoring station in Bayonne. A light easterly wind was moving from Raritan Bay across the heavily industrial Perth Amboy area, past the New Jersey Turnpike and the Garden State Parkway. It passed dozens of other highways, boulevards, and factories. Some of the polluted air was blocked by the 653-foot Watchung Ridge. By midafternoon the smog had engulfed an area 25 miles long and 10 miles wide.

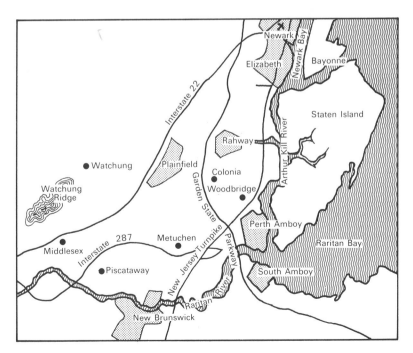

Fig. 1-4. Location of Piscataway in relation to other large industrialized New Jersey and New York areas.

At the Quibbletown Junior High School students practicing football suddenly experienced excessive lacrimation (tearing), reddened throats, breathing difficulties, cough, and considerable pain in the chest on inspiration. They also displayed systemic symptoms such as vomiting, pain in the abdomen, and tingling in the extremities. In several boys the abdominal pains persisted for two days.

At Sayreville High School, 10 miles southeast of Quibbletown School six soccer players and nine football players were similarly affected. Twenty-three miles and 14 miles north of Quibbletown School, at Verona High School and in Millburn, respectively, 16 of 65 football players and 15 of 40 soccer players complained of wheezing and dry throats. The story was about the same on the playing fields of at least 6 other schools within 20 miles of Quibbletown School. For some unexplained reason the athletes at some schools became more seriously ill than at other schools and in some they remained unaffected. No data have been made available so far on the morbidity of populations in the affected area or on the possible increase in mortality caused by the smoke.

On the morning after the incident the only abnormal findings obtained from a large series of tests that were carried out on seven of the afflicted boys were an alkaline phosphatase level of 728 units in one boy (normal, 30 to 85 units); an elevated total bilirubin level of 1.2 to 2.4 mg/100 ml in six boys (normal, 1 mg/100 ml); and high lactic dehydrogenase level of 445 and 559 in two boys (normal, 200 units). The last-mentioned test is indicative of damage to the heart, the others indicate a disturbed liver function.[6] One unusual finding was the low cholinesterase* levels in blood drawn on the day of the incident. The ranges were between 14.73 and 24.20

in red blood cells and between 1.61 and 5.49 in serum (normal, 50 to 100 "number" in red blood cells and 50 to 130 "number" in serum). Although no definite conclusions can be drawn with respect to large populations, it appears that a selected group of individuals had been harmed more than others (see Chapter 18).

EVALUATION OF THE DISASTERS

Numerous scientists have been at work in an attempt to relate the illness encountered in these episodes to one or more particular pollutants. They were handicapped, especially in the two early disasters, because they lacked the tools of assessing the magnitude of many airborne pollutants and the results of their interaction with each other.

In Los Angeles officials of local and state health departments have made great strides in unravelling a highly complicated problem by discovering the intricate photochemical action of the sun on vehicle exhaust gases. Although to date they have not succeeded in eliminating the hazard completely, they have reduced remarkably the daily outpouring of pollutants into the air.

Similarly, in London much progress has been made by limiting the use of soft coal in home fireplaces.[7] In contrast to the Donora and Meuse Valley disasters, where smelting and manufacturing establishments were responsible for the emission of industrial pollutants, the great London air pollution catastrophe of 1952 was precipitated mainly by burning of coal and other fuel in thousands of fireplaces in conjunction with the high moisture content of the London fog. Here, such agents as carbon monoxide, carbon dioxide, sulfur dioxide, and tar were thought to have played a significant role.[8] In view of their delayed action on the respiratory tract and because of the high incidence of respiratory disorders following rather than during the December fog, it is likely that respiratory irri-

---

*An enzyme involved in transmission of nerve impulses.

tants did exact their toll by acting together. In addition, such agents as fluoride, cadmium, mercury, and many other constituents of coal were also escaping from the burning fireplaces. Both coal and wood contain between 50 to 200 ppm fluoride,[9] 0.10 to 0.25 ppm cadmium,[10] and 0.09 to 33 ppm mercury.[11]

Concerning the Piscataway episode, no data on the magnitude of the various air pollutants are, as yet, available. The low content of cholinesterase (an enzyme affected by chlorinated phosphate pesticides [Chapter 18]) in the blood of the afflicted persons suggests that the pesticides that were being manufactured in the area influenced the activity of this enzyme.

Opinions regarding causes of the Meuse Valley and the Donora disasters were and still are sharply divided. The Belgian government had set up a commission with an allotment of 250,000 francs to study the cause of the disaster. They concluded that poisonous products in waste gases emanating from many factories in the valley acted in conjunction with unusual climatic conditions. They placed most of the blame on sulfur dioxide (SO_2), which was detected in the factory smoke.

Several other scientists including the noted lung specialist of the University of Leyden, Holland, Storm VanLeeuwen, expressed the opinion that the disease in question represented acute intoxication by gaseous fluoride compounds, substances about whose effect on health little information was available at that time.

Shortly after the disaster, Kaj Roholm of Copenhagen began a thorough investigation on his own. He had previously studied fluoride intoxication in workers where cryolite, a fluoride-bearing rock, was being mined.

Roholm[12] questioned the likelihood that a local irritant to the lungs, such as sulfur dioxide, was the principal culprit. Although the victims coughed, their eyes watered, and they were short of breath, in the last

10 patients who were autopsied the bronchial tree and the lungs showed relatively little damage and some appeared to be perfectly healthy. No more deaths occurred after the fog in the Meuse Valley and in Donora had lifted, which is in contrast to the London disaster of 1952. In fact, some of the survivors had recovered rapidly as soon as they had climbed the nearby hills, where they were above the fog. Such prompt recovery could not have taken place if sulfur dioxide had done significant damage to the delicate lining of the respiratory tract. Pneumonia would have ensued and more deaths would have occurred at a later date than at the time of the fog. Sulfur dioxide and its related sulfur compound sulfur trioxide (SO_3) attack the respiratory organs but leave little or no remote systemic effect elsewhere in the system. Roholm implicated fluoride as the poison that must have entered the bloodstream and attacked the heart and other internal organs. At least 15 of the 27 factories in the area employed fluoride-containing raw materials in their manufacturing process. The 15 factories included four large iron works with blast furnaces and steel works, three large metal works, four glass works and ceramic factories, three zinc works, and one superphosphate fertilizer factory. Silicon tetrafluoride (SiF_4) and hydrogen fluoride (HF) are by-products of all of these manufacturing processes and are emitted as gaseous materials into the atmosphere.

Steel and metal works employ fluorspar (CaF_2). During smelting, silicon tetrafluoride gas escapes according to the following reaction:

$$3\ SiO_2 + 2\ CaF_2 = SiF_4 + 2\ CaSiO_3$$
(silicon dioxide + fluorspar = silicon tetrafluoride + calcium silicate)

In glass and pottery manufacturing, fluorspar and cryolite are added to raw material in order to facilitate melting and to produce certain properties in the finished product. Zinc ore contains fluorspar, cadmium, and lead. In superphosphate manufacturing, hydrofluoric acid and silicon tetrafluoride are liberated. In addition, in the area where most deaths occurred, window panes and electric bulbs had lost their gloss, a positive sign of the action of corrosive fluoride gases.

Roholm calculated that at least 30 mg hydrofluoric acid per cubic meter of air (a cube with sides the size of a bridge table) had collected in the stagnant air of the valley. This is the minimum fatal concentration for guinea pigs, which are much less susceptible to fluoride damage than are humans. Roholm also reasoned that the polluting agent had been emitted in two widely separated areas: in the wide entrance to the Meuse Valley, with its large metal works, and in the Meuse city of Engis, where the zinc and superphosphate works were located (Fig. 1-1). In the strip of several kilometers between the two regions, no fatalities had occurred. The light easterly winds had concentrated the pollutants southeast of the two regions (principally along the north bank of the river at the north wall of the valley where immense masses of soot and dust had been emitted from the works) and promoted condensation of smoke. The solid fluorine compounds had dissolved partially in the microscopic particles of the water present in the moist air. Thus, they had become unusually active and easily absorbable into the bloodstream from the lungs after inhalation.

Fluorides were also implicated in the Donora disaster by Philip Sadtler,[13] a chemist of Philadelphia and the consultant for the city of Donora. He found over 1000 ppm fluoride in an air-conditioning unit, in conjunction with sulfur dioxide and carbon monoxide. Blood from the diseased and hospitalized patients showed twelve to twenty-five times the normal quantities of fluoride and those who died had displayed symptoms of chronic fluoride poisoning prior to the disaster. A high incidence of "mottled teeth"—white specks on the tooth

enamel, a sign of previous internal damage by fluoride—had been prevalent among the young people of the area. Corn crops had shown typical fluoride damage and most vegetables growing north of the town had been killed. Sadtler reasoned that the acute outbreak had climaxed a long-term pollution problem that had remained unrecognized by the authorities. The U. S. Public Health Service initiated an investigation[14] two months after the disaster. They disagreed with Sadtler's opinion. In pooled urine specimens from 19 adults and children they found an average of 0.2 ppm fluoride, a level that the Public Health Service investigators considered "normal."[*]

Three human ribs from the deceased contained from 174 to 1400 ppm fluoride (fat free). Although some scientists consider these levels "normal," others[16] have reported crippling bone disease at such levels after long-term fluoride consumption.

At the time when the Public Health Service began sampling the air for fluoride and other pollutants, the production of the zinc and steel plants had been considerably curtailed. Even then, the air still contained as much as 5.9 mg of fluoride per cubic meter which, according to what was then considered the "best available information," could not have caused any serious disease. Today however the maximum allowable safe concentration for fluoride in the air for a 40-hour week for a healthy worker is 2.5 mg/meter^3 in the United States, 2 mg in Germany, and 0.5 mg in the U.S.S.R.[17]

Another poisonous agent, zinc ammonium sulfate, is considered a major factor in the Donora air pollution episode by Amdur and Corn[18] scientists at Massachusetts Institute of Technology whose major

---

[*]Recent experiences have shed doubt on the diagnostic reliability of urinary assays for fluoride as well as for many other air pollutants, particularly when a number of specimens are pooled prior to analysis instead of each being studied individually[15] (see Chapter 13).

interest has been the study of sulfur oxides. Zinc, lead, and cadmium are emitted from zinc smelters. In view of the fact that ammonium zinc sulfate is a pulmonary irritant, not a systemic poison, it is not likely to have caused the systemic symptoms manifested by the Donora patients.

Like the Meuse Valley official investigators, the Donora team concluded that a combination of several toxic agents caused the disaster and that not one of these agents by itself could have reached high enough levels in the air to have been responsible for damage. Neither committee, however, recognized the dominant significance of fluorides among these agents. Apparently neither the members of the Donora nor of the Meuse Valley investigating team were aware of Roholm's account of the Belgian disaster, since they made no reference to it in their report.

In the above-described disasters, sudden outbursts of pollution took the lives of many and damaged the health of numerous others. As will be demonstrated in subsequent chapters, this is in contrast to the slow erosion of a person's health by the ever-present pollution in cities, particularly among those residing near industrial establishments or those exposed to automobile exhaust and to the many other contaminants.

Difficult though it was for the appointed scientists to pinpoint the cause of pollution disasters involving large populations, how much more difficult is the task of physicians to relate to its cause or causes an illness that creeps upon one slowly and insidiously with vague, inconspicuous symptoms and with few tangible laboratory or other clinical features. Epidemiologic statistics, that is, surveys on large population groups, are of relatively limited value because numerous variables render controls (populations not exposed to pollutants for comparison) practically impossible to find.

Clothing and faces may become dirty from dust and smoke, ships and automobiles may collide because of smog, vegetation may deteriorate, and domestic animals may succumb to the effects of pollution, yet these experiences are insignificant compared to the risks to which humans are exposed when they inhale or ingest airborne toxic agents year after year for a lifetime. The subsequent chapters, in large part, will be devoted to the diseases to which everyone living in our civilized environment is susceptible to a greater or lesser extent.

REFERENCES

1. Ciocco, A., and Thompson, D. J.: A follow-up of Donora ten years after: methodology and findings, Amer. J. Public Health 51:155-164, 1961.
2. Profile of Air Pollution Control, Air Pollution Control District, County of Los Angeles, 1971, Los Angeles, California.
3. California Health Department Survey: Air pollution: effects reported by California residents, Berkeley, California, 1960.
4. Goldsmith, J. R., and Breslow, L.: Epidemiological aspects of air pollution, J. Air Pollut. Contr. Ass. 9:129, 1959.
5. Jackson, D.: The cloud comes to Quibbletown, Life 71:72-75, 79-82, 1971.
6. Harrison, M. J.: Personal communication, January 27, 1972.
7. Lawther, P. J., and Bonnell, J. A.: Some recent trends in pollution and health in London, and some current thoughts. Presented at the Second International Clean Air Congress, Washington, D. C., December 6-11, 1970.
8. Wilkins, E. T.: Air pollution and the London fog of December 1952, J. Roy. Sanit. Inst. 74:1-15, 1954.
9. Monkhouse, A. C.: The minor constituents of coal, Coke and Gas 12:363-368, 1950.
10. Schroeder, H. A.: Personal communication, 1972.
11. Joensuu, O. J.: Fossil fuels as a source of mercury pollution, Science 172:1027, 1971.
12. Roholm, K.: The fog disaster in the Meuse Valley: a fluorine intoxication, J. Industr. Hyg. Toxicol. 19:126-137, 1937.
13. Sadtler, P.: Fluorine gases in atmosphere as industrial waste blamed for death and chronic poisoning of Donora and Webster, Pa. inhabitants, Chemical and Engineering News 26:3692, 1948.
14. Schrenk, H. H., Heimann, H., Clayton, G. D., and others: Air pollution in Donora, Pa. Epidemiology of the unusual smog episode of Oc-

tober 1948, Prelim. Rep. Pub. Health Bull. 306, 1949.

15. Waldbott, G. L.: Fluoride in clinical medicine, Internat. Arch. Allergy Appl. Immunol. **20**(Suppl. 1):1-50, 1962.

16. Singh, A., Jolly, S. S., Bansal, B. C., and others: Endemic fluorosis, Medicine **42**:229, 1963.

17. Threshold limit values of airborne contaminants, Adopted by ACGIH for 1969, Industr. Hyg. Digest 33:4-13, 1969.

18. Amdur, M. O., and Corn, M.: Irritant potency of zinc ammonium sulfate of different particle size, Amer. Industr. Hyg. Ass. J. **24**:326, 1963.

2
POLLUTANTS AND THEIR SOURCES

Most people identify air pollution with a cloud of smoke emanating from the chimney of a factory or the exhaust of an automobile. These are indeed the principal sources of air contamination, but actually any airborne matter can pollute the air. It might be derived from natural sources such as volcanoes, swamps, and forests; it might originate from a source on the ground; or it might be a so-called secondary pollutant formed in the air by interaction of several agents under the influence of moisture, heat, sunlight, and other forces, some of which are not yet fully understood. Continuous changes that are taking place aloft render the total polluted air mass over a populated area highly unstable.

FORM OF POLLUTANTS

Pollutants occur either as gases or as fine particles, usually referred to as particulate matter. Both forms are present in the atmosphere simultaneously, but gases constitute about 90% of all pollutants. Indeed, pollution of the air by a single agent is nonexistent, although one or a few chemicals may be dominant near a given industrial complex. The kinds of pollutants that are present in the atmosphere are contained in the following list.

Kinds of pollutants

gases Gaseous phase of liquid or solid matter
mists Fine liquid droplets suspended in air
vapors Gaseous state of a volatile solid or liquid
clouds Same as vapors, but formed aloft
fog Same as clouds, based on ground
haze Dust or salt particles suspended in water droplets
dust Solids suspended in air, resulting from fragmentation of matter
smoke Gas-borne solids from incomplete combustion
soot Finely divided carbon particles adhering together
fumes Minute particles from combustion of metals

Particulates are either solids or fine liquid droplets called mists. They vary over a wide range according to size, shape, density, and chemical composition. Even though they make up only 10% of all pollutants of the air, they are very significant in their biologic action.

Many primary pollutants participate in reactions in the atmosphere by producing secondary pollutants, such as ozone and other constitutents of photochemical smog. Water droplets, for instance, combine with acids such as hydrogen sulfide (the gas with the rotten-egg odor) to produce acid aerosols (particles suspended in vapor) that are corrosive. The wide variety of such reactions, which are constantly taking place, is one reason for the difficulties encountered in assessing the biologic effects of an individual pollutant.

Smoke, a mixture of gases with particulate substance, is produced by three processes: burning, vaporization, and dispersion into the air. If smoke is gray or black, it contains much carbon from the incomplete combustion of coal. A brownish-red color indicates a high content of iron oxide particles, usually derived from the steel and coal industry. Other solid particles in smoke are compounds of silica, fluoride, aluminum, lead, and such organic material as hydrocarbons, acids, bases, and phenols. *Soot*, derived from fireplace smoke, for example, consists of finely divided carbon particles.

Dense smoke usually contains an abundance of water vapor. *Fog* rises from the ground, usually from bodies of water; whereas *clouds* are formed in the air. Fog shows no visible downward movement; clouds, unlike fog, have no base on the ground. They provide an excellent vehicle for spreading pollutants. *Haze* consists of suspended dust or salt particles so small that they cannot be seen with the naked eye. Haze has a bluish tinge when viewed against a dark background in distinction to the gray hue of fog. *Fumes*, on the other hand, originate from combustion of metal or oils. They give the smoke an opaque appearance.

Dust is a mixture of particles whose di-

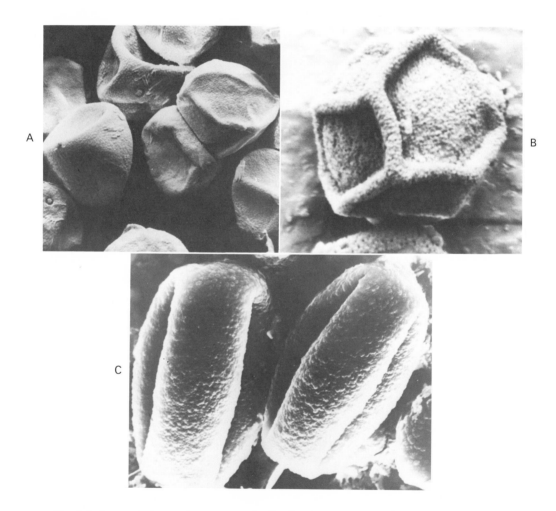

Fig. 2-1. Scanning electronphotomicrograph of pollens. **A,** June grass *(Poa pratensis)*; **B,** eastern cottonwood *(Populus deltoides)*; and **C,** white oak *(Quercus alba).* (Courtesy Allergy Laboratories of Ohio, Inc., Columbus, Ohio.)

ameter is larger than that of a single small molecule ranging from 0.0002 micron (μ) to 500 μ (one micron is one thousandth of a millimeter or 0.000039 inch). It is either of natural or industrial origin. Dust is derived from disintegration of solids. The large-sized dust particles (about 10 μ) are usually not carried far from their source except at times of high winds.

Virtually every human activity and, indeed, every breath of air, regardless of where we are, is associated with some kind of air pollution.

Indoors, in our daily routine, we are continuously exposed to vapors originating in the kitchen; to fumes from cleaning with detergents; to particulates from cosmetics (face powder); to fibrous particles from rugs, draperies, blankets, and clothes; to aerosols in spray cans; to tobacco smoke. The danger from widespread use of pesticides in households and commercial establishments has been brought into focus in recent years. In homes and commercial buildings, heating and cooling systems cause dust to circulate continually.

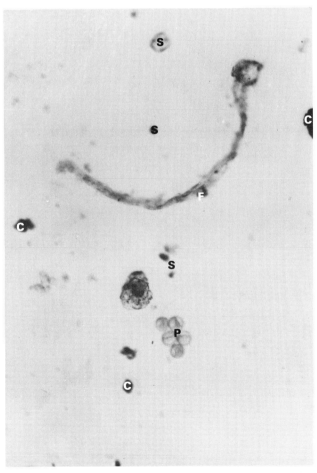

Fig. 2-2. Particles adhering to a Vaseline-coated slide exposed for 24 hours in the inner city of Detroit at a height of about 15 meters. F is a fiber, probably of plant origin; P, a cluster of pollen; C, carbon particles; S, spores of fungi.

Outdoors we are exposed to particles derived from insects, to odors from animal and human excretions, to gases that arise from marshes, and to dusts from fields and streets. During the growing seasons of spring and summer, pollen (Fig. 2-1) adds materially to the burden with which our respiratory organs must cope in a continual chain of seasonal peaks; whereas fungus spores (Figs. 2-2 and 2-3) and constituents of decaying plants and animal matter, bacteria, and viruses, permeate the air throughout the entire year.

"NORMAL" AIR

So-called normal air consists of the following gases: oxygen (O_2) 20.94%, nitrogen (N_2) 78.09%, and argon (A) 0.93%.

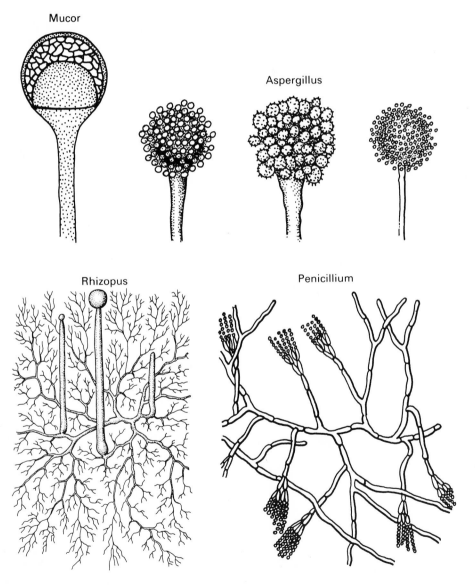

Fig. 2-3. Diagram of four common fungus spores. Their small size and light weight render them readily windborne.

Carbon dioxide (CO_2) is present in the air in the minute concentration of 0.03%. These four components make up 99.99% of the gas mixture by volume. Water vapor represents approximately 1% to 4% by volume of the total mixture.

In contrast to these percentages, sulfur dioxide (SO_2), one of the most common gaseous contaminants, is rarely found in concentrations higher than 0.0001% (1 ppm). Carbon monoxide and nitrogen oxides occur in even more minute concentrations.

Two types of aerosols* are normally present in the atmosphere:

1. Neutral particles, such as dusts and fumes, range in diameter from 0.1 to 30 μ. They tend to precipitate and settle on the ground.
2. Condensation nuclei, which are made up of hydroscopic (moisture attracting) substances, range in size from 0.01 to 0.1 μ.

Natural sources of the nuclei are: (1) volcanic eruption, meteoric dusts, and natural radiation; (2) organic decay (natural combustion); and (3) sea spray.

Volcanoes and meteors. Volcanic eruptions throw into the air tremendous amounts of dusts and gases consisting of a wide array of chemicals. The smallest particles are known to travel thousands of miles and are carried into many parts of the world. They account for high atmospheric levels of noxious agents, particularly carbon dioxide, ammonia, and fluorides.

Minute meteoritic particles are constantly impinging upon the earth's atmosphere, liberating compounds of Na, Mg, Al, Si, K, Ca, Ti, Cr, Mn, Fe, Co, and Ni. These minute particles are sources of condensation nuclei.

In addition to these natural contaminants, sources of natural radiation, namely radioactive material in soil and from cosmic rays,

are forever present in the atmosphere (Chapter 20).

Organic decay. Besides these agents derived from celestial or geophysical sources, numerous natural sources on the earth itself contaminate the atmosphere. Fragments from eroded vegetation and decaying animals and particles from living creatures, especially insects, are present in the air "normally," even where man-made pollution is minimal. Under aerobic conditions, protein from dead tissue is incompletely oxidized to foul-smelling nitrogen compounds, a process termed "putrification." The final products of this process are carbon dioxide, sulfides, methane gas, and nitrogen compounds.

Organic gases, such as ketones, hydrocarbons, and aldehydes occur normally in the air in minute amounts. They originate from organic matter and from green plants as the result of photochemical action. Volatile organic products, released from forests on hot days, often create extensive haze.

Ocean air. Above the ocean, salt is an important constituent of normal air in concentrations ranging from 4 micrograms (μg)/meter^3 to about 22,000 μg/meter^3 (2.2%). The amounts are largely governed by wind velocity.

Fallout of sea salt on the continents amounts to approximately 1 billion tons per year.[1] In conjunction with other aerosols derived from marine life, salt is present in air bubbles that rise to the surface from the depth of the sea. Upon bursting, small film drops of the size of 1 to 20 micrometer (μm) in diameter are formed. When the bubble collapses, larger-sized drops (100 μm) are ejected with considerable force in the manner of a jet at a speed of 10 meters per second from the bottom of the bubble.[1]

A part of the salt's chlorine, approximately 200 million tons per year, is found in the atmosphere in the form of gaseous hydrogen chloride. It is probably derived

---

*A cloud of solid particles or liquid droplets suspended in a gas.

Table 2-1. Particulates in rural air

PARTICULATE	PERCENT
Carbons and soot	46.0
Silicates (constituents of sand)	42.5
Coal dust	2.8
Fibrous matter	3.7
Miscellaneous	7.0

from the reaction of salt with airborne carbon dioxide and sulfur oxides. Released from mist and spray, it is carried long distances inland. When water is deposited on the salt nucleus, the size of the aerosol increases considerably.

The ocean surface is also the source of minute amounts of airborne iodine, either in gaseous or particulate form at magnitudes of 0.05 to 0.8 μg/meter^3 of air.[2] Magnesium chloride, calcium chloride, and bromides are also released from ocean spray. Nitrous oxide and carbon monoxide are produced in sea water by microorganisms and released into the atmosphere.[1] Concentrations of carbon monoxide in ocean air are estimated to range between 0.025 to 0.44 ppm.[3] Near the South Carolina coast, methane concentrations over the ocean were found to be 1.24 ppm.[4] They combine with gases and form acids in the liquid phase.

Rural air. In clear country air, the concentration of particulate matter is about 0.1 mg/meter^3 as compared with that in a manufacturing town of about 2 mg/meter^3. Layne,[5] who reviewed the findings of the 1952 London disaster, recovered particulate matter in country air from an electrostatic filter as shown in Table 2-1.

MAN-MADE POLLUTION OF AIR

The origin of man-made air pollution dates back to ancient times when man began to make use of fire. In the middle ages pollution plagued many European countries, especially in England with its persistent fog. Combustion of fuels has been, and still is, the number one source of pollutants both in industry and in households. Other sources are incineration of waste material, industrial processes, abrasion, and wear from vehicular traffic.

Around 1885 coal began to replace wood as the dominant source of energy in the United States for ships and trains. By 1925 gasoline distilled from oil had become the source of energy for transportation. In the early 1940s diesel engines began to propel trains, trucks, and ships. Today, approximately 40% of all moving vehicles are powered by oil, 40% by gasoline, and less than 20% by coal.[6]

Moving sources

Although transportation accounts for only 20% of the total energy in use in the United States, exhaust from automobiles produces about 60% of the total air pollutants and as much as 90% in certain urban areas.[7] Indirect contributions to air pollution made by the automobile are processing fuel, manufacturing of automobile parts, and scrapping of automobiles.

Automobile exhaust is usually identified with the presence of *carbon monoxide,* a product of incomplete combustion that reduces the body's ability to transport oxygen into tissues; with lead, which increases the burden of this metal in one's system; and with hydrocarbons, some of which are cancer producing. Numerous additives, such as antioxidants and antiknock compounds, antirust and antiicing agents, lubricants, and detergents, give gasoline special characteristics. Each of these agents leads to lesser efficiency in complete combustion and thus to greater emission of contaminants. The *hydrocarbons* contained in gasoline are parafins, olefins, naphthenes, and aromatics.

Other major contaminants emitted by automobiles are *nitrogen oxides.* They are harmful, not only by themselves but also because they produce photochemical smog by their interaction with hydrocarbons un-

Table 2-2. Emission factors*

	AUTOMOBILES[†]	DIESEL ENGINES[†]	JET AIRCRAFT POUNDS PER FLIGHT[‡]
	IN POUNDS PER 1000 GALLONS OF FUEL		
Aldehydes (HCHO)	4	10	4
Carbon monoxide	2300	60	20.6
Hydrocarbons (C)	200	136	19
Oxides of nitrogen (NO_x)	113	222	23
Oxides of sulfur (SO_2)	9	40	—
Organic acids (acetic)	4	31	—
Particulates	12	110	34

*Data from Compilation of air pollutant emission factors. Office of Air Programs, Publication Number AP-42, Research Triangle Park, North Carolina, February 1972, U. S. Environmental Protection Agency.
†Statistical average of rate of pollutant emission from burning of 1000 gallons of fuel.
‡At altitude of 35,000 feet.

der the influence of sunshine. *Ozone,* one of the most dangerous contaminants, is produced in this manner (see Chapter 8). Automobiles also emit *carbon* particles, oil, and nonvolatile products derived from motor oil. A plastic bag held to the tail pipe of an idling car to catch the exhaust yielded more than 100 trillion particles per second.[8]

Petroleum industry. Some high-test gasolines are produced by the use of hydrogen fluoride as a catalyst. Much of the fluorine dissolves in the hydrocarbons and ends up in the finished fuel. It is subsequently released through the automobile exhaust.

Although pollution from stationary sources is usually confined to a relatively limited area, the toxic emissions from automobiles extend into practically every nook and corner of the land and into regions far distant from industrialized territory.

In a classical study in 1962, Larsen and Konopinski[9] measured concentrations of air pollutants at the entrance and exit of Boston's mile-long Sumner Tunnel through which about 35,000 vehicles were passing every day. They calculated that a vehicle, during its 1-mile trip through the tunnel, emitted 358 mg total suspended particulates of which 158 mg were *organic* particles and 31 mg *lead.*

A more recent study in Japan[10] showed a close correlation of concentrations of carbon monoxide, nitrogen dioxide, and dust particles from auto exhaust with traffic conditions inside 19 tunnels ranging from 465 to 2953 meters in length. In highly polluted tunnels the carbon monoxide concentrations reached peaks of about 215 ppm. The highest average for 20 minutes was 85 ppm. Schaefer[8] found particulate levels in the Squirrel Hill and Pitt tunnels of Pittsburgh above 10 million particles per cubic meter of air. Sulfur oxide, the major product of combustion of coal and wood, occurs only in insignificant amounts in automobile exhaust. Concentrations of oxides of nitrogen, aldehydes, hydrocarbons, and organic acids are much higher in diesel oil exhaust than in gasoline fuel exhaust.

A major pollution problem associated with jet airplane traffic occurs inside the passenger cabins on airplane runways and during plane loading, when particulate levels range from 80,000 to 1,000,000 per cubic meter of air.[8] Following takeoff, the cabin air rapidly becomes cleaner when outside air is brought into the cabin.[8] The different magnitudes in the emission factor of automobile exhaust, diesel engines, and jet aircraft are illustrated in Table 2-2.[11]

Table 2-3. Emission factors for vessels*

	STEAMSHIPS		MOTOR SHIPS	
POLLUTANT	UNDERWAY KG/KM	IN BERTH KG/DAY	UNDERWAY KG/KM	IN BERTH KG/DAY
Particulates	0.098	6.8	0.49	7.5
Sulfur dioxide†	1.71 S	136 S	0.37	19.5
Sulfur trioxide†	0.02 S	1.8 S	—	—
Carbon monoxide	0.0005	0.036	0.29	20.8
Hydrocarbons	0.05	4.1	0.22	14.9
Nitrogen oxides (NO_2)	1.13	90.7	0.34	22.7
Aldehydes (HCHO)	0.01	0.9	0.017	1.2

*Data from Compilation of air pollutant emission factors. Office of Air Programs, Publication Number AP-42, Research Triangle Park, North Carolina, February 1972, U. S. Environmental Protection Agency.
†Based on fuel consumption and emission factors for fuel oil.

In addition to pollutants emitted from the exhaust pipes, the automobile disperses a multiplicity of particulates from the highways and unpaved roads because of the turbulence that it produces. The major constituents of road dust are sand (silicates), tar products from asphalt, tire dust, pollen, fungi, salt applied to streets in winter, lead from high octane gasoline, and cadmium, a contaminant of rubber.[12] Steamships and motorboats contribute materially to air pollution nearby or on busy waterways, especially when their engines are idling in berths (Table 2-3).

Stationary sources

An attempt to present a complete list of the many industrial processes from which pollutants are emitted would be futile. There is hardly an industry or occupation in which man is not potentially exposed to the hazards of dirty air. Traditionally, certain kinds of industry have been the principal sources of air contamination, particularly construction materials, the mining and smelting of metals, the production of chemicals, and food processing, as shown in the following outline.

Major pollutants from stationary sources

I. Combustion
  A. Coal, wood
    1. Power plant, industrial pressures, space heating
      a. Particulates
        (1) Carbon
        (2) Silica
        (3) Alumina
        (4) Iron oxide
      b. Gases
        (1) Nickel carbonate
        (2) Aldehydes
        (3) Carbon monoxide
        (4) Hydrocarbons
        (5) Nitrogen oxides
        (6) Sulfur oxides
        (7) Fluoride
        (8) Carbon dioxide
  B. Natural gas
    1. Carbon monoxide
    2. Nitrogen oxides
    3. Aldehydes
  C. Fuel oil
    1. Nitrogen oxides
    2. Carbon monoxide
    3. Sulfur oxide
    4. Hydrocarbons
    5. Particulates (ash, sulfates, cenospheres)
  D. Refuse incineration
    1. Hydrochloric acid
    2. Nitrogen oxides
    3. Fluorides
    4. Sulfur oxides
    5. Aldehydes
    6. Hydrocarbons
    7. Organic (acetic) acid
II. Metallurgical industry
  A. Aluminum ore reduction
    1. Hydrogen fluoride
    2. Particulate fluoride

3. Carbon, alumina
B. Copper smelters
  1. Carbon monoxide
  2. Sulfur oxides
  3. Nitrogen oxides
  4. Cadmium
C. Iron-steel
  1. Carbon monoxide
  2. Sulfur oxides
  3. Iron oxides
  4. Fluorides
  5. Nickel carbonate, silicates, graphite
D. Lead and zinc smelters
  1. Sulfur dioxides
  2. Fluorides
  3. Cadmium
E. Magnesium smelters
  1. Fluorides, chlorine
  2. Barium oxide
F. Secondary° metals industry
  1. Nitrogen oxides
  2. Metal oxides
  3. Hydrochloric acid
G. Brass and bronze smelters
  1. Zinc oxide
  2. Lead oxides
H. Secondary aluminum smelters
  1. Fluorides, chlorides, ozone
  2. Numerous metals
III. Chemical industry
  A. Adipic acid (for synthetic fibers)
    1. Nitrogen oxides
  B. Ammonia plant
    1. Carbon monoxides
    2. Ammonia
  C. Chlorine plant
    1. Chlorine gas
    2. Mercury
  D. Hydrofluoric acid
    1. Hydrogen fluoride
    2. Silicon tetrafluoride
    3. Sulfur dioxide
  E. Nitric acid manufacture
    1. Nitric oxide
    2. Nitrogen dioxide
  F. Paint, varnish
    1. Aldehydes
    2. Ketones
    3. Phenols
    4. Terpenes
    5. Glycerines
  G. Petroleum refinery
    1. Hydrogen sulfide
    2. Selenium
    3. Fluorides
    4. Hydrocarbons

°Smelting of scrap, not of ore.

H. Phosphoric acid
  1. Silicon tetrafluoride
  2. Hydrogen fluoride
I. Phthalic anhydride
  1. Hexane
  2. Maleic anhydrides
J. Printing ink
  1. Acrolein
  2. Fatty acids
  3. Phenols
  4. Terpenes
K. Sulfuric acid
  1. Sulfur dioxide
  2. Sulfur oxides
  3. Nitrogen oxides
L. Synthetic rubber°
  1. Alkanes
  2. Alkenes
  3. Ethanenitrile
  4. Carbonyls
IV. Construction industry
  A. Asphalt roofing
    1. Oil mists
    2. Benzo[a]pyrene
    3. Asbestos
    4. Carbon monoxide
  B. Brick
    1. Fluorides
    2. Sulfur dioxide
  C. Calcium carbide
    1. Carbon monoxide
    2. Acetylene
    3. Sulfur oxides
  D. Cement
    1. Various kinds of dust
    2. Chromium
  E. Ceramic and clay processes
    1. Fluorides
    2. Silicates
    3. Ammonia
  F. Frit (glazing enamel)
    1. Fluorides
    2. Silica
    3. Boron
  G. Glass
    1. Chlorine
    2. Fluorides
    3. Sulfur oxides
    4. Nitrogen oxides
    5. Carbon monoxide

Data from Compilation of air pollutant emission factors. Office of Air Programs, Publication Number AP-42, Research Triangle Park, North Carolina, February 1972, U. S. Environmental Protection Agency.
°See Table 2-5.

V. Food, agriculture, household
    A. Coffee roasting
        1. Smoke
        2. Odors
    B. Cotton ginning
        1. Trash
        2. Dust
        3. Lint
    C. Dry cleaning
        1. Petroleum solvents
        2. Synthetic solvents (perchloroethylene)
    D. Feed and grain mills
        1. Dirt (silicates)
        2. Chaff
        3. Grain dust
        4. Fungi
        5. Mercury
    E. Fish meal processing
        1. Hydrogen sulfide
        2. Trimethylamine
    F. Starch
        1. Starch particles

From some industrial establishments detailed information is available on how pollutants originate and are emitted. Relatively little information can be obtained on others. The pollutants evolve either from the raw materials or from agents added during processing, especially fluxes and other additives. They may also originate during the course of storing and shipping of either raw or finished products. Varying manufacturing processes are employed in a given industry in order to achieve the same results. This fact further complicates the assessment of air pollution near an industrial plant.

Combustion. Burning of coal, gas, oil, and refuse constitutes the principal source of contamination from stationary sources.

Coal. Coal is burned in power plants, in many industrial processes, as well as for domestic and commercial heating in a variety of furnaces. The principal particulates emitted from combustion of coal are carbon, silica, aluminum, and iron oxide. The gases emanating from burning coal are sulfur oxides, nitrogen oxides, hydrogen fluoride, carbon monoxide, nickel carbonate, aldehydes, and other hydrocarbons. Smoke from coal combustion also contains lead,

cadmium, selenium, vanadium, zinc, and numerous other elements.[13] How many of these individual pollutants reach the atmosphere depends on the composition of the coal, the kind of combustion equipment, the method of firing, the size of the combustion unit, and other factors concerned with its operation.

Gas. Burning of gas to heat homes and power plants produces mainly carbon dioxide, water vapor, and oxides of nitrogen, which far exceed all other toxic agents.[11] Emission of particulates and sulfur oxides is insignificant.

Oil. The principal pollutants emitted from burning oil are sulfur oxides, nitrogen oxides, and a high percentage of particulate material, about 17% to 25% of which are sulfates, 10% to 30% ash, and 25% to 50% cenospheres (spherical coal structures). Selenium has been indicted as an important pollutant derived from fuel oils.[14]

Refuse. Refuse is burned in incinerators, in sanitary landfills, or is disposed of through composting. Carbon particles contained in flyash constitute a major contam-

Table 2-4. Composition of typical municipal refuse*

TYPE OF REFUSE	PERCENT
Corrugated boxboard	6
Newspaper	13
Magazines, books	2
All other paper	26
Plastic containers	2
Plastic film	1
Rubber, leather	1
Textiles	3
Wood	3
Food waste	10
Grass, leaves	5
Dirt, under 1 inch	6
Glass, ceramics, stones	12
Metal	10

*Adapted from Carotti, A. A., and Kaiser, E. R.: Concentrations of twenty gaseous chemical species in the flue gas of a municipal incinerator, J. Air Pollut. Contr. Ass. **22:**248-253, 1972.

inant. Relatively little nitrogen oxides and sulfur oxides are found in gaseous emissions from incinerators. Carbon monoxide, aldehydes, and hydrocarbons appear in greater amounts.

A wide variety of gases are emitted from municipal incinerators.[15] Although nitrogen oxides and sulfur oxides have received most attention in the past years, chlorides are now the major constituent of municipal incinerator gas emission because of the combustion of polyvinyl and other plastics, which form hydrochloric acid.[15] Significant concentrations of fluorides are also emitted in conjunction with hydrocarbons, cyanide, phosphates, and aldehydes. As Table 2-4

Table 2-5. Major industrial sources of particulate pollutants*

SOURCE	EMISSIONS IN THOUSAND TONS PER YEAR
Combustion	
Coal-fired boilers	
Electric utilities	5,107
Industrial power generation	2,044
Field burning	1,000
	8,151
Chemical	
Acids (sulfuric and phosphoric)	48
Detergents chemical	2
Phosphate rock	49
Fertilizers (solid)	312
	411
Agriculture	
Forest products	
Forestry operations	6,096
Plywood, hardboard, and particle board	70
Pulp mills	627
Grain elevators	1,210
	8,003
Construction	
Asphalt	95
Cement	1,233
Clay	147
Crushed stone	1,490
Lime	142
Paint and varnish	20
	3,127
Smelting	
Iron and steel (including foundries)	722
Aluminum	80
Copper	61
Zinc	39
Lead	35
	937
Petroleum refining	24
Total	20,653

*Excerpted from Vandegrift, A. E., and others: Particulate pollution in the United States. Presented at the Sixty-third Annual Meeting of the Air Pollution Control Association, 1970, Table 11, pp. 23-24.

indicates, a wide variety of objects are being burned in incinerators and the values of the different pollutants vary considerably.

From open burning of refuse, which is still being practiced especially in rural areas, the major emissions are carbon monoxide, hydrocarbons (hexane), and organic acids (acetic acid).

Wood. In many homes burning of wood in the time-honored fireplace is still a routine household procedure during winter months. Schaefer[8] estimates that an ordinary fireplace emits into the air about 30 trillion smoke particles with an average cross section of about 0.3 μ. The composition of wood smoke is similar to that of coal, with wide variations in the magnitude of elements depending on where the wood was harvested.

Estimates on the emission of some of the major industrial sources of pollutants are presented in Table 2-5.

Carbon dioxide. Scientists have become greatly concerned about the increase of carbon dioxide (CO_2) levels in the air. Because of combustion of coal and oil fuels, they have been rising steadily since the middle of the nineteenth century. At the beginning of the twentieth century the burning of coal produced about 3 billion tons of carbon dioxide a year.[16] About 50% of the current man-made output, which is estimated to be 10 billion tons per year, goes into the atmosphere; the rest is stored in forests (10% to 15%) and in oceans (35% to 40%).[1] During the years 1959 to 1967 there has been a yearly increase of 0.7 parts of carbon dioxide in 1 million parts of air and from 1.0 to 1.2 ppm between 1968 and 1971. At this rate the total in the year 2000 will be above 380 ppm (0.038%), which has been estimated by Machta the Director of Air Resources Laboratories, Silver Spring, Maryland. Carbon dioxide together with ozone and water vapor tend to prevent extension of infra-red radiation from the ground into higher atmospheric levels (greenhouse effect) and influence the heat balance and the climate of the earth. Other scientists feel that the future expansion of the use of nuclear energy and the harnessing of solar heat will counter the heretofore expanding use of fossil fuel combustion and the resulting damage from accumulation of carbon dioxide.

Smelting. Metals are produced either by primary smelting operations, that is, the processing of ore obtained in mines, or by recovery from scrap and salvage material, which takes place in so-called secondary smelters.

In primary smelting the ore must be mined, melted, and impurities removed. The metal must then be processed in the form for which it is desired. Different kinds of alloying agents, such as chromium and manganese, are added to produce specialized types of metal. The major pollutants are those contained in the ore. Impurities are removed from the ore in blast furnaces, which emit a wide variety of gases and particulates both from the ore and from the fuel used in the operation.

The ore from which primary lead is produced contains both lead and zinc, compounds of which usually appear in the air together. Roasting, sintering, and smelting operations release sulfur dioxide, fluorides, cadmium, and numerous other agents. The major pollutant in the aluminum industry is fluoride derived from cryolite, which is used as a flux in the electrolytic reduction of aluminum-bearing ore. Smelting of copper, produced from low-grade sulfide ores, emits carbon monoxide, sulfur oxides, nitrogen oxides, fluoride, and a particulate fume.

At secondary metal smelters the metal is not produced from ore but from scrap such as car pistons, borings, lathings, stampings, and rejected sheet metal much of which has been painted. In order to remove impurities from the melted metal, fluxes and many other agents are employed. In secondary aluminum smelters pure chlorine gas is charged into the furnaces in order to

Table 2-6. Emission factors for synthetic rubber factories*

COMPOUNDS	EMISSIONS KG/METRIC TONS
Alkenes	
Butadiene†	20.0
Methylpropene	7.5
Butyne	1.5
Pentadiene	0.5
Alkanes	
Dimethylheptane	0.5
Pentane	1.0
Ethanenitrile	0.5
Carbonyls	
Acrylonitrile	8.5
Acrolein	1.5

*Data from Compilation of air pollutant emission factors. Office of Air Programs, Publication Number AP-42, Research Triangle Park, North Carolina, February 1972, U. S. Environmental Protection Agency.

†Butadiene emission is not continuous and is greatest immediately after a batch of partially polymerized latex enters the blow-down tank.

remove magnesium from the melted material. The smokestacks emit a wide variety of agents including hydrogen chloride and free chlorine gas, hydrogen fluoride, sulfur dioxide, carbon, hydrocarbons, particulate magnesium chloride, and aluminum chloride.

Manufacturing of chemicals. A vast variety of processes in the chemical industry are sources of pollution. They range from manufacturing simple acids and alkalis to complex organic material, such as plastics, rubber products, and pharmaceuticals.

A publication by the U. S. Environmental Protection Agency[11] names some of the major pollutants emitted in the manufacturing of ammonia, chlorine, nitric acid, phthalic anhydride. Some of these agents are named in the outline on p. 18. Data on emissions from manufacturing of synthetic rubber are presented in Table 2-6.

The construction industry. Paints, concrete, asphalt, glass, asbestos insulating material, bricks, and sawdust are the principal products used in the construction in-

dustry. In manufacturing paints and varnishes, a wide variety of organic agents, such as aldehydes, ketones, phenols, turpentines, and glycerin, is produced. Among inorganic agents present in paints are lead, mercury, titanium, and selenium.

Dust arising from cement plants consists of relatively large particles. In the manufacturing of ceramics and in the clay processing industry, which includes brick, tile, sewer pipe, pottery, and vitreous wares, fluorides and hydrogen fluoride constitute the major pollutants. Fluorides are also the principal pollutant in the glass industry where they are used as a flux and to render glass opaque.[17] Frit, a product employed in enameling iron and steel and in glazing porcelain and pottery, is produced in furnaces that emit, on an average, 10 pounds of fluoride per ton of charge. In the manufacturing of asphalt, tar and other organic products are liberated. They include the carcinogen (cancer-producing) benzo[a]pyrene.

Processing of food. Pollutants emanating from most food-processing establishments can easily be detected by their odors as, for instance, in coffee roasting, meat packing, and fish meal processing. Relatively little information is available about pollution from this source. Meat and fish processing emit trimethylamine and hydrogen sulfide. Atmospheric pollutants released in the feed and grain industry during cleaning, rolling, grinding, and blending the grain are chaff and dust. Fungous spores, particularly rust and smut, are a common source of contamination. Fungicides, especially organic mercury compounds, have caused poisoning through the food chain in Japan (see Chapter 12). In the manufacture of starch, significant dust emissions of starch particles occur.

Processing and preservation of agricultural products such as alfalfa and corn dehydration and canning and packing of poultry and meat produce many kinds of organic contaminants conducive to illness, particularly respiratory diseases. Detailed reports on such cases, which occur not infrequently, rarely reach the medical literature because of the difficulties involved in pinpointing the exact cause of the disease.

Cotton ginning produces a wide variety of contaminants, including dust and lint from gins and particulates from incineration of cotton trash. Whereas in cotton workers a disease caused by atmospheric contaminants is well established, no data on individuals not engaged occupationally in work with cotton have been reported.

Agricultural practices. Farmers are exposed habitually to a multiplicity of sources of pollution. Emanations from manure and dust derived from barns and from harvesting and handling crops induce asthma in predisposed individuals. Silage produces gases, especially nitrogen dioxide, which has given rise to sudden fatal pulmonary disease. In addition, silage and manure increase atmospheric fungous spores that can cause pulmonary diseases. Dust arises, particularly on windy days, from application of lime and artificial fertilizers, from tilling the soil, and from harvesting and combine operations.

Much attention has been given to illness caused by crop spraying with insecticides, rodenticides, herbicides, and fungicides. Chlorinated hydrocarbons, such as DDT, lindane, aldrin, dieldrin, and endrin, as well as organic phosphates, including parathion, malathian, and related inorganic insecticides, such as lead and calcium arsenate, or botanical insecticides, such as pyrethrum and rotenone, are recognized as hazards to human health.

Household activities. In addition to products derived from heating and cooking and to dust and lints derived from fabrics, a housewife is exposed to numerous other airborne agents, some of which can have adverse effects on human health. They include refrigerants and many kinds of sprays that are used habitually by housewives,

such as detergents, deodorants, fumigants, paints, varnish, and polishes. Organic contaminants, food odors, fumes, and gases are also sources of pollution.

Approximately 2 pounds (0.9 kg) of solvents, mainly petroleum and synthetic solvents, per capita per year are emitted into the atmosphere in moderate climates and 2.7 pounds (1.23 kg) are emitted in colder areas of the United States.[11] The extent of damage induced by the use of detergents and cosmetics, particularly in allergic individuals (see Chapter 18), is difficult to assess and is not sufficiently appreciated by the public.

REFERENCES

1. Dyrssen, D.: The changing chemistry of the oceans, Ambio **1**:21-25, 1972.
2. Vought, R. L., Brown, F. A., and London, H. T.: Iodine in the environment, Arch. Environ. Health **20**:516, 1970.
3. Robbins, R. C., Borg, K. M., and Robinson, E.: Carbon monoxide in the atmosphere, J. Air Pollut. Contr. Ass. **18**:106-110, 1968.
4. Swinnerton, J. W., Linnenbom, V. J., and Cheek, C. H.: Distribution of methane and carbon monoxide between the atmosphere and natural waters, Environ. Sci. Technol. **3**:836-838, 1969.
5. Layne, D. A.: A review on smog, Roy. Sanit. Inst. **2**:171-191, 1955.
6. Larsen, R. I.: Motor vehicle emissions and their effects, Public Health Rep. **77**:963-969, 1962.
7. Waste Management and Control, National Research Council, Publication 1400, Washington, D. C., 1965, National Academy of Science.
8. Schaefer, V. J.: The threat of the unseen, Saturday Rev. **54**:55-57, 1971.
9. Larsen, R. I., and Konopinski, V. J.: Sumner tunnel air quality, Arch. Environ. Health **5**:597-608, 1962.
10. Kuroe, T., and Tada, O.: Proceedings of the forty-fourth meeting of the Tokyo, Japan Industrial Medical Society, April 3-4, 1971, pp. 152-153.
11. Compilation of Air Pollutant Emission Factors. Office of Air Programs, Publication Number AP-42, Research Triangle Park, North Carolina, February, 1972, U. S. Environmental Protection Agency.

12. McCaull, J.: Building a shorter life, Environment **23**:2-15, 1971.

13. Halstead, W. D., and Raask, E.: The behavior of sulphur and chlorine compounds in pulverized-coal-fired boilers, J. Inst. Fuel **42**:344-349, 1969.

14. Stahl, Q. R.: Air pollution aspects of selenium and its compounds, Litton Industries Inc., Bethesda, Maryland, 1969, U. S. Department of Commerce, National Bureau of Standards, PB 188 077.

15. Carotti, A. A., and Kaiser, E. R.: Concentrations of twenty gaseous chemical species in the flue gas of a municipal incinerator, J. Air Pollut. Contr. Ass. **22**:248-253, 1972.

16. Air conservation, American Association for the Advancement of Science, Publication No. 80, Washington, D. C., 1965, p. 78.

17. Stockham, J. D.: The composition of glass furnace emissions, J. Air Pollut. Contr. Ass. **21**:713-715, 1971.

3
DISPERSION OF AIR POLLUTANTS

Some people have become their own weather forecasters by watching the vagaries of smoke emitted by chimneys. When smoke rises straight toward the sky, they expect a rise in barometric pressure and clear weather. When the smoke gravitates toward the ground, rain is anticipated.

The agent transporting smoke and other pollutants in a horizontal direction is wind; the forces causing vertical movement are buoyancy and friction. Wind is created by uneven heating and cooling of the air masses covering the rotating earth. Warm air is less dense and has a tendency to rise; cool, dense air remains close to the ground. During air movements, changes in pressure and volume of a given air mass occur principally according to the laws of Boyle and Charles. Boyle's law states that the volume of an air mass decreases as the pressure rises and vice versa at constant temperatures. Charles' law states that the volume of a gas changes directly with the absolute temperature (at constant pressure). This means that the volume doubles when the absolute temperature is doubled.

WIND

Direction. The direction and velocity of the wind dominate the list of factors involved in the distribution of smoke and other contaminants in the atmosphere. Wind tends to clean the air by diluting and dispersing the contaminants. In doing so, wind also extends the pollution. Smoke most often follows the direction of prevailing winds in moving from its source, and areas in its path are prone to pollution. Thus, wind currents can contaminate a single street or a single section of a farm when other nearby places remain unaffected. For instance, in Anchorage, Alaska, the instruments of officials studying air pollution recorded unusually high pollution levels. Subsequently they learned that their instruments had been placed directly in the path of a prevailing wind from one of Anchorage's largest industries.[1]

Forests, a row of evergreens, or even tall grasses not only break the force of the wind, but can protect the land beyond them. Trees at the edge of a parcel of woods situated within 300 feet of an Iowa fertilizer factory, which I surveyed, showed extensive pollution damage; whereas vegetation only a few hundred yards beyond showed no visible damage.

Velocity. The greater the wind's velocity, the larger is the area into which pollution spreads in a given time, whereas in close proximity to their source the contaminants become more diluted (Fig. 3-1). A steady wind can carry atmospheric pollutants long distances: California fishermen 40 to 50 miles at sea were suddenly engulfed by haze shown to have originated in Los Angeles.[1] The same kind of Los Angeles smoke, carried 200 miles by the wind, has damaged farms in Arizona.[1]

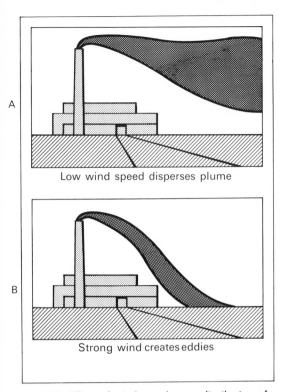

A
Low wind speed disperses plume

B
Strong wind creates eddies

Fig. 3-1. Effect of wind speed upon distribution of smoke.

lution of pollutants, and may account for a rapid build-up of air contamination. In the absence of wind, a cloud of pollutants becomes stagnant and smoke may settle to the surface near the source. A moderately strong wind disperses and dilutes contaminants. As indicated in Fig. 3-1, *A,* wind and buoyancy account for the paradoxical phenomenon that soil and vegetation are usually less contaminated immediately adjacent to a factory than at distant points. This fact is significant in assessing air pollution damage.

Eddies. At times sudden gusts of wind drive pollutants down to the ground (Fig. 3-1, *B*). Such sudden diversions of the wind current are called eddies, or turbulence. They are short counterflows of wind caused by sudden thermal changes or by friction between air masses in the atmosphere. They reverse in direction and break up the plume from a bonfire or a smokestack, or they may divert only a portion of it. In either case they help to disperse the contaminant. When these eddies carrying polluted air approach the ground, however, they may linger and thus enhance the effect of pollution in a given area.

BAROMETRIC PRESSURE

Air pressure and temperature are the other key factors determining the degree of air pollution. At sea level the pressure of air averages 14.7 pounds per square inch or 22,785 pounds per square meter; at 18,000 feet (about 5½ km) above sea level, it is half as high. High-pressure systems move across the continent with dimensions up to 1500 miles across. The high pressure center is generally a region of weak pressure, that is, of weak winds. By eliminating wind, high pressure systems are associated with poor dispersal of contaminants and stagnant air. In the eastern United States they prevail particularly in late summer and autumn, the season when the principal air pollution disasters described in Chapter 1 occurred, namely that in Donora, Oc-

The late Dr. Robert Cooke, the pioneer in allergic diseases in the United States, related to me that three of his patients afflicted with ragweed hayfever, while about 1000 miles east of the United States coastline on a boat returning from Europe, experienced their first hayfever symptoms on a day of high ragweed pollination on the continent. Since ragweed does not grow in Europe and since the patients were not known to be clinically sensitive to other kinds of inhalants, he believed that ragweed carried by the wind from the East Coast of the United States had precipitated their hayfever.

On the ground, winds are usually weaker than they are aloft because of friction with the earth's surface. A low wind velocity on the ground, particularly in foggy or cloudy weather, is often accompanied by slow di-

tober, 1948, and in New York City, November, 1953.

In 1966, on Thanksgiving day (November 24), the eastern part of the United States from New England to Florida was under the influence of a high pressure system that had remained almost motionless for several days. The air aloft was unusually warm and the spread of this warm air in the higher regions restricted vertical dispersion.[2] No exact data are available on the death toll during the 6-day period of November 24 to 30 for the entire area. In New York City alone, an increase of approximately 24 deaths per day above the normal death rate was reported.[3]

TEMPERATURE

Air is normally warmer close to the earth's surface than in the upper atmosphere. When a parcel of air rises, it expands as a result of the decrease in pressure. Furthermore, its temperature commonly drops with the lower pressure.

For every 1000 feet increase in altitude, the temperature is 5.4° F lower (or 1° C for 100 meters).* When the rate of cooling in the environment is greater than 5.4° per 1000 feet, the parcel of air stays warmer and continues to rise. If the rate of cooling is less, the air that began to rise will sink. This atmospheric condition is called "stable."

When warm air rises, carrying with it pollutants from below, it disperses them. In a "stable" atmosphere the air becomes stagnant.

Inversions. Under certain conditions instead of falling, the temperature rises with higher altitudes. This phenomenon is called "inversion." The air fails to rise and clouds of pollutants concentrate near the ground. The inversion acts as a lid and separates layers of air. A layer of warm contaminated air may form a ceiling that prevents the air from flowing into higher regions. This ceiling confines the pollutants into a relatively small space near the ground (Fig. 3-2).

Three major forces enter into the mech-

---

*Provided that there is no significant exchange of heat with its surroundings.

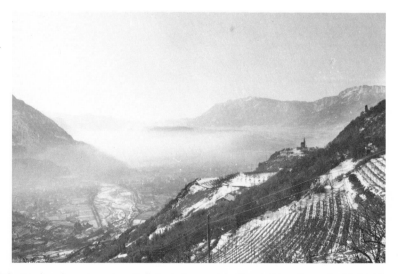

Fig. 3-2. Results of an inversion. Pollutants trapped in the Adiche (formerly Etsch) River Valley at Bolzano, southern Tyrol. Four factories, including an aluminum and magnesium smelter, are responsible for the emission.

anism of an inversion: heat radiation from the ground, solar radiation, and wind. Strong wind currents prevent the cooling of air; conversely, absence of wind makes for greater "stability" and stagnation of pollutants.

After a day when the sun has heated the earth's surface, the ground loses heat by radiation more quickly than the air. This renders the air near the ground cooler than the air aloft and accounts for stability at night. Sunshine tends to rectify this condition the next morning by warming the air near the ground. However, should the sun not pierce through the clouds and the air on the surface fail to warm up, and should

the wind remain light, the inversion persists throughout the day.

Inversions with colder air on the ground than aloft occur during all months of the year but most frequently in the fall and winter (Fig. 3-3).[1] Pollution during inversions in the cold season is further enhanced by furnaces in homes, which emit more smoke from chimneys than at other times of the year.

TOPOGRAPHY

When communities are surrounded by hills or mountains or when an industry or town is located close to a river in a valley, the motion of cold air downward along the

Fig. 3-3. A blanket of dense particulate smog over New York City on Thanksgiving Day, 1966. (Courtesy Atmospherics Incorporated and The Sciences, New York Academy of Sciences, 11:16, 1971.)

DAY

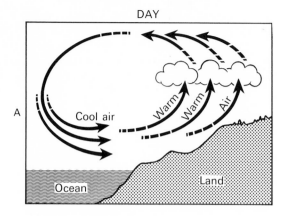

NIGHT

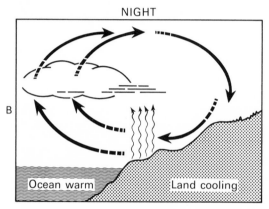

Fig. 3-4. Movements of air at the seacoast.

inates when the sun heats the coastal land at a faster rate than it heats the water (Fig. 3-4, *A* and *B*). During the day the breeze with clean air blows toward the land. At night when air on land is cooler than that above the water the wind blows the contaminants out to sea. A sea breeze, which can extend over 30 miles at a depth up to 1000 feet, thus disperses large masses of polluted air. This is undoubtedly the explanation for improvement of certain respiratory diseases when patients spend their vacations close to the seashore.

PRECIPITATION

One of the most effective cleansers of the atmosphere is precipitation such as rain, sleet, and snow. Lack of rain in southern California is undoubtedly a factor in the occurrence of extended periods of pollution. However, by precipitating airborne pollutants, rain contributes to contamination of soil and particularly of water. Thus the cleaning up of one area of pollution may account for contamination of another. In some rural areas, for example, near a Canadian triple phosphate fertilizer factory, farmers had been using cisterns to collect rain for drinking, for household use, and for livestock. In one of the cisterns as much as 39 ppm of fluoride[4] had accumulated. It had contributed to intoxication of individuals intolerant to this chemical.[5]

Over highly industrialized areas a cloud ceiling effect originates from the exhaust of leaded gasoline: extremely minute particles of lead reacting with iodide form a nucleus upon which water molecules sublimate from water into ice. Ice particles increase in size 100,000 times. When these particles are absorbed by clouds they alter the natural precipitation patterns (Fig. 3-5).

PHYSICAL PROPERTIES OF THE POLLUTANT

In addition to meteorologic factors, the physical properties of a polluting agent, its

mountains at night with accumulation in the valleys becomes significant (Fig. 3-2). Such a kettlelike formation makes escape difficult and the cold air with its contaminants may become trapped. The Meuse Valley and Donora disasters are typical examples of the effect of this kind of inversion. A similar effect holds true in large cities where skyscrapers create virtual canyons and limit dispersion of contaminated air emitted near the ground. However, if pollution originates outside a valley, the mountains often shield the valley's population.

In the flat plains of the Great Lakes and near the sea, the wind disperses contaminants more effectively than in the mountainous and hilly areas. A sea breeze orig-

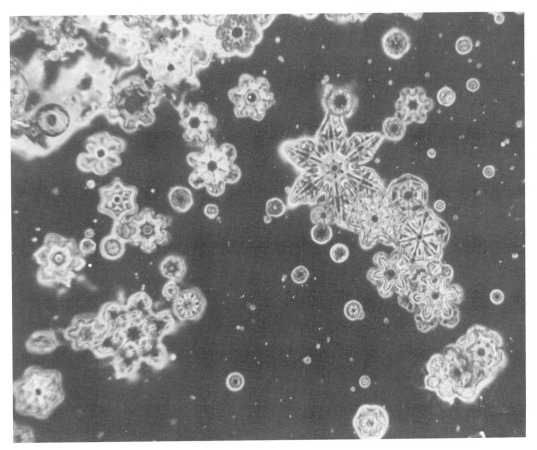

Fig. 3-5. Ice crystals formed in the atmosphere around minute lead iodide compounds derived from automobile exhaust. Reproduced experimentally in a laboratory cold chamber. (Courtesy Dr. Vincent Schaefer, The Sciences, New York Academy of Sciences, **11:**17, 1971.)

size, volume and weight, the configuration of its surface, its tendency to react with other agents, the magnitude of its emission, its distance from the emitting source, all these factors play a role in the polluting potential of a contaminant.

Size. The main mechanism by which particles are removed from the air is through gravitation. Particles of all sizes coagulate, disperse, and grow by condensation. They adsorb and absorb vapors and gases. Gravity causes large particles, with a diameter above 10 μ, to settle rapidly on the ground close to the emitting source. Large particles do not move along with the air currents.[6]

Their settling velocity is in excess of 0.29 cm per second.[7]

Particles in the range of 0.1 to 10 μ in diameter are considered especially significant with respect to their action on the respiratory tract. Those 1 to 10 μ in size clear the air by landing on buildings, trees, and other objects. Rain also precipitates the larger particles but fails to remove those less than 2 μ in diameter.

Particles measuring 0.1 to 1.0 μ in diameter are removed primarily by coagulation. However, they grow more slowly because they move less rapidly in the air and collide less often with other particles.[8]

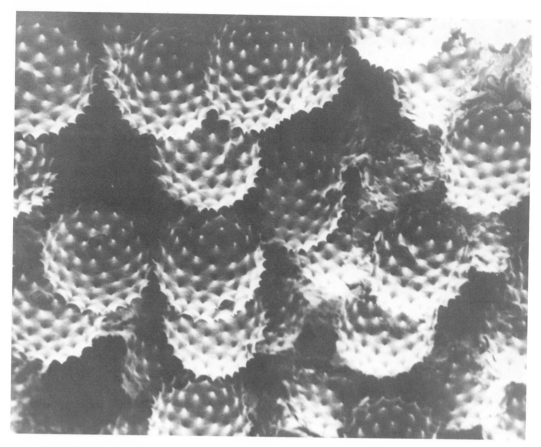

Fig. 3-6. Scanning electronphotomicrograph of short ragweed *(Ambrosia elatior)*. The small size of ragweed compared with other pollens (see Fig. 2-1) and the spiculated surface renders this pollen more windborne and more irritating than others. (Courtesy Allergy Laboratories of Ohio, Inc., Columbus, Ohio.)

Particles of less than 0.1 μ in diameter behave like gases. They move randomly and remain in the air until they grow in size by coagulation through colliding with other particles. Gases are carried much farther by the wind than are solid particles such as flyash.

Moisture. In the reactions between gases and particles, water vapors play an important role. For instance, when gaseous ammonia and sulfuric acid mist form ammonium sulfate at high humidity, the rate of reaction depends on the rate at which ammonia in the air can diffuse into sulfuric acid droplets. Under conditions of low hu-

midity the rate of the reaction is controlled by the rate at which ammonium sulfate formed in the reaction diffuses away from the surface and into the sulfuric acid droplets, thus exposing more surface for reaction by ammonia.[6]

Surface. Pollen, which must be considered a large-sized pollutant, is nevertheless carried long distances from its source. Its buoyancy and wide distribution is accounted for by its light weight and, particularly, the configuration of its surface. Ragweed pollen, the smallest of windborne pollen with a diameter of 19 to 25 μ, has a spiculated surface (thornlike protrusions)

Table 3-1. Factors affecting distribution of pollutants

INCREASE IN	POLLUTION LESS (−) MORE (+)	TYPICAL EFFECT
Precipitation	−	Cleanses the air
Humidity	+	Dissolves many pollutants; renders pollution more visible
Fog	+	Remains the same
Sunshine	+	Initiates oxidation
Wind velocity	±	Less pollution near the source but faster and wider distribution
Wind direction from contaminating source	+	Greater contamination
Increasing temperature with increasing height	+	Less dispersion
Barometric pressure	+	Lighter wind; less dispersion
Height of emitting source	−	Enhances dispersion and dilution of contaminant
Mountains, hills	+	Break force of winds; but promote light winds
Valleys	+	Trap pollutants
Plains	−	Greater dispersion
Distance from contaminating source	−	Remains the same

that lends itself to propulsion by the wind and thus accounts for its wide distribution (Fig. 3-6).

Weight. Large-size pollen such as corn (90 μ) or pollen made heavier by a resinous layer on its surface (flowers and flowering trees) are not windborne. They drop to the ground close to the plant because of their weight. They cause respiratory symptoms only if a person is very close to the respective plant. Spores of fungi that are smaller in size and lighter in weight are carried much farther than pollen.

Because of the interaction of all these factors as summarized in Table 3-1 it is difficult to assess the role of a single one. The problem becomes even more complicated if one takes into account the biologic action of the various contaminants, the interaction of mixtures of pollutants, and particularly their effect on human health, which are discussed in subsequent chapters.

REFERENCES

1. Lewis, H. R.: With every breath you take, New York, 1965, Crown Publishers, Inc.
2. Fensterstock, J. C., and Frankhauser, R. K.: Thanksgiving 1966 air pollution episode in the eastern United States, 1968, National Air Pollution Control Administration Publication Number AP-45.
3. Air Pollution—1966 Hearings before Subcommittees on Air and Water Pollution of the Committees on Public Works, U. S. Senate, 1966, U. S. Government Printing Office.
4. Report to W. C. B. Mills, Medical Officer of Health, Township of Sherbrooke, by Ontario Water Resources Commission, Dec. 6, 1965.
5. Waldbott, G. L., and Cecilioni, V. A.: "Neighborhood" fluorosis, Clin. Toxicol. 2:387-396, 1969.
6. Report by the Subcommittee on Environmental Improvement, Committee on Chemistry and Public Affairs, Washington, D. C., 1969, American Chemical Society, p. 34.
7. Battigelli, M. C.: Particulates: air quality criteria based on health effects. Air Quality Monographs Number 69-2, New York, 1969, American Petroleum Institute.
8. Air Quality Criteria for Particulate Matter, PHS Environmental Health Service, NAPCA, Washington, D. C., 1969, U. S. Department of Health, Education, and Welfare.

4

RECOGNITION OF POLLUTANTS

A lay person can recognize the existence of pollutants by a large number of criteria. For instance when a highway sign "Danger Smoke" (Fig. 4-1) warns a motorist that the image of oncoming cars may be obscured, it is axiomatic that the area is polluted. A housewife can tell by the dirt on her face and on her windowsills and by the appearance of the shirts she washes that the air is unclean. In winter the soiled surface of the snow betrays the presence of pollutants. When the new paint on a building turns black in short order, when outdoor light bulbs turn opaque, and when the window glass of homes becomes etched, certain chemicals in the air must be suspected. Sometimes, however, air pollution is not perceptible to a person who is unaware of its existence.

RINGELMAN CHART

In the late 1800s a professor of engineering, Maximilian Ringelman of Paris, devised a system of assessing the degree of pollution. Called the Ringelman Smoke Chart, it served to standardize the density of smoke emitted into the air (Fig. 4-2). It consists of five squares on a white background with criss-crossing black lines of varying thickness. By holding these charts at a distance from the eye, the thin lines give the appearance of white or gray, the heavy black lines merge together and appear to be solid black. By matching the various shades with those of contaminated atmosphere the degree of pollution can be estimated as "number 1, 2, 3, 4, or 5 Ringelman." Although this device in its day served a useful purpose, obviously it is not an accurate means of evaluating pollution. Nor does it yield information about the composition of the smoke. The Ringelman estimate is largely dependent on the presence of black carbon particles in the atmosphere. Although these particles are harmless by themselves, they indicate that the air is polluted. In spite of the development of many new devices* for recognition of pollutants, on occasion the time-honored Ringelman device is still being utilized as a rough gauge of the extent of air pollution.

ODORS

Our sense of smell can be as sensitive an indicator of existing pollution as our eyesight.

Mode of action

Since malodors are often the first manifestation of air pollution, they can constitute a monitor for contaminated air. They bear no relationship to the toxicity of a pollutant nor are they themselves the cause of an organic disease. They merely indicate the presence and, to some extent, the concentration of a pollutant in the atmosphere. Offensive odors occur even when the odorant is present in very low concentrations.

Unfortunately the interpretation of odors

---

*The principal instruments for sampling pollutants in the air are outlined by Morgan and others.[3]

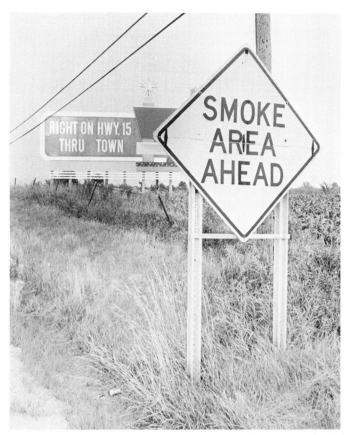

Fig. 4-1. Sign on an Indiana highway warns of smoke from an aluminum smelter ¼-mile distant. It was erected following an automobile accident caused by poor visibility.

is subject to variations from person to person and the description of an odor in words is usually very inadequate. Furthermore, the sensitivity of an individual observer varies from day to day. Under certain conditions the sense of smell becomes rapidly fatigued. Sensitivity to odors reaches its maximum at puberty and decreases with age.[1]

Interactions of several odors may have different effects. Some are synergistic, others counteract each other. A combination of odors of hydrochloric acid and chlorine gas, for instance, is more easily perceptible than either one by itself.[2]

Numerous publications can be cited that suggest that allergic symptoms are aggravated or precipitated by odors. Although it is conceivable that a reflex action, initiated in the olfactory organ, may induce bronchospasm and allergic nasal symptoms, it has never been established that the odor itself rather than the presence of particulates, fumes, or vapors was responsible.

Sources

Odors in air naturally. In nature, odors are produced principally by decomposition through bacterial action[4] of protein-containing material derived mostly from vegetables and animal life. They occur mostly in stagnant and insufficiently aired water, such as swamps and sewers. Dimethyl sulfide and methyl mercaptan, two sulfur com-

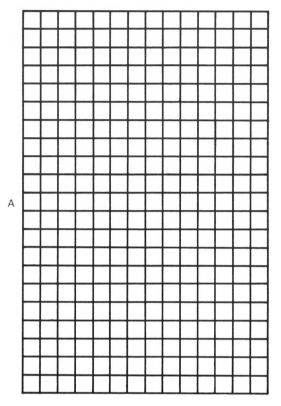

A

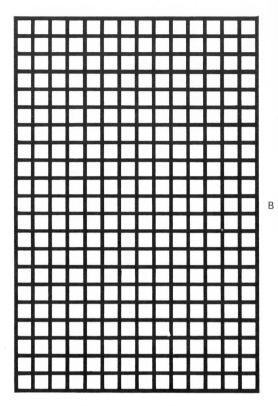

B

Fig. 4-2. Ringelmann's scale for grading the density of smoke. **A,** Equivalent to 20% black.

B, Equivalent to 40% black.

pounds that emanate from marine algae and from certain seaweeds, are the major pollutants causing odors from natural sources. Forest fires and open field burning contribute further to odorants in the environment.

Household odors. Some of the principal odorous substances encountered in a household are named by Sullivan[5] in the following list.

Odorous substances

1. Cleaning fluid
2. Cooking odors
3. Feces
4. Fish
5. Food
6. Formaldehyde
7. Fresh paint
8. Furniture polish
9. Gasoline
10. Lighter fluid
11. Moth balls
12. Newspaper print
13. Oils
14. Perfume
15. Rubber
16. Spices
17. Tobacco smoke
18. Turpentine
19. Wood smoke

Although the odors of certain perfumes and cosmetics may be pleasant to some, to others they are not only undesirable but irritating, particularly to allergic individuals, in whom they may trigger sneezing, cough, and asthmatic attacks at public gatherings.

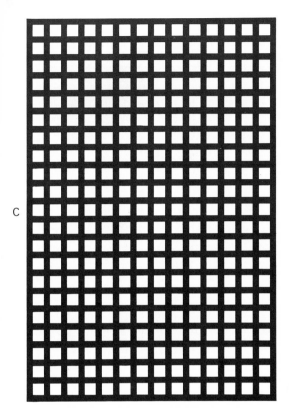

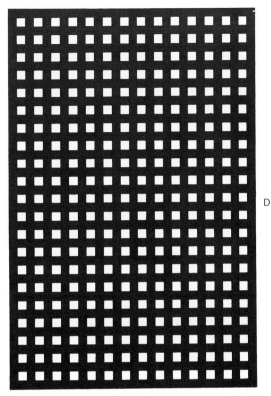

C

D

C, Equivalent to 60% black.

D, Equivalent to 80% black. (Reproduced from U. S. Bureau of Mines Information Circular Number 7718, 1955.)

The principal industries that produce odorants are oil refineries, natural gas, and chemical plants, especially those engaged in the manufacture of sulfur-containing chemicals. Others are paper mills, dye and rayon factories, iron and metal smelters, ovens, cement, fertilizer, and rendering plants, tanneries, and food processing establishments.

Near petroleum refineries, the perceptible odorous emissions consist of hydrogen sulfide, mercaptans (sulfur-containing alcohol), phenolic compounds, organic sulfides and amines, aldehydes, and aliphatic and aromatic compounds.

The most offensive odors from chemical establishments are nitrogen and sulfur compounds associated with organic materials that are evolved in high temperature. Soap manufacturing plants[6] produce aminelike (fishy) odors, that can be detected as far as 5 to 6 miles from the plant.

The rotten-egg odor in the pulp and paper mill industry is caused by hydrogen sulfide, mercaptans, organic sulfides, and disulfides. In coking operations,[7] in the iron and steel industry, and in coal mining[8] hydrogen sulfide is the major malodorous product.

Food processing, such as smoking, drying, baking, frying, boiling, dehydrating, fermenting, distilling, curing, canning, and freezing, induces a variety of obnoxious odors. Both in slaughtering operations and in cutting up the carcasses offensive odors are released. When animal matter is spilled or otherwise exposed to the atmosphere it becomes infested by flies and maggots. The

Table 4-1. Odors characteristic of pollutants*

COMPOUNDS	CHARACTERISTICS
Acrolein (a hydrocarbon in diesel exhaust)	Like burning fat
Ammonia	Sharp, pungent, odor of urine
Chlorine	Pungent, irritating
Hydrogen sulfide	Rotten eggs
Isocyanides (in polyurethane plastics)	Sweet, but repulsive
Mercaptans (sulfur-containing alcohols)	Like decayed cabbage
Selenium compounds	Putrid, garliclike
Ozone	Electric sparks, lightening
Skatole	Odor of fecal matter
Sulfur dioxide	Pungent, like musty rooms
Tars	Rancid, skunklike
Tellurium	Garliclike

*Compiled from Kaiser, E. R.: Odor and its measurement. In Stern, A. C., editor: Air pollution, vol. 1, New York, 1962, Academic Press, Inc., pp. 520-522.

highly obnoxious trimethylamine[9] as well as other amines, ammonium, hydrogen sulfide, skatole, sulfides, and mercaptans are formed. Animal fats produce aldehydes and organic acids. The principal source of fish odors is trimethylamine.[10] Two other major chemicals, putrescine and cadaverine, run a close second. In tanneries, the principal malodorous chemical derived from skins that have become infested with maggots is ammonia.

The odors liberated from automobile exhaust as the result of combustion of gasoline are not as offensive as those of diesel oil. The latter are usually related to aldehyde concentrations.

The characteristic pungent odor of photochemical smog is caused by its acrid component ozone.

Some odors typical of certain chemicals are presented in Table 4-1:

MATERIALS

Several pollutants can be identified by their effect on materials. Carbon dioxide, for instance, affects building stones, especially carbonate rock such as limestone.[12]

Sulfur oxides produce a variety of damage to materials (Table 4-2). On aluminum equipment they create a white powder, aluminum sulfate. On copper they induce the well-known greenish coating, copper sulfate. They are also capable of attacking building material including limestone, marble, and roofing slate. After protracted exposure to sulfur oxides, leather is weakened, paper turns brittle, and its resistance to folding lessens. Sulfur oxides cause natural and synthetic fibers to deteriorate. Damage to women's nylon hose by sulfur oxides has made newspaper headlines.

Hydrogen sulfide tarnishes silver and copper. The discoloration of white paint of homes in humid areas is caused by the formation of *lead sulfide*.

Hydrogen fluoride is noted for attacking metals, glass, and enamel-coated material. It turns window panes opaque and damages the finish of automobiles.

Ozone's ability to crack rubber and rubber products has served as a means of measuring ozone concentrations in the atmosphere. After a certain period of exposure to air the exact depth of the cracks in strips of rubber of precise formulation is determined. The oxidizing power of ozone causes colorfast dyes in textiles to fade.

Carbon, one of the solid particles in the

Table 4-2. Damage to materials by pollutants

POLLUTANT	MATERIAL	DAMAGE
Carbon dioxide	Limestone	Deteriorates
Sulfur oxides	Metals (steel, aluminum, copper)	Corrodes
		Conversion into sulfates
	Building materials	Weakens
	Leather	Turns brittle
	Paper	Damages
	Textiles	
Hydrogen sulfide	Silver	Tarnishes
	Copper	Darkens
	Paint	Blackens
Hydrogen fluoride	Glass	Etches, opaques
Ozone	Rubber	Cracks
	Textiles	Weakens
	Dyes	Fades
Solid particulates	Laundry	Soils
	Building surfaces	Soils

air, tends to soil white surfaces, such as linens; whereas light-colored solids, such as *cement* particles and *gypsum,* render dark surfaces gray.

VEGETATION

In establishing the kind and severity of pollution, a careful assessment of damage to vegetation is more significant than damage to materials. When trees, particularly evergreens, show damage confined to the side facing the prevailing winds in line with an industrial establishment, the presence of a polluting source must be suspected. Although a fungus, a virus, or some kind of nutritional deficiency can account for similar damage to vegetation, certain pollutants elicit highly specific kinds of injuries to a plant. If properly evaluated they permit prompt identification of the kind and range of concentration of the air pollutant involved.[13]*

*Jacobsen and Hill have presented an atlas with colored photographs of the major injuries to plants. They are undoubtedly the most useful source of information on this phase of pollution.

Monitoring

Cultivation of test plants. Assessment of such damage as a means of monitoring for air pollution has extensive practical applications. Officials are cultivating pollutant-sensitive plants at measured distances from a factory in order to determine the extent of pollution damage. The tobacco plant, for instance, is being used to map air pollution by ozone; the pinto bean plant to detect peroxyacetyl nitrate (PAN) and petunias to investigate total oxidants; gladiolus and tulips to identify damage by fluorides; lichens for sulfur dioxide damage. Dahlias and alfalfa are also excellent detectors for sulfur dioxide damage.

Fumigation experiments. In addition, leaf injury is being experimentally reproduced by fumigating plants in especially designed chambers as a model for comparison with plants injured by pollution. On broad-leafed plants (for example, gladiolus, tulips, lilies of the valley) the percentage of the injured leaf surface in relation to the total length of the leaf is measured. Chemical assays for the respective pollutant give

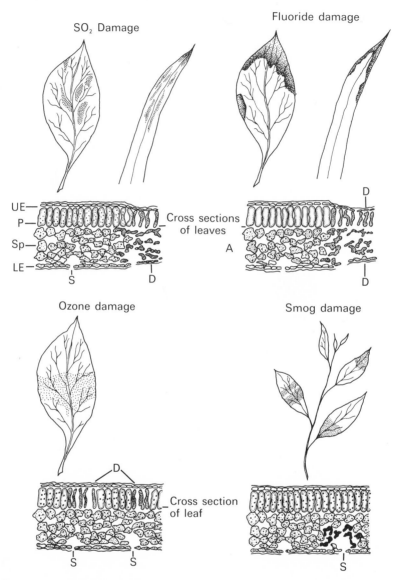

Fig. 4-3. Schematic drawing of damage to leaves caused by sulfur oxides, fluorides, ozone, and smog. SO$_2$ injury mainly affects the spaces between the ribs of the leaf; fluoride involves the tips and margins; ozone and smog produce a stippled lesion. On cross section, fluoride and sulfur dioxide involve the whole leaf with greater shrinkage and collapse of cells by fluoride. In ozone injury, only the palissade layer is affected. Smog produces the initial damage near the stomata. *P,* palissade cells; *Sp,* spongy cells; *S,* stomata through which polluted air enters the leaf; *LE,* lower epidermal cells; *UE,* upper epidermal cells; *A,* air spaces that serve as passage for pollutants; *D,* destruction of cells by pollutants.

further confirmatory information in monitoring for pollutants.

Entry into plants

Airborne particles and vapors are deposited on or enter vegetation either in natural state by dry deposition, for example, impaction or sedimentation, or by wet deposition if they are incorporated in falling rain drops and in droplets of clouds.[14] Such pollutants enter the plant either through its aerial parts (above the soil's surface) or through absorption by roots from the soil. From the soil, pollutants are taken up mainly by root hair and they are translocated through the vascular system along with nutrients and other chemicals to its stem, leaves, and fruits. Uptake of air contaminants is more sustained and intense above the ground than from roots. It takes place through the leaves, fruits, stem, or bark.

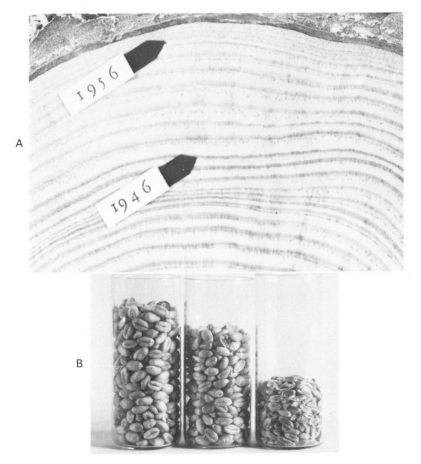

Fig. 4-4. A, Effect of fluoride emissions on growth of pine trees. Note disturbance in growth of pine tree. An almost complete standstill in growth is indicated by the narrowed growth rings after 1956, the year a fluoride-emitting fertilizer factory started its operation. **B,** Comparison of winter wheat grown at various distances from an aluminum factory. Specimens left to right composed of 1000 grains harvested 2.5 km, 300 meters, and 50 meters east of an aluminum smelter. They contained 0.02, 0.16, and 2.99 mg% fluoride and weighed 50.2, 42.0, and 17.1 gm, respectively. (Courtesy Dr. H. Bohné, Bonn-Bad-Godesberg, Germany.)

Mode of injury

The major kinds of damage by air pollutants to plants are destruction of leaf tissue and chlorosis (fading of the natural green color [chlorophyll] of a leaf) and stunting in growth of the plant.

Leaf necrosis and chlorosis. The cross section of a leaf is composed of several layers of cells. The epidermis lines its upper and lower surfaces. A row of elongated cells standing on end, called palisade cells, lies below the upper epidermis (Fig. 4-3). Between their lower edge and the lower epidermal layer, irregularly shaped cells with large air spaces between them form the parenchyma. The epidermis contains stomata (small openings between cells), which are capable of opening and closing. Through these so-called stomata, gases and particulates enter the leaf. The stomata of most plants close at night. Therefore plants appear to be more resistent to pollutants in the dark.

The degree of humidity is a vital factor in the uptake of pollutants by plants. Loss of water in the cells, caused by atmospheric pollutants, leads to their disintegration. When injury is the result of oxidants, this

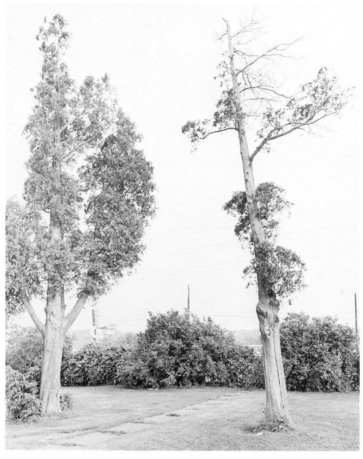

Fig. 4-5. Hydrochloric acid and fluoride damage to trees ½-mile northeast of a secondary aluminum smelter in Indiana. Leaves showed 104 ppm fluoride. Greater damage to leaves occurred on side down wind from the factory.

process takes place in the parenchymal cells near the stomata. Ozone damages the palisade cells. Injury by sulfur dioxide begins in the spongy parenchymal cells. Fluoride damage originates mainly in the central portion of a leaf.

Changes in growth. Air pollution can cause stunted growth in plants, lack of normal vigor, and early senescence (aging).[15] Small fruit and reduced yield is common in citrus groves exposed to pollution. Reduction in the growth of rings in forest trees (Fig. 4-4, *A*) and lower wheat yields (Fig. 4-4, *B*) follow injury to leaves by fluoride.[16] Mohamed[17] demonstrated defects in chromosomes of tomato plants, which resulted in stunted growth following experimental fumigation with hydrogen fluoride at a concentration as low as 3 μg/meter^3 of air.

Fluoride damage to trees is usually reversible.[18] During temporary closure of a factory, a dying plant can recuperate promptly. Upon resumption of operations the damage recurs (Fig. 4-5).

Assessment of plant damage

In assessing damage to vegetation, one must keep in mind that each species and each plant, indeed each portion of a plant, reacts differently to a damaging pollutant. Young growing plants, for instance, are more susceptible to fluoride than older ones; turgid leaves are more susceptible than wilted ones. Certain varieties of gladiolus or tulips are relatively resistant to fluoride. They can accumulate considerable amounts of the halogen in leaftips[19] with little or no apparent damage. The kind of fertilizer used on a plant, the amount of water that it receives, the soil, temperature, light intensity, and many other factors alter its response to a pollutant. All these facts must be taken into account in assessing damage to vegetation by air pollution.

Certain bacteria, fungi, viruses, insects, nematodes, as well as excessive water loss associated with hot winds, can induce symptoms that closely resemble those caused by air pollutants and thus camouflage an otherwise characteristic pollution injury. Symptoms similar to sulfur dioxide injury can be induced by frost or by mineral deficiency. Viruslike symptoms are sometimes confused with ozone injury.[20] The problem is further complicated, since air pollution injury, particularly one caused by ozone, predisposes certain plants (ponderosa pine) to bark beetle infestation.[21] Table 4-3 presents the typical damage caused by and the major plants resistant and sensitive to the five most important pollutants.

Kind of damage

Fluorides, which some consider the most noxious of all phytotoxic pollutants,* promptly diffuse with the normal nutrients and flow of water from the stomata of the leaf to the margins and tips.[15] In distinction to many other pollutants, fluorides remain anchored in the leaf tissue. The affected cells dry out and turn deep brown to tan. A sharp reddish-brown demarcation line between the healthy and the diseased leaf tissue is characteristic of fluoride damage (Fig. 4-6). Occasionally the diseased tip drops off the leaf. In tulips and gladiolus, the length of the injured portion of a leaf and its fluoride content provide a clue to the degree of air pollution.[18] As little as 1 ppb of hydrogen fluoride in the atmosphere will mark gladiolus leaves within a few days.[18]

In apricot orchards and vineyards exposed to fluoride pollution in the Swiss Rhone Valley, damage to leaves was limited to particular plots that had been fertilized with a boron-containing fertilizer.[23] Fluoride levels in leaves ranged up to 600 ppm (dry matter) in plots where a boron-containing fertilizer had been applied[23];

---

*Zimmerman[22] graded the toxicity to green plants of the five most important gases in the following order: HF, Cl_2, SO_2, NH_3, H_2S.

Table 4-3. The most significant pollutants toxic to plants

| | MARKINGS | LEVEL PPM | INDICATOR PLANTS | |
			SENSITIVE	RESISTANT
Sulfur dioxide	White to brown, bleaching, blotching between veins	0.1 to 3.0	Pumpkin Barley Squash Alfalfa Cotton Wheat Apple	Potato Onion Corn Maple Most trees
Fluoride	Necrosis on tips and edges of leaves, sharply demarcated by dark brown-red band	0.0001	Gladiolus Tulips Prunes Apricots Pine	Alfalfa Roses* Tobacco Tomato Cotton
Ozone	Red-brown flecks	0.15	Tobacco Tomato Bean Spinach Potato	Mint Geranium Gladiolus Pepper Bean
Oxidant smog	Silver or bronzelike on underside of leaf; banded pattern	0.2	Petunia Lettuce Pinto bean Bluegrass	Cabbage Corn Wheat Pansy
Chlorine	Bleaching, necrosis on margins and between veins, scattered spotting	about 1.5	Radish Alfalfa Peach Cosmos Buckwheat	Eggplant Tobacco Begonia Pepper
Ethylene	Withering and drying of flowers; growth retardation, loss of flower buds	0.01	Orchids Carnations Azalias Tomatoes Cotton	Grasses Lettuce

*Cut roses are sensitive to fluoride.

these values were much higher than those in leaves in the nonboron fertilized area.

Another approach in assessing the extent of air pollution by fluoride is the determination of the percentage of defoliation (falling of leaves) of a plant.[17]

The margins of fruit tree leaves often curl so that the leaves assume a "boat or spoonlike" appearance. Corn and citrus trees, damaged by fluoride, exhibit chlorosis (a yellowish-pale color) before the edges and tips are adversely affected. On evergreens, especially on ponderosa pines, fluoride damage starts at the tips of the needles. This injury by fluoride is similar to that caused by cold temperature.

Sulfur oxides tend to dry up the plant, which then assumes a light ivory or tan color. The injury to leaves originates and concentrates between their veins (Fig. 4-7). Often the veins themselves begin to bleach out. Grasses, which have two layers of palisade cells, collapse throughout the thickness of their blade. On evergreens, sulfur oxides induce a reddish discoloration either at the tips of the needles or as a band over their entire length; subsequently the dead tissue shrivels up. Sulfuric acid, which is formed in the atmosphere by sulfur oxides (SO_3) in the presence of moisture, produces small necrotic (dead) areas simulating burns. They are surrounded by a black ring with its edges slightly erased.

Oxidants precipitate tissue collapse in the parenchymal cells surrounding the space into which the stomata open (Fig. 4-6). Cheeseweed and annual blue grass are some of the most delicate indicator plants for oxidants. Atmospheric concentrations, as low as 0.11 ppm of ozone, lead to a characteristic silvery-bronzing of the upper leaf surface. Tiny white and brown spots involve the whole thickness of the leaf (Fig. 4-8). When such lesions appear on tobacco leaves, they are often mistakenly described as "weather spots." Chlorosis is usually quite pronounced.

Damage resulting from oxidants is somewhat similar to that caused by sulfur oxides. However, the oxidants induce a cross-the-leaf band rather than blotches or streaks, which characterize the sulfur oxide lesions.

Many other pollutants are injurious to plants. Their concentrations in the air, however, are rarely high enough to cause visible injury.

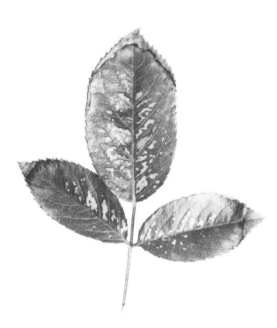

Fig. 4-6. Rose leaves injured by sulfur dioxide (lesions in between ribs of leaves) and fluoride (sharp demarcation line between the wilted and green tissue). (Courtesy Dr. I. J. Hindawi, Environmental Protection Agency, Research Triangle Park, North Carolina.)

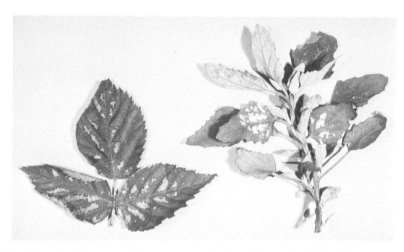

Fig. 4-7. Sulfur dioxide injury of lambsquarter (right) and bramble (left), with spoon formation of the left lower leaf. (Courtesy Dr. I. A. Leone, New Jersey Agriculture Station, Rutgers University.)

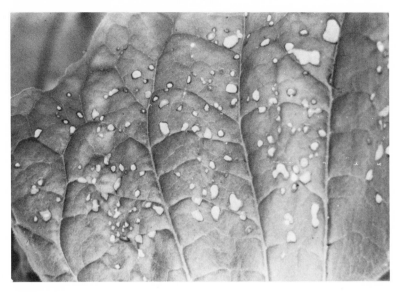

Fig. 4-8. Ozone injury to a tobacco leaf. (Courtesy Dr. I. J. Hindawi, Environmental Protection Agency, Research Triangle Park, North Carolina.)

Chlorine gas, for instance, is three times as noxious to plants as sulfur dioxide but only limited damage has been reported in the literature. Chlorine gas that escaped from a cylinder used to chlorinate a swimming pool near Yonkers, New York[24] and from accidental leaks in the vicinity of sewage treatment installations in California caused damage to plants. Necrotic (dead) areas appear along the veins of broad-leaved plants, generally toward the center of the leaf. In some plants, especially tomatoes, tobacco, and cucumbers, chlorine causes necrotic areas all over the leaf blade. Chlorosis develops on either side of the veins, although the veins themselves remain green.

Hydrogen chloride induces damage that resembles the damage caused by sulfur dioxide and ozone. Its typical lesion consists of necrosis on leaf margins with dark reddish-tan spots. The damaged area on the leaf margin is narrower and less severe than that caused by fluoride. Randomly distributed necrotic spots appear over the leaf surface. A concentration of approximately 7 ppm of hydrochloride for a few hours damages plants.

Hydrogen sulfide, the obnoxious gas with the rotten-egg odor, is relatively harmless to vegetation. It causes slight damage with light tan to white markings on plants. Cosmos, radishes, and clover, some of the plants most susceptible to hydrogen sulfide, serve as indicator plants.

Hydrogen cyanide is occasionally found in manufactured gas at concentrations of 200 to 300 ppm. It is rarely injurious in the open atmosphere.

Ammonia escapes into the atmosphere while being applied to crops, as a source of nitrogen, with irrigation water. A silvery glow on the underside of leaves resembling the markings of oxidents, is its hallmark. The leaf damage, often described as "cooked green," turns brown on drying. Mustard plants and sunflowers are among the most sensitive indicator plants for ammonia. On corn and grass it causes streaks at the leaf's edges and lesions between the veins.

Mercury causes more damage to flowers

than to leaves. On peach trees and privet hedges, which are very susceptible to the metal, fading and subsequent browning of interveinal tissue of old leaves occurs. Early abscission (falling of leaves) is noted following mercury exposures at the ppb range.[13]

Ethylene, a hydrocarbon gas of the olefin series derived from automobile and truck exhaust and widely used in the chemical industry, injures plants without directly attacking plant tissues; it undergoes photochemical reactions with nitrogen oxides and with ozone. Ethylene interferes with the activities of plant hormones and thus causes growth retardation. Concentrations as low as 0.05 ppm impaired normal development of leaves and blossoms of marigolds, tomatoes, and pepper plants. Great economic losses have been reported through injury to orchids, a very sensitive crop.[25]

The above-described evidence of damage to vegetation and material can give only a rough impression regarding the presence of and the degree of air pollution. In recent years highly sophisticated apparatus and equipment to trap the air and to analyze its constituents have been developed and employed to great advantage.[2] Indeed an entirely new technologic industry has arisen to cope with this subject. It is not the intent of this book to deal with this phase of pollution. However, recent advances along this line have led to important knowledge serving both industry and, particularly, those engaged in controlling pollution.

INTOXICATION OF ANIMALS

Animal life, like plants and materials, constitutes a monitor for damage caused by air pollution. In general, mammals and insects are much more resistant to pollutants than plants. Animals, both domestic and wildlife, as well as humans are subject to acute and chronic illness as the result of air pollution.

In early May 1970, the volcano Hekla, a 4747-foot peak in Southern Iceland, erupted

and sent a huge smoke cloud high into the air. Sections of the Greenland icecap, 300 miles away, were blackened by ashes (Fig. 4-9). Farmers within a 130-mile radius of the eruption reported that their sheep on pasture lost their appetite and that their wool became shabby.[26] One farmer lost 21 sheep; on another farm, at least 100 ewes gave birth to dead lambs. Over 6000 lambs and 1500 ewes died of fluorosis (chronic fluoride poisoning). Cattle and horses also were adversely affected. Iceland's chief veterinarian, Pall A. Palsson, urged farmers to have their lambs and calves boarded out on farms in distant areas. Although the volcano emitted many pollutants, fluoride was held principally responsible for the damage.

To the people of Iceland, disaster as the result of volcanic activity, is an old story. Following a severe eruption of Hekla in the eleventh century[27] fluorosis in cattle and sheep was rampant. Records from 200 years ago show that another eruption led to the worst famine in Iceland's history. Exactly to what extent the farmers themselves were adversely affected in these and in the 1970 disaster has not been investigated.

Acute poisoning

During the acute air pollution disasters in the Meuse Valley and London, animals died in acute distress with pulmonary disease and heart failure[28] as established by postmortem examinations.

Short-term episodes of severe pollution damage to animals are not uncommon in areas close to factories. I observed severe damage to pigs on a farm in Indiana, situated about one-third mile from a secondary aluminum smelter. On several occasions, epidemics of cough developed in the herd. At first the veterinarian suspected, but ruled out, an infectious disease. With increased production at the plant, the coughing became more severe and several animals died. In a sow autopsied at Purdue University, the lining of the throat was

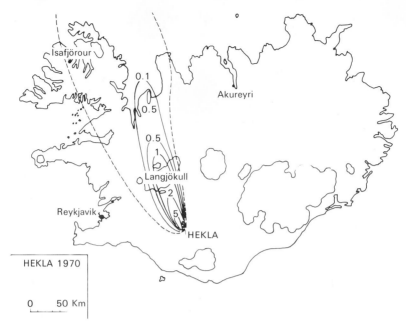

Fig. 4-9. At the outbreak of volcano Hekla in Iceland in 1970, flyash was dispersed farther than 250 km from its source. (Courtesy Dr. G. Georgsson, University of Iceland.)

found to be virtually "burned off." The diagnosis made by the veterinary pathologist was pulmonary edema. When surviving hogs were kept inside the barns, away from the smoke, most of them recuperated within a few days, but they remained unproductive. Three boars and a group of sows that had produced young could not reproduce again. Newly bred sows, brought into the affected area, gave birth to pigs but subsequently were infertile.

Chronic intoxication

Acute episodes of poisoning such as that resulting from inhalation are less common than chronic intoxication caused by feeding on contaminated forage and by continuous inhalation of contaminated air. Certain animals, especially cows, sheep, and goats on pasture take up with their forage substantial quantities of contaminated soil, about equal in amount to the forage itself.[29]

Arsenic. As far back as 1902, 625 of a herd of 3500 sheep died within 15 miles of a copper smelter in Montana.[30] Grass and moss on which they were feeding contained up to 405 ppm of arsenic trioxide (AS_2O_3) and up to 1800 ppm copper. In their organs, arsenic levels ranged from traces in the liver to several hundred ppm in hair and up to 1015 ppm in an ulcer on a horse's nose. In a similar episode in Saxony in the 1930s[31] deer in the area lost their hair; the upper layer of their skin turned unusually thick, a condition called scleroderma. Dead deer were found with malformed bones and swollen joints. Several years earlier an unexplained mortality of bees had stumped the farmers and agricultural scientists until they recognized the disease as arsenic poisoning caused by emissions from the same plant. The bees contained about 1 μg arsenic. The minimum lethal dose for bees is 0.1 to 0.2 μg.

Lead. Lead poisoning was encountered in cattle and horses grazing within 5 km of a German lead and zinc smelter.[32] The animals became emaciated, their joints

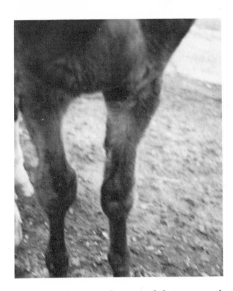

Fig. 4-10. Arthritis in knee at left in one of ten horses observed in the Trail, British Columbia area near a lead smelter. Besides lead, fluoride, cadmium, and zinc were contributing factors.

painful and swollen (Fig. 4-10). Some had palsy of the recurrent nerve, which affected their vocal cords: a peculiarly hoarse voice, and a characteristic roaring was accompanied by shortness of breath, especially after mild exercise. Dust from the area contained up to 45% lead and up to 32% zinc combined with traces of arsenic and fluoride. Cadmium was undoubtedly another major constituent for which no tests were made at that time. More recently similar damage to horses was reported near a lead smelter in Trail, British Columbia.[33]

Hamond and Aronson[34] described a similar outbreak of lead poisoning near a smelter outside of St. Paul, Minnesota, which recovered lead from discarded batteries. Lead poisoning in domestic animals also occurs when cattle drink water from discarded paint buckets or lick flaking paint from barns.

Captive animals in zoos[35] are subject to damage from air pollution. In eastern zoos, jaguars died in convulsions; their bodies were "loaded with lead" believed to have been derived from automobile exhaust. Lions, tigers, and other cats have a tendency to lick their fur, which accumulates lead and other heavy metals from the atmosphere.

The Detroit Zoo has lost six seals and sea lions in two years as a result of lead poisoning. Tigers and jaguars at the Staten Island Zoo have elevated levels of lead in their digestive systems. Death of an orangutang at Chicago's Brookfield Zoo was attributed to lead ingested by the animal when paint chips were scraped off the walls of its quarters. The lead-laced strips of Polaroid film dropped thoughtlessly in zoo ponds and yards where animals nibble or lick them are believed to contribute to poisoning.[37]

Fluoride. According to the U. S. Department of Agriculture fluorides "have caused more world-wide damage to domestic animals than any other air pollutant."[38] The extensive body of data that has accumulated from many countries is summarized by Lillie.[37]

Bardelli and Menzani[38] presented one of the earliest and most complete descriptions of fluoride damage to animal life near an Italian aluminum smelter in the deep oval valley of the Adice (Etsch) river, extending over 7 km in length and 2 km in width. They noted two distinct periods of illness in cattle. During the first stage the cows appeared ill; they lay down frequently; their hide was less elastic; pressure on their ribs and lumbar spine induced pain. In the second stage, sudden lameness developed often preceded by stiffness of movements. Swellings appeared below the hide, which could be flattened out and which disappeared in 10 to 24 hours (Fig. 4-11). Milk production was reduced. Intermittent bowel disturbances, often of short duration, were noted. As the disease progressed further, gradual emaciation took place. The vertebral column became rigid, the lameness permanent; protrusions on the metacarpal and metatarsal (foot) bones were

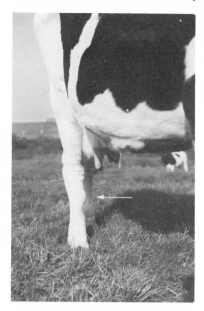

Fig. 4-11. Leg of a cow showing protrusion (arrow) indicative of arthritis and bone apposition caused by fluoride. (Courtesy Professor Cohrs, Hannover Veterinary University, Germany.)

painful. Ultimately, the animals died of chronic wasting (Fig. 4-12, *A* and *B*).

Disturbances in sexual function of the cattle were not apparent, but the calves showed poor body development. At autopsy, major changes in the cattle were found in the pituitary and thyroid glands and in the skeleton.

Bardelli and Menzani also reported a 100% mortality in silkworms that were raised in the valley. The trouble began shortly after the aluminum factory started its operations in 1929. The larvae were smaller and their development was retarded. In the advanced stage, a marked reduction in or total elimination of fatty tissue was associated with an excessive reduction in the silk-producing gland. The intestinal tract was usually empty. The mulberry leaves on which the worms had been feeding contained 4 to 20 times greater quantities of fluoride than mulberry leaves in other regions.

Among other nonmammalians, death of bees has produced serious economic hardship in France's Rhone Valley and, more recently, in industrial areas of East Germany.[40] When fluoride levels on plant surfaces were above 100 ppm and on pollen between 9 and 28 ppm, the fluoride values in dead bees varied between 2 to 33 μg per bee. The lethal concentration for bees ranges between 4 and 5 μg.[37] Fluoride has replaced arsenic as the most serious cause of death to bees.[39]

In 1970 analysis of a number of insects by Carlson and Dewey[21] showed marked accumulation of fluoride in a wide variety of other insects near an aluminum plant in Montana (Table 4-4).

Selenium. Prior to the early 1930s, farmers in South Dakota had serious trouble with livestock as a result of selenium poisoning.[40] A farm, known locally as the "Reed Farm," changed owners repeatedly. Usually a law suit was filed by the new owners charging misrepresentation by the previous ones. Horses and cattle became sick and valueless. Chicks from incubated eggs failed to hatch; they were so grossly deformed that they were incapable of breaking their way through the shell. It was established eventually that the chick malformations occurred only in eggs from hens fed wheat grain that contained excess selenium and that poisoning was caused by the wheat's high selenium content derived from soil.[41] Purchase of the farm by the Federal Government in the mid-1930s ended the "Reed Farm" tragedies. It is now a subagricultural experiment station.

Animals suffering from chronic selenium poisoning lose weight and fail to respond to good care. Prominent among symptoms are loss of hair and abnormal hoof growth. Postmortem examination reveals damage to the liver, kidney, and heart. The disease is caused by daily ingestion of cereals and grasses containing 5 to 20 ppm selenium.[40]

Molybdenum. In the mid-1950s, cows grazing within 100 meters of a Swedish steel plant showed degenerative changes in

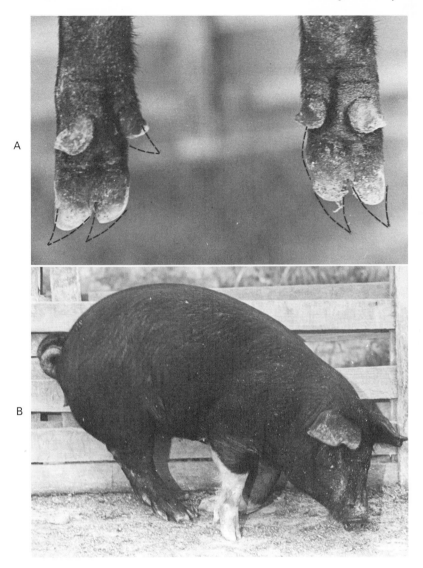

Fig. 4-12. A, Stunted (short, stubby) toes and protrusions on hoofs in young pigs ¾-mile west of a secondary aluminum smelter in the Midwest. This finding was observed throughout the entire herd, July 8, 1970. In another herd 10 miles southeast of the smelter, no abnormalities were found. **B,** Typical fluoride damage in hogs (same herd as in **A**). Painful forelegs caused by spontaneous fractures and arthritic changes.

liver cells and inflammation of the small bowels. Molybdenum was established as the cause. The cows' blood contained 25 times more molybdenum than that of normal cattle.[42] Stiffness in legs and back, below normal copper levels in the blood, and changes in the color of the hide from black to rusty or from red to yellow are other symptoms of molybdenum poisoning.[37] Horses appear to be much more resistant to the disease than cattle.[42]

Organic mercury. On November 28, 1967, three of a herd of 49 mixed-breed pigs on a farm in New York state were found dead.[43]

Table 4-4. Effects of fluoride on insects*

FLUORIDE ACCUMULATION LEVELS IN INSECTS	PPM	CONTROL INSECT SAMPLES PPM
Pollinators		
Bumblebee (*Bombus* species)	406.0	7.5
Sphinx moth (*Hemaris* species)	394.0	—
Honey bee *(Apis mellifera)*	221.0	10.5
Skipper butterfly *(Erynnis)*	146.0	—
Foilage feeders		
Grasshoppers (*Melanoplus* species)	31.0	7.5
Cambium feeders		
Engraver beetles (*Ips* species)	52.5	—
Predators		
Ants	170.0	—
Damselflies (*Argia* species)	21.7	9.2

*Compiled from Carlson, C. E., and Dewey, J. E.: Environmental pollution by fluorides in Flathead National Forest and Glacier National Park, Appendix VI, October, 1971, U. S. Department of Agriculture, Forest Service.

They became listless, uncoordinated, blind, and developed fever and vomiting for 3 to 5 days before they died in coma. The diagnosis of mercury poisoning suggested at autopsy was subsequently confirmed when 2 mg of mercury per 100 gm of tissue (20 ppm) was found in the liver of one of the deceased pigs. On November 29, seven pigs had been removed for sale as slaughter animals. Eventually the whole herd died. Of 5 litters of between 50 to 70 piglets, only five were born alive. They too died soon after weaning. The poisoning was caused by seed wheat fed to the animals, which had been dressed with Panogen, a preservative containing mercury dicyandiamide (see Chapter 12).

Pesticides. Bird life in certain areas has been reduced to a minimum by pesticides, and their reproductive capacity has been affected to such an extent that whole species have been nearly wiped out. Numerous instances of fish kills and damage to other aquatic life have reached the public press (see Chapter 22). In 1966, for instance, of 9,115,000 fresh-water fish reported killed by identifiable pollution sources in 46 states, 217,000 had succumbed to insecticides and poisons used on farms to increase productivity of crops[45] (Table 4-5). The primary sources were water contaminated by wastes and drainage from mines and over-enriched with organic material from municipal sewage.

At the Snake River in Idaho, 500,000 fish suffocated when organic wastes from potato-processing plants reduced the level of dissolved oxygen in water to below 0.5 ppm, encompassing a 7-mile stretch above a dam.[44]

In a recent survey[45] scientists investigated the possibility of using English sparrows, which are nonmigratory, as a biologic indicator of atmospheric pollution. Histologic studies of samples from grossly polluted Davis and Sacramento, California were compared to those obtained along California's Sonoma Coast where the air is swept clean by westerly winds. Far more black pigment-laden macrophages were found in lungs of inland sparrows than in those of the coastal group; the liver showed minimal fatty degeneration in the former group, none in the latter. These birds constitute an ideal biologic air sampler because they remain in the same area the entire year around, they are plentiful, and they live close to man.

Table 4-5. Sources of the 1966 fish kill in the United States*

SOURCES	NUMBER KILLED
Industrial pollution	4,622,790
Waste from cities	1,347,248
Agricultural operations	1,259,599
Transportation accidents	102,631
Insecticides	217,000
Miscellaneous (building and highway construction, airplane washing, illegal disposal of poisons in water)	1,410,569

*Compiled from Fish kills by pollution 1966, seventh annual report, Washington, D. C., 1967, Federal Water Pollution Control Administration, U. S. Department of the Interior.

When an epidemic of cough develops overnight in a herd of hogs, sheep, or cows; when their skin is covered with flydust; when cows that had been perfectly healthy prior to being exposed to smoke and dust can no longer be bred successfully; when spontaneous abortions, stillbirths, and reduction in milk productivity occur in cattle, sheep, or goats; and when health departments and veterinarians have ruled out other causes for the disease, especially chronic infections: then one must suspect damage from airborne pollutants. Under certain conditions, such damage might occur even though the source of pollution is many miles away. The multiplicity of causes renders the identification of individual sources most difficult.

Nevertheless there are numerous ways to identify pollution even by those not equipped with the sophisticated instruments available to scientists. The major pollutants can sometimes be identified by a careful look at vegetation, animal life, and materials.

REFERENCES

1. Horstman, S. W., Wromble, R. F., and Heller, A. N.: Identification of community odor problems by use of an observer corps, J. Air Pollut. Contr. Ass. **15**:261-264, 1965.
2. Stayzhkin, V. M.: Hygienic determination of limits of allowable concentrations of chlorine and hydrochloride gases simultaneously present in atmospheric air, translated by Levine, B. S., U.S.S.R. Literature on Air Pollution and Related Occupational Diseases, **9**:55, 1962.
3. Morgan, G. B., Ozolins, G., and Tabor, E. C.: Air pollution surveillance systems, Science **170**:289-296, 1970.
4. Monganelli, R. M., and Gregory, C. J.: The effect of hydrogen sulfide on various surfaces, Atmospheric Pollution Technical Bulletin No. 25, New York, 1965, National Council for Stream Improvement, Inc.
5. Sullivan, R. J.: Air pollution aspects of odorous compounds, Litton System, Inc. Bethesda, Maryland, 1969, U. S. Department of Commerce, Nat. Bureau of Standards, PB 188 089.
6. Molos, J. E.: Control of odors from a continuous soap making process, J. Air Pollut. Contr. Ass. **11**:9, 1961.
7. Kirk-Othmer, Encyclopedia of Chemical Technology, New York, 1954, Interscience.
8. Sussman, V. H., and Mulhern, J. J.: Air pollution from coal refuse disposal areas, J. Air Pollut. Contr. Ass. **14**:279-284, 1964.
9. Summer, W.: Methods of air deodorization, Amsterdam, 1963, Elsevier.
10. Danielson, J. A., editor: Air pollution engineering manual. Air Pollution Control District County of Los Angeles, U. S. Public Health Service, Bureau of Disease Prevention Environmental Control, Cincinnati, Ohio, 1967, National Center for Air Pollution Control.
11. Kaiser, E. R.: Odor and its measurement. In Stern, A. C., editor: Air pollution, vol. 1, New York, 1962, Academic Press, Inc., pp. 520-522.
12. Yocom, J. C.: Effects of air pollution on materials. In Stern, A. C., editor: Air pollution, vol. 1, New York, 1962, Academic Press, Inc., pp. 199-219.
13. Jacobson, J. S., and Hill, A. C., editors: Recognition of air pollution injury to vegetation: a pictoral atlas, Pittsburgh, 1970, Air Pollution Control Association.
14. Particulate controls: A must to meet air quality standards, Environ. Sci. Technol. **3**:1149-51, 1969.
15. Garber, K.: Effects of air contamination, Berlin, 1967, Gebrüder Bontraeger.
16. Bohne, H.: Fluorides and sulfur dioxides as causes of plant damage, Fluoride **3**:137-142, 1970.
17. Mohamed, A. H.: Cytogenetic effects of hydrogen fluoride on plants, Fluoride **2**:76-84, 1969.
18. MacLean, D. C., McCune, D. C., Weinstein,

L. H., and others: Effects of acute hydrogen fluoride and nitrogen dioxide exposures on citrus and ornamental plants of central Florida, Environ. Sci. Technol. 2:444-449, 1968.

19. Spierings, F.: Factors determining the sensitivity to HF in plants, Fluoride 1:34-36, 1968.

20. Hindawi, I. J.: Air pollution injury of vegetation, Raleigh, N. C., 1970, U. S. Department of Health, Education, and Welfare, Public Health Service National Air Pollution Control Administration.

21. Carlson, C. E., and Dewey, J. E.: Environmental pollution by fluorides in Flathead National Forest and Glacier National Park. October, 1971. U. S. Department of Agriculture, Forest Service.

22. Zimmerman, P. W.: Chemicals involved in air pollution and their effects upon vegetation, Boyce Thompson Institute 3:124, 1955.

23. Bovay, E.: Fluoride accumulation in leaves due to boron-containing fertilizers, Fluoride 2:222-228, 1969.

24. Stahl, Q. R.: Air pollution aspects of chlorine gas, Litton System, Inc., Bethesda, Maryland, 1969, U. S. Department of Commerce, National Bureau of Standards, PB 188 087.

25. Stahl, Q. R.: Air pollution aspects to ethylene, Litton System, Inc., Bethesda, Maryland, 1969, U. S. Department of Commerce, National Bureau of Standards, PB 188 069.

26. Thorarinsson, S.: Hekla: a notorious volcano, Reykjavik, Iceland, 1970, Almenna Bokafelagid.

27. Roholm, K.: Fluorine Intoxication, Copenhagen, 1937, Arnold Busck.

28. Stokinger, H. E.: Effects of air pollution on animals. In Stern, A. C., editor: Air pollution, New York, 1962, Academic Press, Inc., pp. 282-286.

29. Oelschläger, W.: Errors in fluoride analysis, Fluoride 1:2-8, 1968.

30. Harkins, W. P., and Swain, R. E.: The chronic arsenical poisoning of herbivorous animals, J. Amer. Chem. Soc. 30:928, 1908.

31. Prell, H.: Die Schädigung der Tierwelt durch die Fernwirkungen von Industrieabgasen, Arch. Gewerbepathol. Gewerbehyg. 7:656, 1937.

32. Hupka, E.: Über Flugstaub Vergiftungen in der Umgebung von Metalhütten. Wiener Tierärztl A. 42:763, 1953.

33. Schmitt, N., Brown, G., Devlin, E. L., and others: Lead poisoning in horses, Arch. Environ. Health, 23:185-197, 1971.

34. Hammond, P. B., and Aronson, A. L.: Lead poisoning in cattle and horses in the vicinity of a smelter, Ann. N. Y. Acad. Sci. 111:595-611, 1964.

35. Bazell, R. J. Lead poisoning: zoo animals may be the first victims, Science 173:130-1, 1971.

36. No more sore throats, editorial, Pollution abstracts, 2:6-7, 1971.

37. Lillie, R. J.: Air pollutants affecting the performance of domestic animals: a literature review, Agriculture Handbook No. 380, Washington, D. C., 1970, U. S. Department of Agriculture, p. 41.

38. Bardelli, P., and Menzani, C.: La fluorosi (fluorosis), part II, Atti Ist. Veneto Sci. 97:623-74, 1937-38.

39. Müller, B., and Worseck, M.: Bienenschäden durch Arsen und Fluorhaltige Industrieabgase, Mschr. Veterinar. Med. 25:554-6, 1970.

40. Lakin, H. W.: Selenium accumulation in soils and its absorption by plants and animals. Publication authorized by the Director, U. S. Geological Survey, 1971.

41. Franke, K. W., Moxon, A. L., Poley, W. E., and others: Monstrosities produced by the injection of selenium salts into hen's eggs, Anat. Rec. 65:15-22, 1936.

42. Hallgren, W., Kerllson, N., and Wramby, G.: Molybdenosis in cattle, Nord Veterinarmed 6:469, 480, 1954.

43. Kahrs, R. F.: Chronic mercurial poisoning in swine: a case report of an outbreak with some epidemiological characteristics of hog cholera, Cornell Vet. 58:67-75, 1968.

44. Fish kills by pollution 1966, seventh annual report, Washington, D. C., 1967, Federal Water Pollution Control Administration, U. S. Department of the Interior.

45. Wellings, S. R., Boardman, M., McArm, G. E., and others: Pulmonary pathology of English sparrows from gross polluted atmospheres, Fed. Proc. 30:293, 1971.

5
THE TOXIC ACTION OF POLLUTANTS

In humans the toxic action of a pollutant is rarely, if ever, the same in two individuals because of widely varying factors, which are discussed in this chapter.

This fact was vividly brought to mind when I observed a family of six residing on a farm within 1½ miles of a Canadian lead and zinc smelter. The father and a 4-year-old boy had had frequent episodes of abdominal colics simulating such diseases as bowel obstruction, "intestinal flu," and acute pancreatitis. Their physician had not arrived at a diagnosis. Two other children had had convulsions, a common feature of lead poisoning. Another child had a disturbance of the glucose metabolism simulating diabetes. The mother had a brain disease for which no diagnosis had been made. All these conditions are clinical features of, and pointed to, chronic lead poisoning (see Chapter 12). This diagnosis was supported by high lead levels in their food and in body tissues,* by lead poisoning encountered in horses near the smelter,[1] and by the fact that most of the vegetables and fruits consumed by the family were raised on their farm.

Before discussing the many factors that account for such a variation in the health effects of a toxic pollutant, the mechanism of its action should be considered.

MECHANISM OF ACTION

A pollutant exerts its injurious effect upon an organ by either depressing or stimulating normal metabolic function of that organ. In fact, minute amounts of many toxic agents stimulate the function of an organ, whereas large doses impede or destroy its activity.

Three principal mechanisms dominate the toxic action of pollutants:

1. Their influence upon enzymes that are involved in an organ's activity
2. Direct chemical combination with a cell constituent
3. Secondary action as a consequence of their presence in the system[2]

Effect of pollutants on enzymes

Enzymes are complex proteins that catalyze (alter the rate of) metabolic activities of the body without themselves undergoing changes. Many are highly specific and selective. The substance upon which the enzyme acts is termed the substrate. The enzyme requires so-called cofactors or activators that are either a metal, a vitamin, or both. Two of the most important activators are magnesium and manganese. A toxic pollutant that inactivates the cofactor metal will also render the enzyme inactive. Cyanide, for instance, inhibits the activity of an iron-dependent enzyme by combining with its ion.[2]

Another mode by which a toxic substance can inactivate an enzyme is by combining with active groups of the enzyme structure. Mercury and arsenic, for instance, attach themselves so tightly to the active group of certain enzymes that the enzyme activity is blocked. Such toxic agents as ozone, fluo-

---

*A gallstone contained 39.9 ppm lead.

rine, or iodine destroy the function of an enzyme by converting some of its constituents to nonfunctioning groups. Similarly, a large number of pesticides, namely the organophosphates, destroy the important enzyme acetylcholinesterase, which regulates nerve-muscle action.

Besides combining with the active constituent of an enzyme, a toxic substance can compete with the cofactor, that is, with the metal or vitamin essential for the enzyme's action. Such metal to metal competition, for instance, is believed to be the basis of the poisonous action of beryllium. This metal has the capacity to compete for the site of magnesium and manganese on the structure of certain enzymes in the test tube.[2] Similarly cadmium inactivates certain enzymes by replacing zinc.[3]

Finally, interference with enzyme activity can be brought about by synthesis of new toxic agents. The new compound in turn exerts its deleterious effect on organ tissues. A typical example of this mechanism is the effect of sodium fluoroacetate, the well-known rat poison 1080. In the human or animal organism, enzyme action converts fluoroacetate into fluorocitrate. The latter produces serious damage because it breaks the metabolic chain of activity involved in respiration of organ tissue.

Combination of pollutants with cell constituents

Certain poisons affect the cells of an organ directly by chemical action rather than by interfering with the functioning of enzymes. After carbon monoxide, for instance, has penetrated the alveolar tissue and is absorbed into the bloodstream from the inhaled air, it combines with the hemoglobin of blood cells. It displaces oxygen in the blood's hemoglobin and interferes with the transport of oxygen to the tissues. It can thus cause serious damage, especially to brain and heart tissue, which are most vulnerable to oxygen deprivation.

Secondary action of pollutants

Under the influence of certain pollutants other substances are released, which damage cells. This is the well-known mechanism underlying the effect of pollen in hayfever. The damaging intermediary substances are histamine, serotonin, and similar products. Tolylene diisocyanate (TDI), the constituent of polyurethane plastic, is believed to act in a similar manner. Carbon tetrachloride, on the other hand, is responsible for massive discharge of epinephrine from sympathetic nerves, a condition believed to be the cause of liver damage encountered in carbon tetrachloride poisoning.[4]

Another chemical process accounts for secondary action of a toxic pollutant, namely the combination of an organic structure with a metal, a process called chelation. The metal becomes firmly bound to the new structure. In this manner, biologically active metals are removed from the system whereas others, such as iron, are absorbed and retained in the body at levels that may cause damage.

Other ways by which the human body attempts to dispose of or detoxify a noxious agent is through oxidation, reduction, or synthesis. By chemical changes, the toxic agent itself becomes a new substance. Many of these processes are not understood. In subsequent chapters some of these mechanisms bearing on the understanding of diseases caused by pollutants are discussed.

INTERACTION OF MIXTURES OF AIR POLLUTANTS

The unpredictable biologic response to some pollutants has been demonstrated in animal experiments. Frequently the presence of other pollutants in the atmosphere accounts for widely varying effects. Two different agents can interact to produce either a synergistic or an antagonistic action. Under certain conditions the presence of other agents even enhances an animal's tolerance to a pollutant. A large number of such interactions has been thoroughly studied experimentally in recent years. Thus, important facts in furtherance of our understanding of the action of pollutants have been brought to light.

The lethal effect of nitrous oxide fumes, for instance, in acute exposures is materially reduced when mice inhale particulates simultaneously with nitrogen oxides.[5] Welding fumes containing acidic nitrogen oxides are less toxic when particles of iron oxide are present.[5]

Oil mists afford protection in mice against the acute effects of ozone and nitrogen dioxide. Interestingly, this protection reaches its peak if exposure to the gases occurs 18 hours following exposure to the oil. When animals are exposed to the oil and the oxidant simultaneously, they are afforded no protection by the interaction of the two.[6] Indeed, such simultaneous exposure even enhanced the damaging effect of the two agents. Mineral oil appears to convey greater protection than motor oil. Stokinger[6] believes that the beneficial effect of the oil-ozone interaction does not represent a true antagonism of the two chemicals but that changes in the animal's defense system induce a tolerance in its response to the pollutants. Such tolerances can also develop in animals following repeated exposures.

On the other hand, when nitric oxide and carbon monoxide (two gases present in automobile exhaust) combine at high concentrations they are more than twice as deadly to experimental cats than when inhaled separately.[7] Hydrogen fluoride in the presence of beryllium sulfate is considerably more dangerous than either one of the agents by itself.[8]

Hydrogen peroxide at concentrations above 1.5 ppm combined with 1 ppm ozone were lethal to some animals; whereas hydrogen peroxide by itself in a concentration of 200 ppm produced only a slightly toxic response.[9]

Even more significant is the interaction of sulfur dioxide with other gases and solids. In the lungs, sulfur dioxide is oxidized to sulfur trioxide, which produces sulfuric acid upon reaction with water. Sulfuric acid acts as a carrier for sulfur dioxide gas, which rides into the alveoli. As the result of this phenomenon, it has been shown[10] that sulfuric acid mist at 8 mg/meter^3 and 89 ppm sulfur dioxide together produce greater retardation of growth, greater damage to the lungs, and greater impairment of respiration than anticipated from exposure to either one alone. When sulfur dioxide is adsorbed to sodium chloride as, for instance, on city streets in winter, the combination not only carries greater amounts of sulfur dioxide into deeper portions of the lungs but also increases the level of pollution in a given area.

A similar and probably much more complex situation takes place inside the body. For instance, arsenic, itself a poison, tends to neutralize the effect of cadmium, magnesium, calcium, and fluoride.

FACTORS GOVERNING TOXICITY

It has already been shown how a pollutant acts on the body and how its effect becomes modified in the presence of other agents. In the following discussion some of the many features that determine its effects on humans are discussed.

The nature of an environmental poison, its concentration in the atmosphere, and the length of time during which a person is exposed to it are paramount in determining its toxicity; an individual's state of health and nutrition is another significant factor.

Dose and length of exposure

Damage from air pollution may range from a slight irritation of the eyes to sudden death. Obviously, a massive dose of an airborne contaminant will induce a much more severe and more acute illness than exposure to the same agent in minute amounts over long periods of time.

Acute illness. The well-known disaster of Poza Poca is a classical example of an acute epidemic caused by lethal doses of a single agent, hydrogen sulfide, which escaped into the air for 20 to 25 minutes.

On November 24, 1950, at 5 A.M. the citizens of the little town of Poza Poca, the center of Mexico's biggest natural gas field, were seized suddenly with severe respiratory and neurologic symptoms. A new plant had just been opened that was to remove hydrogen sulfide from natural gas and convert it into commercially useful sulfur. Something went wrong with a valve in the pipes. Hydrogen sulfide, released inadvertently into the atmosphere, spread into the town. On that day, because of a heavy fog, absence of wind, and an atmospheric temperature inversion, the gas did not disperse. The stench of rotten eggs awakened some of the people. In their attempt to escape from their homes, some fell unconscious on the ground and died. Others lapsed into convulsions prior to death. Twenty-two persons died of hydrogen sulfide poisoning and 320 had to be hospitalized. Those who survived developed headaches, eye irritation, cough, and shortness of breath. They lost their sense of smell for several weeks. The gas killed all of the canaries in the area and about 50% of commercial and domestic animals, among which were chickens, cattle, pigs, geese, dogs, and cats.[11]

Chronic effects. In contrast to such acute episodes, illness caused by long-term exposure to minute concentrations of hydrogen sulfide or any other contaminant follows a much less spectacular course. Illness develops slowly and insidiously. Such vague symptoms as general weakness, loss of appetite, muscle pains, and loss of energy are common clinical features of diseases caused by air pollution. Whereas a sudden massive exposure to a respiratory irritant will precipitate pulmonary edema (water-logging of the lungs) and acute heart failure, long-term exposure to the same agent in minute doses induces a slowly developing cough with shortness of breath, which gradually gives rise to emphysema and pulmonary fibrosis (scarring). Up to 20 years may elapse before exposure to minute doses of asbestos, beryllium, lead, or fluoride precipitate overt symptoms of poisoning. Even more prolonged periods are required for a pollutant agent to induce cancer.

Interrupted exposures to pollutants

Another determinant factor in the action of an environmental poison is whether exposure to it is continuous or intermittent.

When laboratory animals[12] were exposed to 7,800 μg/meter^3 (4 ppm) of ozone repeatedly for 30 minutes, intervals as brief as 15 to 20 minutes between exposures reduced substantially the edema of the lungs and the animals' mortality. Animals subjected intermittently to fluoride inhalation developed a resistance that enabled them to withstand otherwise lethal doses of the gas.[13]

Similarly in a person working only a part of the day in a polluted atmosphere or in one taking frequent vacations, a disease caused by an occupational pollutant is likely to be less severe than in one exposed continuously.

On the other hand, intermittent exposures give rise to recurrent sudden episodes of illness as, for instance, following massive emissions of contaminants from a factory.[14]

Age

That age affects the tolerance to a toxic agent is well established. Young growing animals are much more susceptible to adverse effects by fluoride than are older ones. Similarly, the acutely toxic effect of ozone[12] and sulfur dioxide[15] is more pronounced in young animals than in older ones by a factor of 2 to 3. Newborn children and infants appear to be more susceptible to lead and mercury poisoning than adults (Chapter 12).

However, in the major air pollution disasters, the older age group of the population was most seriously affected because cardiovascular and respiratory diseases of other origins render these people less able to withstand the superimposed effects. Furthermore, an aging lung loses some of its elastic recoil[16] and its ability to withstand disease.

Activity and stress

The toxic effect of most respiratory agents is markedly enhanced when a person undergoes physical exertion, mainly because increased demand for oxygen occurs at the same time that oxygen consumption is impeded. Exposure of rats to 1 ppm (1,960 μg/meter³) of ozone, a level that does not cause obvious acute effects, proved fatal when the animal was forced to be active in a rotating cage for a few minutes each hour during exposure to the gas.[17] Cows under the stress of pregnancy or lactation are more susceptible to fluoride intoxication than others.[18] Women who had undergone multiple pregnancies developed cadmium poisoning more readily than other members of a Japanese population group.[19]

Health status

Each person's system copes with a toxic pollutant in a different manner. In persons with an inherited tendency to pulmonary disease, a respiratory irritant causes much more damage than in a person with healthy lungs. In some individuals the ciliary activity in the upper air passages is reduced because of an inherited deficiency. A constitutional tendency to allergy or a special disposition to malignancy of the lungs may prevail. A lack of alpha$_1$-antitrypsin in the blood,[20] the enzyme that regulates trypsin levels in the lungs, predisposes a person to emphysema.

Patients with diseases of the heart or blood are more susceptible than others to carbon monoxide poisoning. In an alcoholic with brain and liver damage, the toxic effect of fluoride is vastly different from that in an otherwise normal individual[21] (see Chapter 13). Even a relatively low-grade exposure of a smoker to an environmental contaminant may tip the scale and disable him. Poor nutrition, lack of vitamins, sedentary occupation, and poor eating habits, are likely to affect the course of an illness caused by air pollution.

REFERENCES

1. Schmitt, N., Brown, G., Devlin, E. L., and others: Lead poisoning in horses, Arch. Environ. Health **23**:185-197, 1971.
2. Stokinger, H. E.: Occupational diseases: a guide to their recognition. In Gafafer, W. M., editor: United States Public Health Service Publication No. 1097, 7-26, 1964.
3. Simon, F. P., Potts, A. M., and Gerard, R. W.: Action of cadmium and thiols on tissue enzymes, Arch. Biochem. **12**:283-291, 1947.
4. Brody, T. M.: Mechanism of action of carbon tetrachloride, Fed. Proc. **18**:1017, 1959.
5. LaBelle, C. W., Long, J. E., and Christofano, E. E.: Synergistic effects of aerosols, Arch. Industr. Health **11**:297-304, 1955.
6. Stokinger, H. E.: Toxicologic interactions of mixtures of air pollutants, Int. J. Air Pollut. **2**:313-326, 1960.
7. Stokinger, H. E.: Effects of air pollution on animals. In Stern, A. C., editor: Air pollution, vol. 1, New York, 1962, Academic Press, p. 325.
8. Stokinger, H. E., Ashenberg, N. J., Devoldre, J., and others: Acute inhalation toxicity of beryllium: Part II, the enhancing effect of the inhalation of hydrogen fluoride vapor on beryllium sulfate poisoning in animals, Arch. Industr. Hyg. **1**:398, 1950.
9. Svirbely, J. L., Dobrogorski, O. J., and Stokinger, H. E.: Enhanced toxicity of ozone-hydrogen peroxide mixtures, Amer. Industr. Hyg. Ass. J. **22**:21-26, 1961.
10. Amdur, M. O.: The physiologic response of guinea pigs to atmospheric pollutants, Int. J. Air Pollut. **1**:170-183, 1959.
11. Katz, M.: Effects of contaminants other than sulfur dioxide on vegetation and animals: background papers prepared for the National Conferences on Pollution and Our Environment, Montreal, Canada, October to November, 1966, Canadian Council of Resource Ministers.
12. Stokinger, H. E.: Ozone toxicology: a review of research and industrial experience, 1954-

1964, Arch. Environ. Health **10:**719-731, 1965.

13. Keplinger, M. L.: Effects from repeated short-term inhalation of fluorine, Toxicol. Appl. Pharmacol. **14:**192-200, 1969.

14. Waldbott, G. L., and Cecilioni, V. A.: "Neighborhood" fluorosis, Clin. Toxicol. **2:** 387-396, 1969.

15. Thomas, M. D., Hendricks, R. H., Gunn, F. D., and others: Prolonged exposure of guinea pigs to sulfuric acid aerosols, Arch. Industr. Health **17:**70-80, 1958.

16. Turner, J. M., Mead, J., and Wohl, M. E.: Elasticity of human lungs in relation to age, J. Appl. Physiol. **25:**664-671, 1968.

17. Stokinger, H. E., Wagner, W. D., and Wright, P.: Studies in ozone toxicity: Part I, potentiating effect of exercise and tolerance development, Arch. Industr. Health **14:**158, 1956.

18. Rosenberger, G., and Gründer, H. D.: The effect of fluoride emissions near a hydrogen fluoride factory, Fluoride **1:**41-49, 1968.

19. Tsuchiya, K.: Causation of ouch-ouch disease (Itai-Itai Bye): Part I, nature of the disease. Part II, Epidemiology and evaluation, Keio J. Med. **18:**181-194, 195-211, 1969.

20. Laurell, C. B., and Eriksson, S.: The electrophoretic a_1 globulin pattern of serum in a_1-antitrypsin deficiency, Scand. J. Clin. Lab. Invest. **15:**132-140, 1963.

21. Soriano, M.: Periostitis deformans due to wine fluorosis, Fluoride **1:**56-64, 1968.

6
THE BODY'S DEFENSES

In order to be able to evaluate the action of the major air pollutants on the human system, a brief review of the organism's defense mechanism is in order.

The organs involved in diseases caused by inhalation of toxic materials are the nose, sinuses, pharynx, larynx, bronchial tree, and lung tissue. The other principal ports through which pollutants enter the body—the intestinal tract and, to a lesser extent, the skin—can also be targets for acute or chronic disturbances. The kidneys, the main organs of excretion, are especially vulnerable to damage by toxic agents. Pollutants can also affect individual organs not involved in their uptake or excretion, such as brain, liver, muscles, as a part of a systemic disease by specific action upon the respective target organ.

RESPIRATORY TRACT

The three sections of the respiratory tract, the nasopharynx, the tracheobronchial area, and the lung tissue proper, that is, the alveoli (air sacs) (Fig. 6-1), are remarkably well equipped to cope with harmful invaders through three processes: filtration, inactivation or destruction, and removal.

Nasopharynx

The turbinates and septum of the nose warm and moisten the air and the hair at the entrance of the nose. They filter and remove the largest particles from the in-haled air current.[1] Mucous glands imbedded in the lining of the nose, the sinuses, and the upper bronchi produce and eject a constant slow stream of mucus,[2] which, like the tears in the eyes, wash out the larger-sized (above 10 μ) particles such as dust, carbon, and pollen spores. The ciliae, the hairlike brush system lining the cells on the surface of the bronchial and nasal passages (Fig. 6-2) function like a broom to sweep the noxious agents out of the system with as many as 1300 beats per minute.[3] Under certain conditions, as for instance in an allergic nasal disease, this mechanism breaks down and particles such as pollen grains enter the tissue of the nasal passages. (Fig. 6-3, A). They wander towards the cartilage through the lymph spaces and remain embedded in the tissues for weeks until they disintegrate (Fig. 6-3, B and C).[4]

Bronchi

A large portion of the bronchial tree is surrounded by muscular layers that contract the bronchi (Fig. 6-4) when they are invaded by such substances as coal dust, charcoal, india ink, or aluminum powder. The contraction of bronchial muscles narrows the lumen of the bronchi (Fig. 6-5). Thus, lesser amounts of particulate matter are permitted to enter the lower portions of the bronchial tubes.[5]

Like the sneeze reflex in the nose, the cough reflex assists in this process in the

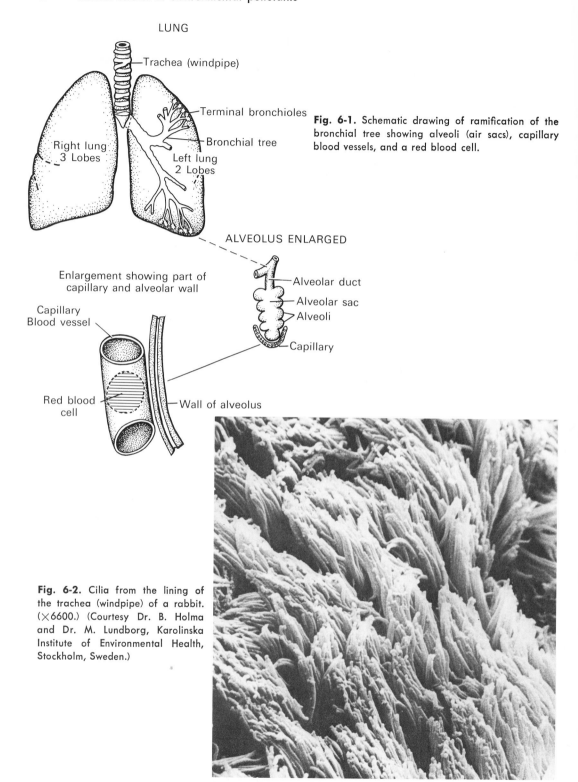

LUNG

Trachea (windpipe)

Terminal bronchioles

Bronchial tree

Right lung
3 Lobes

Left lung
2 Lobes

Fig. 6-1. Schematic drawing of ramification of the bronchial tree showing alveoli (air sacs), capillary blood vessels, and a red blood cell.

ALVEOLUS ENLARGED

Enlargement showing part of capillary and alveolar wall

Alveolar duct

Alveolar sac

Alveoli

Capillary
Blood vessel

Capillary

Red blood
cell

Wall of alveolus

Fig. 6-2. Cilia from the lining of the trachea (windpipe) of a rabbit. (×6600.) (Courtesy Dr. B. Holma and Dr. M. Lundborg, Karolinska Institute of Environmental Health, Stockholm, Sweden.)

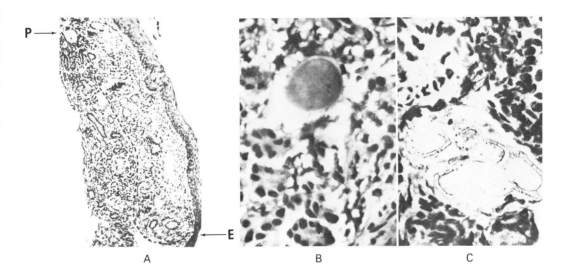

A   B   C

Fig. 6-3. A, Route of a rye pollen grain inside nasal tissue of a guinea pig on its way toward the cartilage during the course of 1 hour. *E, entry; P, present position.* (×360.) **B,** Rye pollen lying inside the nasal tissue of a normal guinea pig 15 minutes after the animal was exposed to it. The light space surrounding the pollen represents mucus. (×720.) **C,** Remnants of several grains of partially disintegrated rye pollen lying for more than a month in the nasal tissue of a guinea pig previously made sensitive (allergic) to it. (×720.) (Courtesy Dr. Olf Strömme, Studies on the histology of pollinosis, Oslo, 1952, Thronsen and Co.)

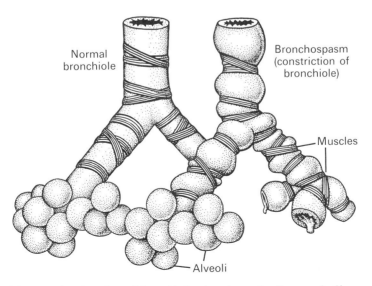

Fig. 6-4. Schematic drawing of small bronchi showing the contracting muscle fibers and alveoli. (Courtesy Riker Laboratories, Inc., Northridge, Calif.)

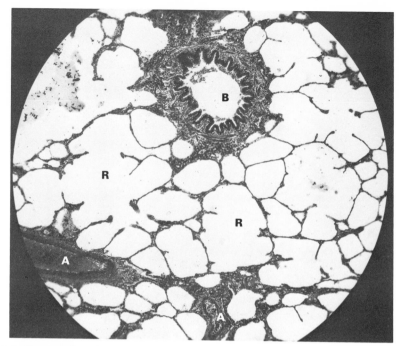

Fig. 6-5. Cross section of a normal lung showing *A,* blood vessels, and *B,* bronchus containing some mucus. Some of the alveolar walls are ruptured, *R.* Between alveolar cavities lies interstitial tissue containing blood vessels and lymphoid structures.

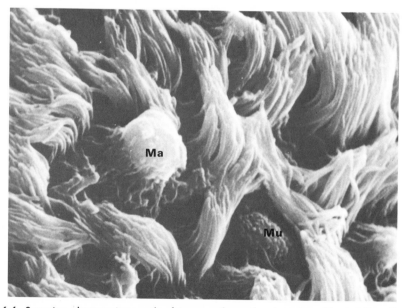

Fig. 6-6. Scanning electronmicrograph of inner surface of a bronchus. The hairlike cilia sweep intruding particles into the upper air spaces. *Ma,* macrophage; *Mu;* droplet of mucus. (×2900.) (Courtesy Dr. C. B. Boyd, Wayne State University School of Medicine, Detroit, Mich.)

bronchial tree. Cough eliminates the mucus that has accumulated in the bronchi and in the alveoli in which the foreign invader is lodged together with white blood cells and with other scavenger cells that the body has mobilized (Figs. 6-6 and 6-7). They enter the bronchi from the bloodstream and from the lining of the alveoli. A spasm of the bronchi tends to prevent the invading agents from reaching the tiny balloonlike air sacs (Fig. 6-8) that are located at the alveolar duct, the terminal branches of the bronchial tree. However, this very defensive action, in conjunction with the mucus present in the bronchi, impedes a victim's ability to breathe; it causes obstruction of the airspaces in the bronchi and thus leads to respiratory distress.[2]

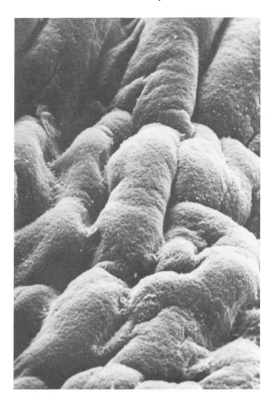

Fig. 6-7. Inside lining of a terminal human bronchiole showing a ridged surface. (×60.) (Courtesy Dr. C. B. Boyd, Wayne State University School of Medicine, Detroit, Mich.)

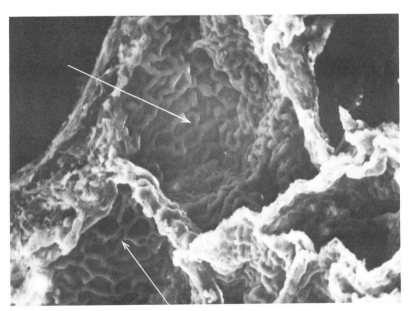

Fig. 6-8. Scanning electronphotomicrograph of alveolar surface (normal lung) showing the inner lining of the alveoli (air sacs). Ridges on the concave surface constitute minute capillaries covered with an extremely thin membrane (arrows). (×530.) (Courtesy Dr. C. B. Boyd, Wayne State University School of Medicine, Detroit, Mich.)

Alveoli

In the alveolar sacs, the number of which is estimated to be about 300 million,[6] man's innermost contact with air and with environmental pollutants takes place. Here, a delicate tissue only 0.0001-inch thick, separates the air from the blood that flows through the alveolar surface layer (Fig. 6-9).[1] The total surface of the alveoli through which the gases reach the bloodstream has been calculated to be as large as the size of a tennis court. Life depends on this contact of the tiny cap-illaries with the alveoli. In this way a steady flow of oxygen enters the blood vessels and is carried, linked to the blood's hemoglobin, as oxyhemoglobin to the heart and to the body tissues.

Another exchange takes place in the opposite direction. Carbon dioxide, the product of human metabolism, leaves the blood and diffuses into the air via the alveoli.

In addition to this mechanism, designed for exchange of gases, the alveolar tissue is endowed with various protective properties. It absorbs and filters pollutants. It

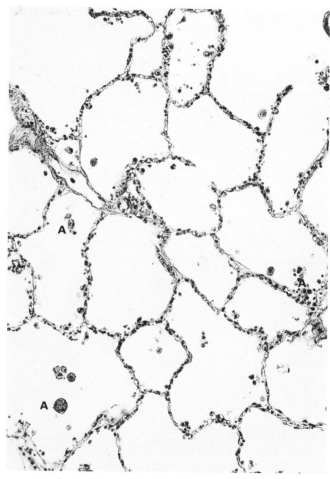

Fig. 6-9. Cross section of normal lung tissue showing extremely thin walls of the alveoli, which contain capillary blood vessels carrying red blood cells. Other cells lie inside the air spaces, A. (×40.) (Courtesy Dr. C. B. Boyd, Wayne State University School of Medicine, Detroit, Mich.)

possesses a uniquely effective cellular defense apparatus. Among the four types of cells present in the alveoli, the alveolar epithelial cells (type 1) and the alveolar endothelial cells are primarily concerned with providing the surfaces required for gas exchange. The large alveolar cells (type 2) and especially the alveolar macrophages, which are found free in the alveolar lumen, participate in a number of basic oxidative and synthetic processes designed to defend the lungs against invading organic and inorganic material (Fig. 6-10).[7]

Mechanism of respiration

The movements of the lungs during inspiration and expiration depend on the action of the muscles of the chest and diaphragm. When these muscles alternately compress and expand the lungs, the alveolar pressure rises or falls. During inhalation, air flows into the alveoli through the bronchi because the pressure of the alveoli becomes slightly negative compared with that of the atmosphere, namely about −3 mm Hg. Conversely a rise of pressure in the alveolar sacs during exhalation causes the air to flow out.

A continuous tendency of the lungs to recoil away from the chestwall and to collapse the whole lung is caused by two major factors: (1) a multitude of elastic fibers, which permeate the lungs, are being persistently stretched and are endeavoring to shorten; (2) surface tension of the fluid lining the alveoli reduces the surface areas of the individual alveoli. All the forces working together tend to collapse the whole

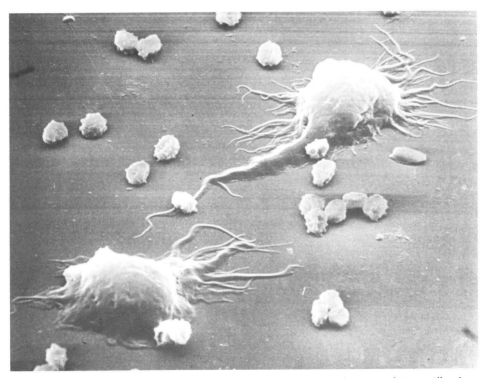

Fig. 6-10. Lung macrophages in rabbit cultured outside of body and spores of *Aspergillus fumigatus* (a common fungus) during the process of phagocytosis (dissolving the spores). (×4200.) (Courtesy Dr. B. Holma and Dr. M. Lundborg, Karolinska Institute of Environmental Health, Stockholm, Sweden.)

lung in the expiratory phase of respiration. The elastic fibers account for about one third of the recoil tendency, the surface tension for about two thirds.[1]

The surface tension in the alveoli is largely dependent on the presence of a lipoprotein mixture called surfactant, which is secreted into the alveoli and into the lining of the respiratory passages. Dipalmityl lecithin, a phospholipid, the major constituent of surfactant, is mainly responsible for lowering the surface tension at the alveolar fluid-air interface. Surfactant forms a layer between the cells of the alveoli and the air. It thus prevents contact of the fluid lining the alveoli with the air in a manner similar to that of a detergent. The decrease in surface tension of fluids that line the alveoli facilitates inflation of air sacs with relatively small changes in air pressure. In the absence of surfactant it is difficult for the lungs to expand—a condition responsible for the respiratory distress syndrome of human newborns, especially premature babies.[8]

Pulmonary function

On the basis of its function, the lung can be divided into two parts—the conducting system and the combined conducting and respiratory system. The former includes the bronchial tree to the level of the terminal bronchioles and the latter, the respiratory bronchioles and the alveolar ducts and alveoli (Fig. 6-11).[9] The conducting system permits no exchange of oxygen and carbon dioxide through its walls. It is therefore considered dead space.

Between the mouth and the alveoli the pressure of the incoming air decreases. This pressure gradient is brought about by the resistance of the airways, mainly of the bronchi, which range in diameter from 3 to 8 mm, decreasing in size from the center of the lung to the periphery. In normal individuals, the drop in pressure induces an average flow rate of inspired air of about one liter per second. The peripheral portions of the bronchial tree smaller than 2 mm in diameter constitute only 10% of the total airway resistance.[9]

Below the conducting airways are the terminal branches of the bronchial tree, called respiratory bronchioles, and the alveolar ducts. This segment of the airways accounts for only a small total of the airway resistance, but the constriction of the alveolar ducts can contribute significantly to the decrease of the breathing capacity of the lungs.[9]

Action of pollutants in the respiratory tract

Particulates. The action of particulates on the lungs differs from that of gases.

The deposition of particles in the lungs is governed mainly by their size, their density, their shape, their tendency to aggregate, and by the force of their impact upon the lining of the lungs and upper respiratory tract. Solid particles whose diameter is larger than 5 μ are removed almost completely from the nose and bronchial tree.[10] The smaller the size, the further the particles reach down into the peripheral branches of the bronchial tree, where little mucus is formed (Fig. 6-7). Particles of 1 μ or less in diameter are usually deposited in

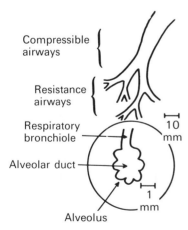

Fig. 6-11. Schematic drawing of the ramification of the bronchial tree. (Courtesy Dr. S. Ayres, New York University, New York.)

the alveoli. Those smaller than 0.5 μ behave like gases. They settle in the alveolar air spaces where they may be retained.[11] A hygroscopic particle, such as sodium chloride, dissolves in the moisture of the upper air passages from which it can be eliminated more readily than coal dust of equal size.[12]

Three forces determine the action of particulates in the lungs:

1. In the upper air passages where the air pressure is high, a centrifugal force deposits them into the bronchial wall especially where the airstream meets the areas where the bronchi branch off from the main stems of the bronchial tree.

2. A second force governing the movements of particles in the respiratory tract is sedimentation, that is, fallout caused by gravity. This occurs especially in the lower portion of the bronchi where the pressure of the incoming air is reduced.

3. In the alveoli the so-called Brownian motion* largely determines the movements of small particles and gases. They are subjected to a constant bombardment by the molecules of air, which keeps them in continuous motion until they are deposited at the alveolar walls.

A particulate air pollutant that has reached the alveolar spaces either remains intact or is engulfed by the macrophages, the body's scavenger cells (Fig. 6-10). Eventually it is moved with the mucous sheath higher up into the ciliated areas of bronchi, nose, and pharynx where it is either expectorated with mucus or swallowed. Soluble particulates, deposited in the nonciliated alveolar sacs, usually dissolve and enter the bloodstream. The less

soluble particles that remain within the alveoli eventually penetrate the alveolar ducts and lodge either in the interstitial tissue (connective tissue that holds the lung together) (Fig. 6-9) or enter the lymphatic spaces and lymph glands, the body's sewer system, which eventually drains into the bloodstream. Fractions of coal dust that are not eliminated remain in the lungs permanently and are responsible for what is called the "black lung" (Fig. 8-2, A). Lungs of city dwellers at autopsy are blacker than those of rural residents[13]; however, the "black lung" is not necessarily associated with illness. The entry of minute particulates into the bloodstream depends on their ability to diffuse into the capillary system and lymph spaces, on the rate of a person's breathing, and on his "respiratory flow rate," that is, the absence or presence of an anatomical obstruction of the bronchial tree that interferes with the passage of air.

Gases. In contrast with solid particles, the size of which largely determines their fate in the lungs, the action of an airborne gas is dependent mainly on its ability to dissolve in water.

The most soluble gases, such as ammonia and sulfur oxides, are promptly adsorbed to the surface of the upper airways because of their strong attraction to their moist surfaces. Other gases, such as nitrogen dioxide and phosgene, are less soluble and therefore reach the lower airways and the terminal branches of the bronchial tree where conditions for their entrance into the bloodstream are more favorable.

Gaseous and particulate interaction. Frequently, gases and particulates interact and form a compound, the action of which differs greatly from that of the original agents. Formaldehyde, for instance, attaches itself to particulates and is carried by them down into the alveolar spaces, where it produces inflammation (Fig. 6-12). The interaction of a gas condensed on a particulate may either enhance or de-

---

*Brownian motion is the main means for deposition and expiration. Particles below 0.5 μ are under bombardment by air molecules and are thus continuously in motion.

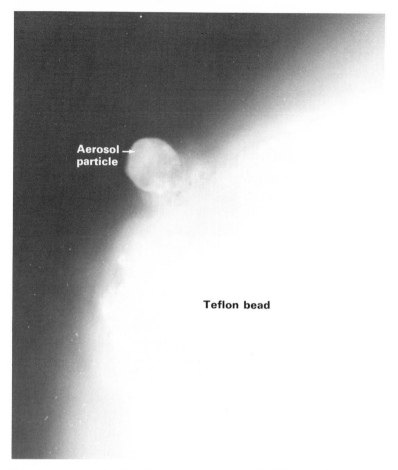

Fig. 6-12. Photomicrograph of a 2.5 μm copper chloride ($CuCl_2$) aerosol particle adhering to a 350 μm Teflon bead demonstrates the manner in which minute atmospheric particles adhere to larger sized particles. (Courtesy Dr. R. T. Cheng, Dr. J. O. Frohliger, and Dr. M. Corn, University of Pittsburgh; from J.A.P.C.A. **21**:138, March 1971.)

crease the toxicity of a pollutant (see Chapter 5).

Diseases caused by respiratory pollutants

The principal respiratory diseases elicited by pollutants are bronchiectasis, emphysema, pulmonary fibrosis (scarring of lung tissue), pulmonary edema, and partial atelectasis (collapse of lung tissue). Pneumothorax and cystic lungs are less common.

Emphysema. Lungs that can no longer expand properly manifest a decrease in their elasticity. They lose their capacity to exchange oxygen for carbon dioxide in the blood. This condition is encountered in emphysema, a disease characterized by overexpansion of alveolar sacs and rupture of their walls (Fig. 6-13). Loss of surface and of functional tissue results. The lungs exhibit increased airway resistance, increased pressure of the pulmonary blood vessels, and overloading of the right heart with subsequent heart failure. Smoking and chronic exposure to other air pollutants are causes of emphysema.

Pulmonary fibrosis. Scar formation of the

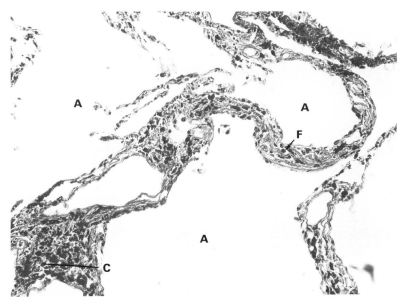

Fig. 6-13. Cross section of emphysematous lung showing chronic fibrosis (scarring). Note thickened walls with fibrotic tissue, *F,* and marked enlargement of the alveolar spaces, *A.* Capillaries in the walls are partially replaced by scar tissue. Width of walls is 8 to 12 times that of normal. Large carbon particles, *C,* are visible in the left lower corner. (×40.) (Courtesy Dr. C. B. Boyd, Wayne State University School of Medicine, Detroit, Mich.)

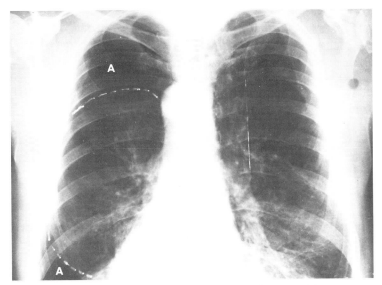

Fig. 6-14. Pneumothorax. Collapsed left lung caused by perforation of lung tissue at its surface and by air escaping from the lung into the pleural space, which is normally under negative pressure. (Note air, *A,* between lung and chest wall.) Five similar cases of this rare disease were observed among persons residing close to a secondary aluminum smelter that emitted chlorine gas and hydrofluoric acid.

interstitial (connective) tissue, which holds the lung structure together, is another common effect of certain pollutants. Shortness of breath and decreasing lung capacity with subsequent damage to the right heart characterizes this disease as outlined in Chapter 10.

Atelectasis. A less common disease, occurs when the mucus formed in the bronchi is so abundant and thick that it cannot be expectorated; it can completely obstruct a branch of the bronchial tree. The vacuum created between the point of obstruction and the lung tissue served by the obstructed bronchus causes the particular area of the lung tissue to collapse, a condition called atelectasis. It is similar to what happens when a food particle is "swallowed wrong," that is, when it lodges in the trachea or in the bronchus instead of passing through the esophagus into the stomach. If the mucous plug is not promptly removed by the cough reflex or by means of a bronchoscope, the involved portion of the lung becomes infected and eventually damaged to the point that it can no longer function at all.

Pneumothorax. In some individuals the connective tissue that holds the lungs together is weakened so severely from coughing or perhaps by irritation of atmospheric chemicals that a hole is virtually blown into the surface of the lung. The lung collapses like a punctured balloon. This condition, termed pneumothorax, is rare compared with most other lung diseases (Fig. 6-14). Since it usually occurs in one lung, it is not necessarily a fatal disease, but, in extreme cases, it can result in death. I observed five individuals afflicted with this relatively rare disease residing within 3 blocks of a secondary aluminum smelter, which spewed hydrochloric and hydrofluoric acid, two agents with a strong corrosive action on the lining of the bronchi.*

---

*No other such cases occurring near secondary aluminum smelters have been reported in the medical literature.

Cystic lungs. Inside of the lungs the pressure caused by strenuous cough may rupture portions of the thin, tautly stretched alveolar walls and produce blebs or cysts. The latter may be as small as a cherry or so large that they actually crowd out much of the functioning lung tissue and lead to marked functional impairment. Surgical removal of the overstretched lung tissue can aid in the reexpansion of the intact portions of the lungs and thus provide considerable relief.

Pulmonary edema. When highly concentrated amounts of an irritant or corrosive pollutant reach the lungs suddenly, the immediate effect is startling. The lining of the lungs and of the nose and sinuses becomes irritated and waterlogged. Bronchial tissue and alveolar capillaries pour out large amounts of fluid and blood in an apparent attempt to dilute the toxic agent. They may virtually "drown" all available respiratory tissue in fluid. If this serious condition, called pulmonary edema, is not fatal, it leads to secondary inflammation of the lungs by bacteria that settle in the diseased tissue, a process that simulates pneumonia. Occasionally such areas of "pneumonitis" fail to heal and result in permanent destruction of the alveolar tissue in the involved portion of the lungs. Small defects in the fine ramifications of the bronchial tree ensue, and the affected areas fill up with mucus or pus. In conjunction with accompanying spasm of the bronchi, they materially restrict a patient's breathing.

Other pulmonary diseases caused by air contamination will be discussed in subsequent chapters.

GASTROINTESTINAL TRACT

Certain airborne toxic agents, such as lead, fluoride, mercury, and cadmium compounds, reach the system largely through ingestion of contaminated food or water via the gastrointestinal tract. The polluting poison settles on leaves and fruits of edible plants[14] and enters the leaves through the stomata as outlined in Chapter 4. Flydust deposited in soil is also taken up by a plant through its fine hair rootlets. Fruit, vegetables, and grain contaminated in this manner constitute a major portion of a person's body burden of a poison. When contaminated hay and grain is fed to domestic animals, their meat, eggs, and milk contribute additional poison to a person's daily menu. In this manner, the intestinal tract becomes an important portal of entry for air pollutants.

The main part of the gastrointestinal tract from which a toxic agent is adsorbed into the bloodstream lies between the stomach and the upper portion of the bowels. The inner layer of this part of bowel tissue is lined with millions of so-called villi; fingerlike projections about 0.5 to 1 mm long, which contain a lymphoid capillary surrounded by a network of blood capillary vessels (Fig. 6-15). The villi rep-

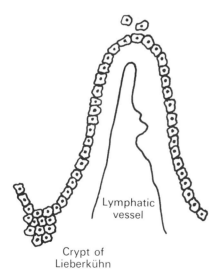

Lymphatic vessel

Crypt of Lieberkühn

Fig. 6-15. Fingerlike projections of the mucous membranes in the upper bowels, called villi, serve to absorb the end products of digestion. The core of the villus is made up of lymphatic vessels, which is surrounded by a network of capillary blood vessels, and the crypts of Lieberkühn, containing mucous-secreting glands.

resent an enormous total surface area. They thus render the absorptive capacity of the inside lining of the small intestines remarkably efficient. In this manner, a surface of about 300 square meters is ready to take up both nutrients and toxic agents contained in our diet. Like the lungs, the bowels are also equipped with mucus-producing glands. Similar to the cough reflex of the lungs, spastic movements in the stomach and bowels tend to eliminate noxious agents either by inducing vomiting or through speedy propulsion of fecal matter through the entire intestinal tract.

The readily soluble poisons are promptly absorbed into the bloodstream. Less soluble ones are carried into the lower portions of the bowels where they are eliminated with the feces.

In passing through the intestinal tract, a toxic agent can induce diarrhea, spastic pains, or constipation, mucus, and blood in the stool. If the poisoning extends over protracted periods, chronic changes arise. Certain types of chronic enteritis or mucous colitis, or both, can ensue, diseases of the bowels for which, thus far, relatively few satisfactory causes have been established. Low-level intake of lead, mercury, fluorides, and arsenic can induce such chronic illness as will be shown in subsequent chapters. Interference with the normal function of the lower bowels inhibits absorption of water, sodium, other vital minerals, and vitamins, some of which are synthesized in the lower portions of the intestinal tract by bacterial action.

KIDNEYS

The kidneys, the major organs of elimination for most absorbed toxic agents, are liable to be damaged by inhaled or ingested air pollutants.

The human kidney contains about one million functional units, called nephrons, which clear the blood plasma of unwanted substances. Each nephron begins with a glomerulus, a tiny tuft localized in the kidney's outer portion, the cortex, and ends in a collecting tubule located toward the kidney's central part (Fig. 6-16).

The glomeruli constitute the system that filters fluid from tiny capillary blood vessels into the minute tubules together with normal constituents of blood, waste substances and toxic agents, except for proteins and some lipids (fats). The energy for this process is furnished by the heart, which maintains sufficient blood pressure to filter these agents through the capillary walls. A resting adult's kidney receives about 1.2 liter of blood or 25% of the heart's output per minute.[1]

The tubules undergo a series of convolutions and then empty the urine into a central collecting system for its eventual elimination through the bladder (Fig. 6-17). A

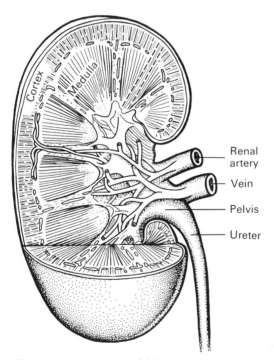

Fig. 6-16. Cross section of kidney showing the cortex, which contains the glomeruli (filtering system), the tubules in the medulla radiating toward the center, and the pelvis (the urine collecting system) from which the urine flows to the bladder.

part of the tubules reabsorbs water, sugar, sodium, potassium, and other vital electrolytes from the tubular fluid in order to maintain the necessary homeostasis (equilibrium) of these vital agents in the blood. Another portion of the tubules in the kidneys is equipped with cells that secrete toxic agents into the tubular fluid for their elimination with the urine. The tubules thus separate the agents needed in the blood from those that are unwanted.

Most chemical poisons exert a selective action on the kidneys by injuring the tubules much more than the glomeruli. Mercury, for instance, causes kidney damage by destroying some of the vital cells in the tubular system. Others, like cadmium, are believed to attack the kidney's tiny blood vessels.

Minor portions of such agents as iodide, bromide, fluoride, and mercury leave the system with the saliva through the salivary glands or with the sweat through the sweat glands in the skin. Persistent irritations, even ulcers of the mouth and chronic sore throats in persons intolerant to halogens, may thus manifest themselves as a part of low-grade systemic poisoning.

A pollutant can adversely affect the skin either by direct contact with the air or through being carried to the skin via the bloodstream. The passage of halogens, particularly iodine, through the sweat glands precipitates certain skin diseases, especially acne.

TARGET ORGANS

The bulk of a toxic agent that has entered the bloodstream through the respiratory and intestinal tract, is carried, mainly by the albumin fraction of the blood serum, into such target organs as the liver, the kidneys, the heart, the bones, and the brains, where it either remains intact or undergoes changes that may lead to functional disturbances. Little is known about the exact mechanism of action of most toxic pollutants inside of the respective organs es-

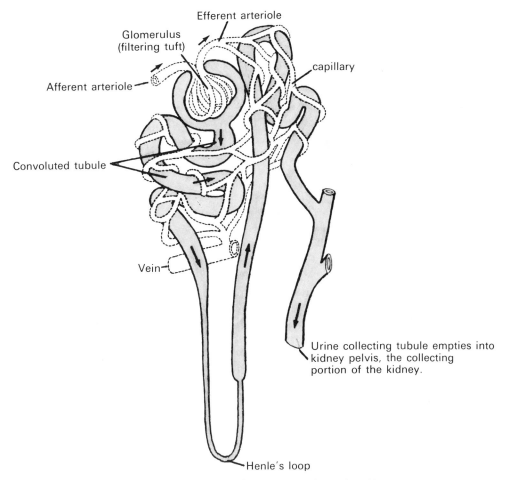

Efferent arteriole

Glomerulus
(filtering tuft)

capillary

Afferent arteriole

Convoluted tubule

Vein

Urine collecting tubule empties into
kidney pelvis, the collecting
portion of the kidney.

Henle's loop

Fig. 6-17. Schematic drawing of a nephron showing the glomerulus (filtering system) with the afferent arteriole (incoming blood) and efferent arteriole (outflowing blood), convoluted tubules collecting the urine, Henle's loop, in the ascending limb of which reabsorption of vital substance takes place, and urine collecting tubule, which empties into the kidney's pelvis from which the urine flows into the bladder. (Courtesy Dr. A. T. Guyton, Department of Physiology and Biophysics, University of Mississippi School of Medicine; Basic human physiology: normal function and mechanisms of disease, Philadelphia, 1971, W. B. Saunders Co., p. 340).

pecially in relation to other biologic agents with which they are associated.

Some environmental poisons are known to have special preferences for certain organs as, for instance, methyl mercury for the brain, iodine and cobalt for the thyroid, strontium for bones, cadmium for blood vessels and kidneys, and chlorinated hydrocarbons (DDT) for fatty tissue.

Although these are the principal targets, intoxication by most air pollutants is associated, like any other chronic illness, with a variety of systemic symptoms not characteristic of any particular agent, especially during the early stage of the disease. Since these manifestations are common to numerous other illnesses, it is difficult to relate them to specific pollutants.

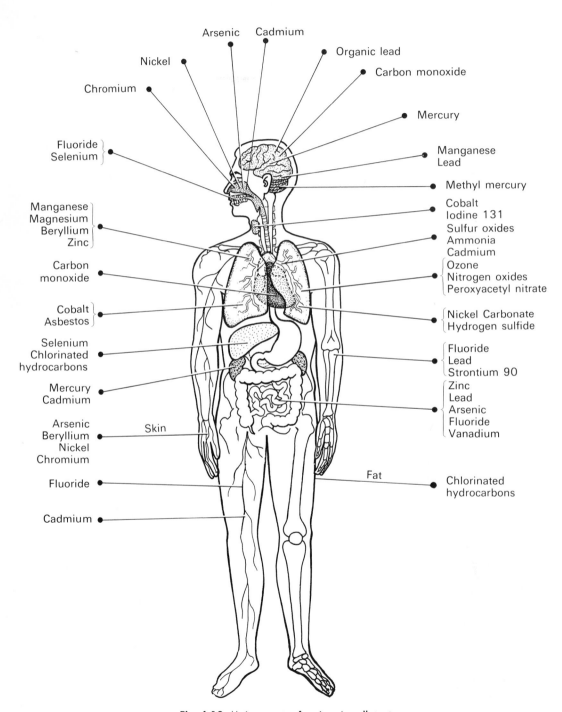

Fig. 6-18. Main targets of major air pollutants.

CLASSIFICATION OF POLLUTANTS ACCORDING TO THEIR HEALTH EFFECT

In the following discussion the major atmospheric contaminants are classified according to their effect on human health. This task is difficult, since most toxic agents elicit a variety of changes in the human organism, and overlapping between the individual groups is unavoidable. Therefore, their main toxic action upon the human organism will form the basis for the classification (Fig. 6-18).

In pursuing this aim, one can readily distinguish between respiratory and systemic pollutants on the basis of whether or not their impact and major effect upon human tissue takes place in the respiratory tract or in other organ systems.

Regardless of whether a pollutant causes an acute or a chronic disease, reversible or irreversible changes, systemic or localized illness, two other significant factors determine its effect on the human body—namely one pertaining to the pollutant itself, the other to the human host. Although most, if not all, pollutants attack the human organism in their own particular manner (Table 6-1), specific host responses are also involved. The latter are essentially the same regardless of the kind of pollutant. They are allergic reactions, the development of malignant cells, and interference with cellular growth in the case of mutagens.

In pursuance of these considerations we recognize three main groups of air pollutants: (1) respiratory, (2) systemic, and (3) host-specific.

Respiratory pollutants can be divided into five subgroups according to the pattern of their deposition and their fate in the respiratory tract, namely:

1. Pulmonary irritants (Chapter 7)
2. "Dusts" (Chapter 8)
3. Granuloma-producing agents (Chapter 9)
4. Fever-producing agents (Chapter 10)
5. Asphyxiants (Chapter 11)

The pulmonary irritants affect the surfaces of the nasopharyngeal and tracheobronchial structures and of the alveolar bed. The "dusts," such as silica, carbon, and iron oxide, either remain in the interstitial lung tissue and the adjoining lymphoid structures or are transferred to lymph and blood. Other agents, such as beryllium, form focal lesions in the lungs, so-called granulomas, whereas certain metals, such as zinc and manganese, produce changes in the lungs that are characterized clinically by sudden short-lived episodes of fever. The asphyxiants penetrate instantaneously through the alveolar walls into the bloodstream, where they interfere with respiration of cells. Carbon monoxide inhibits the oxygen-carrying power of the blood, whereas hydrogen sulfide tends to paralyze the respiratory center.

The *systemic pollutants* affect more than one organ system. They are taken into the system mainly through the gastrointestinal tract and are distributed through the bloodstream to various organs. The most common manifestations are stomach and bowel disorders, diseases of the central nervous system, and urinary tract involvement.

The *host-specific pollutants* are comprised of allergenics, carcinogens, and mutagens. They include both respiratory and systemic pollutants. The allergenic agents induce specific lesions mainly in the nose, sinuses, lungs, and skin but are liable to affect any other organ of the body. The agents producing cancer and birth defects can attack any body organ. Their target organ seems to be determined to a large extent by the host's individual susceptibility.

In evaluating the health effects of atmospheric pollutants in the subsequent chapters, it should be emphasized that there is relatively little clinical material available on their long-term effects at the minute concentrations at which these air pollutants appear in the atmosphere. It is therefore mandatory to include in the following discussions data on acute intoxication caused

Table 6-1. Examples of specific effects of pollutants

GROUPS		AGENT	PRINCIPAL AFFECTED ORGANS
Respiratory pollutants			
Pulmonary irritants	7*	Sulfur oxides Nitrogen oxides Ozone Chlorine Ammonia	Lining of the respiratory tract
Dusts	8	Quartz Silica Carbon Asbestos Cobalt Iron oxides	Pulmonary interstitial tissue
Granuloma-producing agents	9	Beryllium	Lungs
Fever-causing agents	10	Zinc Manganese Hemp, cotton	Alveoli
Asphyxiating pollutants	11	Carbon monoxide Hydrogen sulfide	Hemoglobin Respiratory center
Systemic pollutants	12	Lead Mercury	Nerve tissue Brain, bowels
	13	Fluoride Cadmium	Bones, teeth Blood vessels, kidneys
	19	Chlorinated hydrocarbons	Fat tissue, liver
	18	Organophosphates	Nerve-muscle synapsis
Host specific agents			
Allergenics	15	Thiocyanate Formaldehyde	Respiratory tract Skin, lungs
Carcinogenics	16	Strontium ^{90} Iodine ^{121} Nickel carbonate Chromium Asbestos Selenium Arsenic	Bones Thyroid Lungs, sinuses Nose Pleura Testicular tissue Skin
Mutagens	17	Most systemic pollutants; organic mercury, lead, chlorinated hydro- carbons, arsenic, fluoride, cadmium	

*Numbers indicate the chapter dealing with the respective agents.

by much higher levels than those in the ambient air. Furthermore occupational exposures must be taken into consideration, that is, data on workers who are exposed for prolonged periods of time to doses much larger than those inhaled or ingested by the average urban or rural residents. Although such accounts furnish the pattern of illness that follows inhalation of high levels of air pollutants, they cannot be extrapolated indiscriminately to minute levels of air pollutants.

REFERENCES

1. Guyton, A. C.: Basic human physiology: normal function and mechanisms of disease, Philadelphia, 1971, W. B. Saunders Co.
2. Reid, L.: Experimental study of hypersecretion of mucus in the bronchial tree, Brit. J. Exp. Path. 44:437-445, 1963.
3. Dalhamn, T.: Mucous flow and ciliary activity in the trachea of healthy rats and rats exposed to respiratory irritant gases, Acta Physiol. Scand. 36(Suppl. 123):1-161, 1956.
4. Strömme, O.: Studies on the histopathology of pollinosis, Oslo, Norway, 1952, Thronsen and Co.
5. DuBois, A. B., and Dautrebande, L.: Acute effects of breathing inert dust particles and carbachol aerosol on the mechanical characteristics of the lungs in man: changes in response after inhaling sympathomimetic aerosols, J. Clin. Invest. 37:1746-1755, 1958.
6. Mitchell, R., and Tomashefski, J. F.: Aerosols and the respiratory tract, Battelle Technol. Rev. 13:3-8, 1964.
7. Bertalanffy, F. D.: Dynamics of cellular populations in the lung. In Liebow, A. A., and Smith, D. E., editors: The lung, Baltimore, 1968, The Williams & Wilkins Co., pp. 19-30.
8. Scarpelli, E. M.: The surfactant system of the lung, Philadelphia, 1968, Lea and Febiger, p. 269.
9. Ayres, S. M.: Response of airway to nebulized isoproterenol in chronic airways obstruction: acute and chronic observations. Presented at the Twenty-eighth American College of Allergists, Scientific Congress, March 1972.
10. Van Wilk, A. M., and Patterson, H. S.: The percentage of particles of different size removed from dust-laden air by breathing, J. Industr. Hyg. Toxicol. 22:31-35, 1940.
11. Hatch, T. F., and Gross, P.: Pulmonary deposition and retention of inhaled aerosols, New York, 1964, Academic Press, Inc.
12. Deposition and retention models for internal dosimetry of the human respiratory tract, Task Group on Lung Dynamics, Health Physics 12:173-207, 1966.
13. Battigelli, M. C.: Air Quality Monographs No. 69-2. Particulates: air quality criteria based on health effects, New York, 1969, American Petroleum Institute.
14. Garber, K.: "Luftverunreinigung und ihre Wirkungen." Gebrüder Borntraeger, Berlin, 1967, Verlag.

7
PULMONARY IRRITANTS

Subgroup 1 (Table 6-1), which features damage to the mucous lining of the respiratory tract, includes nitrogen and sulfur oxides, ozone, chlorine, formaldehyde, acrolein, and ammonia. Other irritants such as nickel and chromium with carcinogenic properties are discussed in Chapter 16.

Each respiratory irritant exhibits a different action. Sulfur dioxide and other acid mists increase the acidity of the respiratory tissues, ozone causes intense oxidation and irritation, ammonia fumes decrease the acidity of the alveolar lining.

CHRONIC VERSUS
ACUTE INTOXICATION

For years allergy specialists in Michigan have encountered patients from the industrial Midland-Saginaw-Bay City area who had been referred to them as patients with "allergies of the upper respiratory tract" but their illness failed to fulfill the criteria of an allergic disease. The patients complained of cough, irritation of the nose, more or less continuous sore throats and bloodshot eyes and, occasionally, of wheezing suggestive of the beginning stage of asthma. A review of recent records of 42 patients from the same area revealed 9 who presented the above-described condition. In most of these cases, by means of laboratory and clinical studies, roentgenograms, blood and skin tests, a relationship between allergy and their illness was ruled out. Constant irritation in the throat and upper respiratory tract was the outstanding

feature of their disease. When these individuals were absent from the area for a few weeks, invariably their ill health improved remarkably; upon their return the illness recurred.

So far it has not been possible to pinpoint the exact nature of the responsible pollutant in that area where numerous chemicals are constantly being ejected into the air.

In many respects the condition resembles an illness I described in the *Journal of the American Medical Association* in 1953[1] called "smoker's respiratory syndrome." Because of the irritating effect of cigarette smoke on the mucous membranes of the respiratory tract, it subsequently proved to be the initial phase of emphysema. Although a rise of temperature is rare, antibiotic drugs often provide temporary benefit because they control the infections that are superimposed upon the primarily irritated mucous lining of the nose, throat, and bronchial tubes.

That chemical irritants rather than microorganisms were responsible for the disease was further indicated by the fact that repeated cultures of mucus from the nasal and pharyngeal areas showed only the common harmless bacteria that usually inhabit the respiratory organs.

In contrast to this slowly developing, unspectacular disease, which is relatively little disabling and sometimes impossible for a physician to attribute to its cause, the following sudden acute episode demonstrates the effect of a different kind of pollution. Here, inhalation of a massive dose of a single respiratory irritant made detection of its cause a relatively simple task.

On July 4, 1965, a 42-year-old librarian was trying to remove a stain from a laminated plastic countertop. She used a common chlorine-containing cleansing agent. When the stains failed to disappear, she added vinegar and rubbing alcohol to the cleaning fluid. Almost immediately she experienced extreme irritation in the eyes, ear, nose, and throat and a violent cough. Tears virtually poured out of her eyes. She left the room immediately but returned soon to flush the material into the sink. The actual exposure time could not have been more than 3 minutes. An hour later she developed severe shortness of breath and wheezing and felt her heart beat rapidly. She became extremely fatigued, but with frequent interruptions and resting she managed to get dressed. On the ½-mile drive to her physician's office she had to stop her car repeatedly and rest. The physician gave her injections of epinephrin and cortisone, which relieved her shortness of breath, but her condition gradually deteriorated. She was obliged to spend 14 days in the hospital, much of the time in an oxygen tent, and a period of 6 weeks at home. Fortunately, she was able to return to her job.[2] She had no further respiratory symptoms. The highly oxidative property of the chlorine was believed to have removed hydrogen from surface and tissue water, thus releasing nascent oxygen or ozone. The latter along with hydrochloric acid was believed to be responsible for the irritating and corrosive action on the respiratory tract.

SULFUR OXIDES

Sulfur oxides have been more extensively investigated than any other pollutant. As the oldest known air pollutants, they are foremost in nearly every comprehensive study on the subject. Their presence in the atmosphere has served as an indicator of the degree of pollution, mainly because they are largely responsible for bluish-white plumes and for the reduction of visibility in a polluted area after conversion into sulfuric acid.[3] In recent years, however, sulfur oxides have become relegated into a role of lesser significance because they have been shown to cause much less damage to human health than was formerly assumed. Amdur[4] classifies sulfur dioxide as only a "mild respiratory irritant." Recent experiments on monkeys[5] indicate that sulfur dioxide in concentrations up to 1 ppm does not alter pulmonary function nor is it detrimental to pulmonary tissues on microscopic examination. In experiments at the Hazelton Laboratories, Inc.[6] at Falls Church, Virginia, guinea pigs exposed to sulfur dioxide concentrations of 5 ppm for 1 year survived longer and were less affected by pulmonary disease than animals inhaling pure air. The concentration of 5 ppm is the so-called threshold limit value for healthy workers for a 40-hour week. Although such studies require further confirmatory research, the available data indicate that sulfur dioxide cannot be regarded as an indicator of air pollution by multiple agents.

Sources

Sulfur dioxide and small amounts of sulfur trioxide are generated by burning of wood, coal, and petroleum products, mostly for space heating and for production of electricity. These fossil fuels contain a great deal of sulfur as inorganic sulfides or as organic compounds. Lesser amounts of sulfur oxides originate from refinery operations, from smelting of sulfur-containing ores (copper, lead, and zinc), from manufacture of paper and sulfuric acid, and from refuse incineration (Table 7-1). The total man-made contribution of sulfur dioxide to the world's atmosphere is estimated to be about 100×10^6 tons per year of which 93.5% is produced in the Northern Hemisphere and only 6.5% in the Southern

Table 7-1. Sources of sulfur dioxide emission in the United States, 1966 (29.6 million tons)*

SOURCE	PERCENT
Combustion of coal	58.2
Combustion of residual oil and other petroleum	19.6
Refining of petroleum	5.5
Smelting of sulfur-containing ores	12.2
Manufacturing of sulfuric acid	1.9
Burning of refuse	0.4
Smoldering coal refuse banks	0.4

*Adapted from air quality criteria for sulfur oxides' Washington, D. C., 1970, United States Department of Health, Education, and Welfare, Public Health Service Environmental Health Service, Publication Number AP-50

Hemisphere.[7] The principal natural sources of sulfur oxides are decomposition of organic matter, volcanoes, and sea salt over the oceans.[7]

During combustion most sulfur present in the burning substance is oxidized by photochemical catalytic action to sulfur dioxide and about 40 to 80 times less to sulfur trioxide.[8]

Properties

Sulfur dioxide is a colorless gas with a pungent irritating odor detectable at concentrations of about 0.5 to 0.8 ppm.[8] It is much more soluble in water than most other pollutant gases. Under conditions of high humidity (clouds or fog droplets), of sunlight, and in the presence of such particulate catalysts as charcoal, ferric oxide, and graphite, conversion of sulfur dioxide to sulfur trioxide takes place.

Sulfur trioxide combines immediately with water vapor to form sulfuric acid (H_2SO_4) and these molecules form droplets of sulfuric acid solution. When sulfur trioxide is converted to sulfuric acid, its irritant response on a molar basis in animals increases three to fourfold and four to twentyfold more than sulfur dioxide.[8] Indeed sulfates, which account for 5% to 20% of all particulate matter in urban atmo-

sphere, determine the irritant action of sulfur oxides.[9]

Mean annual atmospheric concentrations of sulfur dioxide from 1962 to 1967 ranged from 0.01 ppm in San Francisco to 0.18 ppm in Chicago.[8] However, near a coal-fired power plant, hourly averages were recorded as high as 2.9 ppm within a ½-mile distance.

About 80% of all sulfates constitute particles below 2 μ in diameter. These particles suspended in the atmosphere account for reduction of visibility, a characteristic feature of sulfur oxide pollution.

Health effects

There is an abundance of data on the health effect of sulfur oxides on animals compared with relatively little exact information on humans. In statistical studies on this subject, no clear distinction is made between the effect of sulfur dioxide and that of smoke in general.[10]

More than 90% of the inhaled gas is absorbed in the airways above the larynx.[11] The degree of irritation of sulfur dioxide, sulfuric acid, and sulfates to the respiratory tract is dependent largely on their concentration in the atmosphere and the size of the particles. The size that causes most irritation to the respiratory tract is about 1 μ in diameter or slightly less; but even larger sulfuric acid particles, which do not reach the lower airways, induce constriction of bronchi associated with severe coughing, probably as the result of reflex action.[12]

Detectable responses in humans begin at atmospheric concentrations of about 0.25 mg/meter^3 or 0.06 ppm[11] but, in general, at 0.3 to 1 ppm, sulfur dioxide is hardly noticeable by taste. At 3 ppm a sulfurlike odor suggestive of breathing dusty air is perceptible. When Frank[11] exposed eleven healthy volunteers to sulfur dioxide concentrations of 5 ppm for 10 to 30 minutes, he recorded an increase in air flow resistance in nine. He observed wide variations in tolerance from person to person. According to Pattle and Collumbine,[13] about 1% of a population encounters bronchospasm even at about 1 ppm. At a concentration of 20 ppm the damage to the respiratory organs is reversible when exposure ceases.[14] Concentrations above 20 ppm cause waterlogging of the lungs and larynx, a tendency to pulmonary edema, and, eventually, respiratory paralysis.[15] Damage is considered to be more dependent on the concentration than on the duration of exposure.[9]

During the 2-day period of the 1952 London disaster, the average concentration of sulfur dioxide was only 1.7 ppm, which is well within the industrial threshold limit value of 5 ppm.

Although it is difficult in an acute air pollution episode to pinpoint damage to health by a single agent such as sulfur dioxide, even greater difficulties arise in interpreting epidemiologic statistics that are designed to establish the effect of airborne sulfur oxides on mortality and morbidity of populations. Such surveys have been made in the United States and in other countries. In many of these studies, cigarette smoking has not been considered as a variant. Other studies have been limited to oxides of sulfur without consideration of other atmospheric pollutants that contribute significantly to morbidity and mortality.

In long-term studies on mortality of populations, there are numerous peaks both in the death rates and in the air pollution levels that are unrelated to sulfur oxides.

One of the most thorough epidemiologic investigations was carried out by Carnow[16] in the Chicago area. On the basis of three morbidity and two mortality studies, this investigator noted a much higher rate of acute respiratory illness, such as cough and shortness of breath, in smokers than in nonsmokers at increasing levels of sulfur dioxide. He considered smokers the "high risk populations." Even the elderly and

the very elderly without cough and phlegm, who were non or mild smokers residing in a large polluted city, are considered "low risk" compared with smokers. Such variables as age, sex, socioeconomic status, and race proved to be significant in the appraisal of data concerned with air pollution.

It has been suggested that certain individuals might actually be allergic to sulfur oxides, since asthma, chronic bronchitis, eye, and nasal symptoms have for years been identified with sulfur oxides. However, narrowing of air passages, swelling of mucous membranes, and increased secretion of mucus closely simulate the clinical picture of allergic asthma rather than constitute genuine asthma.

Interaction with other contaminants

An important feature of the biologic behavior of sulfur oxides is their interaction with other pollutants. Aerosols of soluble salts of iron, manganese, or vanadium in concentrations of 0.7 mg/meter^3 to 1 mg/meter^3 induce a threefold increase in airway resistance in experimental animals.[17] These substances form droplets in the humid respiratory tract and thus permit solution of sulfur dioxide. Furthermore, they are catalytic agents for the oxidation of sulfur dioxide to sulfuric acid.[5] Sulfuric acid mist at 8 mg/meter^3 combined with 89 ppm of sulfur dioxide produced greater injury to lungs, greater alterations in respiration, and greater retardation of growth than either one alone.[18]

The combination of sulfur dioxide with hydrogen peroxide (H_2O_2) at concentrations of 0.29 mg/meter^3 for 5 minutes, with particle size of 4.7 μ, induced a synergistic effect.[19] However, when hydrogen peroxide was associated with the same concentration of sulfur dioxide but of reduced particle size (11.8 μ), no potentiating effect occurred.

Inhalation of sulfur dioxide together with fine particles of sodium chloride 0.04

μ in diameter accounted for greater airway resistance than inhalation of sulfur dioxide alone.[20] However, no such synergism occurred when the size of sodium chloride particles was increased to 2.5 μ at the same concentrations.

The interaction of particulates with sulfur dioxide in animals is a highly complex process and does not always parallel that in humans. Experiments with normal human volunteers, for instance, have failed to demonstrate consistent potentiation of the response to sulfur dioxide by sodium chloride particles.[20]

In Detroit on January 22, 1970, cold, dry weather was combined with heavy traffic. Salt that had been poured on the city's streets to melt snow and ice was blown into the air. The average sulfur dioxide level in the city's air had more than doubled. Droplets of sulfuric acid coalesced with sodium chloride particulates to form the highly irritating hydrochloric acid,[7] and the residue was sodium sulfate.

In the London disaster of 1952 animals in pens that had not been cleaned regularly were remarkably free from untoward effects compared with those kept in clean surroundings. Ammonia fumes, emanating from the animal's excreta, were believed to have neutralized sulfur dioxide by forming ammonium sulfate, which is considerably less harmful than sulfuric acid.[9] This theory was supported by Pattle and Collumbine,[13] who observed the protective effect of ammonia in guinea pigs when the two gases occur together. Amdur[9] points to the need for cleanliness in experimental exposure chambers.

As a major constituent of tobacco smoke, sulfur oxides probably contribute to the production of emphysema caused by cigarettes.

In a home, damage caused by sulfur dioxide exposure can be prevented and treated effectively by spraying rooms with 2% sodium bicarbonate, which will neutralize the acid. This solution can also be used in 5% glycerine for inhalation.[21] Inhalation of steam, on the other hand, will help convert sulfur dioxide into the more irritating sulfuric acid.

NITROGEN OXIDES

A pollutant derived mainly from automobile exhaust but present in practically all combustion processes as well is nitric oxide (NO).

At normal temperatures air contains 79.02% nitrogen (N_2) and 20.94% oxygen (O_2), which are relatively nonreactive. In fact, we inhale about 11,000 quarts (about 10,500 liters) of elemental nitrogen daily without untoward effects.

In the presence of a burning flame as, for instance, in a furnace or in the cylinder of an automobile, specifically at a temperature in excess of 1093° C (2000° F), the two gases combine and form nitric oxide, a gas of little significance as an air pollutant. However, when it is vented into the air and cools rapidly, a fraction is converted into nitrogen dioxide (NO_2). Further complex reactions in the presence of hydrocarbons and of sunshine result in formation of ozone (O_3), nitrogen dioxide, and other oxidants,[22] which are discussed later.

Nitrogen dioxide, a reddish-brown, highly toxic, and irritating gas with a pungent odor, is one of seven known nitrogen oxides. It reduces visibility and changes the color of the horizon.

Sources of nitrogen oxides

Nitrogen oxides, usually designated by the symbol NO_x, occur in the atmosphere naturally. Nitric oxide, the major portion of natural NO_x emission, is produced by bacterial action, particularly during rainy periods, and is usually oxidized to nitrogen dioxide. The atmospheric concentrations in nonurban regions average about 8 μg/meter^3 (4 ppb) for nitrogen dioxide and 2 μg/meter^3 (2 ppb) for nitric oxide.[23] In urban areas, nitrogen oxide concentrations are 10 to 100 times higher.

Table 7-2. Summary of nationwide nitrogen oxides emissions, 1968*

SOURCE	EMISSIONS		
	10⁶ TONS/YEAR		PERCENT
Transportation	8.1		39.3
Motor vehicles	7.2		
Gasoline		6.6	
Diesel		0.6	
Aircraft (below 3000 ft.)		†	
Railroads		0.4	
Vessels		0.2	
Nonhighway		0.3	
Fuel combustion in stationary sources	10.0		48.5
Coal		4.0	
Fuel oil		1.0	
Natural gas		4.8	
Wood		0.2	
Industrial processes	0.2		1.0
Solid waste disposal	0.6		2.9
Miscellaneous	1.7		8.3
Forest fires		1.2	
Structural fires		not reported	
Coal refuse		0.2	
Agricultural		0.3	
	20.6		100%

*Adapted from Nationwide inventory of air pollutant emissions, 1968, Raleigh, N. C., August, 1970, National Air Pollution Control Administration, Publication No. AP-73, pp. 14-16.[25]
†Estimated less than 0.05 × 10⁶ tons/year.

The principal man-made sources of nitrogen oxides, which in the United States amounted to 20.6 million tons in 1968, are coal, oil, natural gas, and motor vehicle fuel combustion (Table 7-2). Of 10 million tons generated by stationary combustion sources, power plants emit 4 million tons, industry 4.8 million tons, and home and office heating plants the remaining 1.2 million tons.[24] Relatively small quantities of nitrogen oxides are emitted from noncombustion industrial processes, namely the manufacturing and use of nitric acid, electroplating, engraving, welding, metal cleaning, explosive detonations and the use of liquid nitrogen dioxide-based rocket propellants.[26]

In a city the nitrogen oxide levels follow a regular pattern dependent on motor traffic and sunlight. Shortly after dawn the concentration of nitric oxide begins to rise. When ultraviolet energy from the sun becomes available, nitrogen dioxide concentration increases until nearly all nitric oxide is converted into nitrogen dioxide. In late afternoon when the sun begins to set, solar energy no longer converts nitric oxide into nitrogen dioxide, consequently, nitric oxide concentrations increase. Whereas nitric oxide concentrations in the atmosphere display marked seasonal variations with higher values during late fall and winter, nitrogen dioxide levels show no distinct pattern from month to month.[24] Peak concentrations of nitrogen dioxide in urban areas rarely exceed 0.5 ppm (0.94 mg/meter³).

Experimental poisoning

Nitric oxide. The medical literature[24] contains little information on human poisoning caused by nitric oxide. In animals, exposure to extremely high concentrations of the order of 2500 ppm (3075 mg/meter³) for 12 minutes induces fatal paralysis and convulsions.[27] However, when animals survive exposures to such high concentrations, they recover rapidly. In experimental poisoning, nitric oxide increases the blood levels of methemoglobin up to 30% to 45% of the total hemoglobin and thus reduces the oxygen carrying capacity of the blood. Normal levels range from 0 to 8%.

A large array of experiments on various animals indicates that nitrogen oxides exert their primary toxic effect on the respiratory system.

Nitrogen dioxide. Nitrogen dioxide is considered to be about four times as toxic as nitric oxide.[28] Since nitrogen dioxide is not very soluble in water, it passes through the relatively dry trachea and bronchi into the moisture-laden alveoli of the lungs where it forms nitrous acid (HNO_2) and nitric acid (HNO_3). Both are very irritating and corrosive to the mucous lining of the lungs.

The product of the concentration of nitrogen dioxide in the atmosphere and the duration of exposure determines the morbidity in animals. Investigators emphasize the reversibility of the damaging effect of nitrogen dioxide after exposure to the gas has ceased.

In rats, high concentrations of nitrogen dioxide of 30 to 1000 ppm for 10 minutes to several hours cause waterlogging of the lung tissue (pulmonary edema) and, in some animals, pneumonitis.[28] Long-term exposures to small doses elicit a cumulative, sustained effect suggestive of a pre- emphysematous condition.

Rats subjected to continuous inhalation of 2 ppm (3.8 mg/meter³) nitrogen dioxide for 3 days[29] lose the lining of the cilia, show changes in the epithelial cells (the lining) of the bronchi, and develop certain crystalloid rod-shaped inclusion bodies in the smallest bronchi. Distention of the alveoli with a tendency to emphysema occurs with

exposures to as little as 0.5 ppm (940 mg/meter³) for 4 hours.[30] When animals are exposed to 0.5 to 25 ppm nitrogen dioxide for 3 months or longer, lung changes similar to those of human emphysema develop.[31]

Both short- and long-term exposures to nitrogen dioxide enhance susceptibility to infections. They impair the ability of the lungs to clear inhaled infectious organisms.[32] Nitrogen dioxide increases mortality and shortens survival time following infections.

In addition to the respiratory symptoms, systemic changes believed to be secondary to those in the lungs have been observed in the kidneys, liver, and hearts of monkeys in proportion to the length of exposure and the dose. Loss of weight, an increase in the concentration of red blood cells, and increased methemoglobin formation has also been reported in long-term experiments.[24]

Nitrogen dioxide intoxication in man

Experimental exposure. The odor of nitrogen dioxide is perceptible to humans at concentrations of 1 to 3 ppm, which are known to occur in polluted air.[33] Experimental exposure of humans to 5 ppm (9.4 μg/meter³) of nitrogen dioxide for 10 minutes produces a temporary increase in airway resistance. At 13 ppm, irritation of the respiratory mucous membranes takes place. Thirty to sixty minute exposures to concentrations of 100 to 150 ppm are believed to be fatal. Death results from edema of the larynx, which closes the air passages and causes asphyxiation.

Acute poisoning. Acute nitrogen dioxide poisoning, leading to instant pulmonary edema and death, has been recognized during the past 3 decades in farmers filling silos. It occurs especially during the early weeks after filling if the farmer happens to be inside the silo. Nitrogen dioxide is derived from moldy silage.[34] In hermetically sealed silos, nitrogen oxides, caused by decaying silage, concentrate at the bottom. Similar accidents have occurred in power plants, in individuals working with boilers, and with industrial gases and in welders.

Nitrogen dioxide that evolved from burning x-ray films was believed to be the major cause of death in the Cleveland Clinic fire of May 1929, when 97 persons died within 2 hours and 26 additional persons within less than 1 month.[35] Neither carbon monoxide nor hydrogen cyanide were believed to be the primary cause of death. By 1965, no effect of the fire on mortality rates of survivors compared with nonexposed controls had become manifest.

An accident in September 1966, yielded a well-rounded picture of the immediate and late effects of acute nitrogen dioxide intoxication. Pure nitrogen dioxide was present without essential interference by other agents and the patients involved were carefully followed. Four fire fighters were overcome by nitrogen dioxide fumes that escaped from a leak in a chemical plant.[36] One of them, age 49, experienced only a mild and transient headache with a dry, hacking cough for about 10 minutes following exposure to the fumes. Twenty hours later, however, he had to be hospitalized because of extreme shortness of breath, a temperature of $102°$ F ($38.9°$ C), wheezing and rattling throughout the lungs, and features indicative of pulmonary edema. The increased burden of pushing the blood through the water-soaked lungs had produced a life-threatening strain on the right heart. He became semicomatous, and his condition continued to deteriorate. Prompt emergency treatment including cortisone, intravenous aminophyllin for the relief of bronchospasm, and digitalis to counteract failure of the heart action helped him rally.

Unexpectedly on the twelfth day following the exposure he abruptly developed fever, chills, and shortness of breath with cough and expectoration of blood. A roentgenogram of the chest revealed fine nodules of the size of cherries distributed throughout the lungs. They persisted for another 5 weeks during which the patient received intensive treatment. Subsequently, he con-

tinued to complain of shortness of breath; his breathing capacity had decreased and pulmonary emphysema had developed.

In his three companions, who were exposed approximately for the same length of time, the overall clinical picture was similar, although an individual difference in their response to nitrogen dioxide was in evidence.*

One of them developed only a slight "sinus" irritation with minor pulmonary symptoms that responded promptly to treatment. Subsequently, he remained free of disease.

In the other two individuals, the disease followed the same pattern as in the first case: following the initial acute phase, with only a slight irritation of the nose and upper bronchial tree and a brief latent period, pneumonia developed. After a time lapse of 2 to 6 weeks' relative quiescence another acute phase occurred.

The initial latent period has been attributed to the low solubility of nitrogen dioxide, which bypasses the relatively dry nasal and bronchial membranes and settles in the terminal portions of the bronchi. Serious damage does not occur until the gas is dissolved in the moist portions of the terminal bronchial tree, where the highly irritating nitrous and nitric acids originate and produce many uniformly distributed tiny foci of inflammation.

Chronic poisoning. There is a great paucity of information on chronic nitrogen dioxide poisoning because damage develops slowly and insidiously and because nitrogen dioxide is usually associated with many other pollutants, which render assessment of its action difficult. In whatever accounts are available the nitrogen dioxide levels exceed those usually present in ambient air. According to the intensity and duration of exposure, respiratory illness ranges from slight irritation, burning and pain in the

---

*Whether or not the difference in doses received by the three individuals accounted for their differing responses could not be determined.

throat and chest, to violent cough and shortness of breath.

Soviet scientists[37] have observed chronic pulmonary disease and blood changes (decreased granulation of basophil cells)* in 127 workers of a sulfuric acid plant exposed for 3 to 5 years to concentrations of nitrogen dioxide up to 2.6 ppm (4.9 mg/meter³).

An elaborate epidemiologic study has been carried out by the U. S. Public Health Service in Chattanoga, Tennessee, where the mean range of daily nitrogen dioxide concentrations, measured over a 6 months' period, was 0.062 and 0.109 ppm (117 and 205 μg/meter³). The mean suspended nitrate level during the same period was 3.8 μg/meter³ or greater. Among infants and school children, a high incidence of acute bronchitis was noted.[38]

Interaction of nitrogen dioxide with other pollutants. Regarding the interaction of nitrogen dioxide with other atmospheric pollutants, sulfur dioxide is known to have an additive effect on pulmonary function in healthy adults.[39]

Nitrogen dioxide is also an ingredient of cigarette smoke. Cigarette, pipe tobacco, and cigar smoke contain approximately 300, 950, and 1200 ppm nitrogen dioxide, respectively.[40] Smokers employed in an environment polluted by automobile exhaust are believed to be particularly vulnerable to harm from nitrogen oxides.

In hamsters exposed to concentrations of 15 ppm nitrogen dioxide for 2 hours followed by exposure to tobacco smoke, irreversible changes in the lining of the bronchi and secondary airways were produced.[41]

OZONE

Ozone (O_3) is an unstable blue gas with an oxidizing power that is surpassed only by that of fluorine. It owes its name to its

characteristic pungent odor, which is derived from the Greek "Ozein," to smell. Sometimes described as "electrical odor" it can be detected instantaneously at concentrations between 0.2 to 0.05 ppm.

In the past, ozone was considered beneficial in that it was believed to assist in oxygenation of blood. As late as 1942, Hill[42] claimed that "pure ozone is not poisonous in any sense of the word." Physicians have even prescribed ozone for respiratory disease because of its bactericidal action. Although it has also been used to "destroy" odors and to "freshen" the air, actually, in this capacity it only masks the air by lowering the perceptibility to odors. Now it is recognized as one of the most dangerous irritants to eyes, throat, and lungs. It damages plants and even cracks rubber.

Ubiquity of ozone

Ozone is by far the most ubiquitous oxidant. Within the past 2 to 3 decades it rose to significance when it became recognized as the key component in oxidant smog created by interaction of hydrocarbons, nitrogen oxides, and sunlight (see Chapter 19). At times, ozone constitutes as much as 90% of the oxidants in smog. In urban areas, ozone concentrations have been found to be 0.001 to 0.03 ppm. In Los Angeles smog, the levels of ozone have reached up to 0.9 ppm.[43]

In the air naturally, ozone can be a threat to aviation personnel at altitudes above 30,000 feet (9144 meters), particularly over the polar region where its presence is most abundant. Fear has been expressed for the health of passengers in supersonic air transportation in which ambient air from outside the plane, used for cabin pressurization, contains high levels of ozone. At 80,000 feet, ozone concentrations in the air are 10 to 12 ppm, which constitute *lethal dose* levels; inside plane cabins, ozone levels are estimated at about 2.5 ppm.[44]

Man-made sources of ozone are high-

---

*White blood cells that stain readily with basic dyes.

voltage electrical equipment, such as x-ray apparatus, spectrographs, electrical insulators, brushes of motors, and ultraviolet-ray quartz lamps. Ozonizing equipment has been used for purification of water and sugar and for control of fungi and bacteria in cold-storage plants.

One source of ozone pollution not generally appreciated by the public is electrostatic air cleaners.[43] In concentrations of 0.001 to 0.002 ppm, it is produced by all electrostatic cleaners, but higher concentrations occur when ionizing wires are incorrectly spaced and produce an invisible corona, when there is arcing against bent corrector plates, or when the plates need cleaning because of heavy coating with particulates. A defective unit can produce as much as 1 ppm or more ozone; 0.05 is the maximum allowable concentration (MAC) in industry for an 8-hour exposure for healthy humans and 0.5 ppm is the "first alert" level in Los Angeles, California.[45]

The dryer the air, the more ozone is being produced. Prompt service to the electronic air cleaner will prevent high concentrations of ozone from this source.

Mode of action

Ozone, like sulfur dioxide, acts upon the respiratory tract and is not absorbed in the general circulation. About three fourths of inhaled ozone is destroyed in the upper respiratory structures, where it reacts rapidly with organic substances with which it comes into contact.[46] Ozone impairs the function of the pulmonary macrophages and induces thickening of the walls of small pulmonary arteries,[47] thus leading to chronic pulmonary disease, to emphysema, and to right heart failure.

Although primarily an irritant to the respiratory organs, ozone acts as a depressant to nerve endings in the portion of the brain that controls the rate of respiration. In this manner, it interferes with the normal ventilation of the lungs and the exchange of oxygen and carbon dioxide in the blood.

In lung tissue, ozone interferes with two important enzymes, namely, alkaline phosphatase, which splits phosphate from organic phosphate compounds under alkaline conditions, and 5-ribonucleotide phosphohydrolase, which splits phosphate off RNA. Activity of succinic dehydrogenase, another important enzyme, is also reduced. Urinary acidity increases in test animals exposed 4 hours daily to 0.8 to 1.5 ppm ozone for 18 weeks.[48]

A characteristic feature of experimental ozone poisoning is the development of tolerance to its acute effects following exposure to it. This tolerance provides no protection against the chronic effects of bronchitis and bronchiolitis (inflammation of the smallest portions of the bronchial tree), which follow massive exposure to ozone.[49]

Short-term exposures

Some persons may detect the odor of ozone at a level as low as 0.001 ppm. In the somewhat higher concentrations of 0.05 to 0.1 ppm, the odor becomes more pronounced and disagreeable.[50] At such levels, a disturbance of the eye muscle balance, a decrease in visual acuity and in adaptation of the eyes to dark become noticeable[51] (Table 7-3).

In 1957, Griswold and others[52] reported the experience of a person who was voluntarily exposed to ozone at 1.5 ppm for 1½ hour followed by 2 ppm for 1½ hours. Besides the typical pungent odor, the person experienced dryness of the mouth and throat, an altered taste sensation, and reduced ability to concentrate and think. He had constrictive pain below the breast bone; his hands and feet felt as though they were "falling asleep." After the exposure was terminated, the chest pains returned in the evening. The patient spent a sleepless, uncomfortable night. Two days later he developed cough and expectorated clear mucus, a condition that persisted

Table 7-3. Effects of ozone in man

CONCENTRATION	DURATION	SYMPTOM	OBSERVER
0.05 to 0.1 ppm	Immediate	Odor noticeable	Jaffe[50]
0.1 to 1.0 ppm	2 weeks	Odor; shortness of breath; headache	Wilska[53]
		Visual disturbances	Lagerwerff[51]
0.6 to 0.8 ppm	2 hours	Substernal cough, irritation in trachea	Young and others[54]
0.94 ppm	1½ hours	Cough; dyspnea, exhaustion	Jaffe[50]
0.1 to 1.0 ppm	1 hour	Increased airway resistance	Goldsmith and Nadel[45]

for 2 weeks. The chest pain recurred periodically for 2 days after which it subsided completely.

Objectively, the subject's vital capacity had been reduced by 13% by the end of the exposure. The reduced level returned to normal after 22 hours. His maximum breathing capacity, which is the total amount of air taken into his lungs by deep breathing, showed only a slight reduction, namely 3%.

This experiment demonstrated that short-term exposures to high concentrations of ozone lead to vague and unspectacular symptoms of the kind similar to those caused by other kinds of chronic respiratory irritants.

In four individuals exposed to lower doses of 0.1, 0.4, 0.6, and 1 ppm for 1 hour for a period of 75 days, Goldsmith and Nadel[45] observed an increase in airway resistance. These results were not related to the dose and appeared to be less pronounced than in healthy persons inhaling smoke from a single cigarette. Edema of the lungs appears at concentrations of ozone above 1 ppm.[55]

In laboratory animals death occurs from a single 4-hour exposure to ozone at 1 to 3.2 ppm.[56] At lower levels, ozone causes a wide variety of respiratory disorders ranging from bronchitis, bronchiolitis, bronchopneumonia, atelectasis, lung abscess, hemorrhages, and focal necrosis (destruction of lung tissue).

Chronic toxicity

From repeated exposures to ozone in experimental animal studies, three long-term effects are recognized:

1. *Chronic pulmonary disease*, especially emphysema and fibrosis of the lung tissue, have appeared in small laboratory animals exposed daily to a concentration slightly above 1 ppm.[49] In humans, this condition is particularly treacherous because patients do not develop active symptoms such as cough and expectoration like they do from most other pulmonary irritants. Furthermore the progress of the disease is slow and insidious.

2. *Premature aging* is a second effect of chronic low-level exposure to ozone experimentally, which, however, has not been verified in humans. In rabbits, there was a progressive breakdown of the tissue of the alveolar wall as exposure progressed.[49] Although the animals develop a tolerance to acute pulmonary episodes, nevertheless the lung tissue that comes in contact with ozone gradually deteriorates. Calcifications of the cartilage of the thorax, depletion of body fat, and such signs as a dull cornea and sagging conjunctivae (the membrane lining the outer surface of the eye) were observed in animal experiments.

3. *Lung tumors* in animals is a third effect of exposure to ozone. Adenomas (tumors) of the lungs were produced in a strain of mice prone to lung tumors following daily exposures to about 1 ppm ozone. After 15 months, 85% of the exposed animals had developed the tumor compared with 38% of the control mice.[57] Werthamer and others[44] induced tumor growth in the lungs in 23% of mice exposed to 4.5 ppm of ozone for 2 hours every third day for 75 days. In interpreting these experiments one must be aware that different animal species vary in their response to ozone. Rodents appear to be most sensitive, dogs least, and man's sensitivity lies between.[54] The experience gained in animal experimentation cannot be applied uncritically to human toxicology.

Another likely action of ozone that has not as yet been fully established is its possible ability[58] to mimic radioactivity, that is, to damage cells in a manner similar to injury by radiation.

Aggravating factors

A number of factors alter an animal's response to ozone. The synergistic effect of exercise, presence of infection and early age have already been outlined in Chapter 5. Increased thyroid activity renders mice highly susceptible to ozone and nitrogen oxide.

A rise in temperature from 75° to 90° F doubles the susceptibility of rats and mice to ozone.[57]

Animals with respiratory infections *(Klebsiella pneumoniae)* prior to ozone exposure have a shorter survival time and increased mortality.[59]

Protection against ozone toxicity

On the other hand, damage by ozone was lessened substantially when animals were given prophylactically such reducing agents as ascorbic acid either alone or in combination with glycuronate or sulfur compounds, especially cysteine (a sulfur-containing

amino acid). Recently as the result of animal experiments two additional antioxidants have been suggested as protection against ozone toxicity, namely, vitamin E[60] and para-aminobenzoic acid (PABA).[61]

CHLORINE

Chlorine (Cl_2), a green-colored gas with a sharp odor, is 2.47 times as heavy as air and 20 times as toxic as hydrogen chloride gas. It became notorious as a poisonous gas in World War I. When it reaches the lung tissue, it combines with the hydrogen of water to form the highly corrosive hydrochloric acid (HCl).[62] During this process ozone, another strong irritant, and free oxygen are also liberated according to the following formulas:

$$Cl_2 + H_2O \longrightarrow HCl + HOCl$$
$$8\ HOCl \longrightarrow 6\ HCl + 2\ HClO_3 + O_2$$

(In sunlight or bright light, HOCl decomposes mainly as follows:

$$2\ HOCl \longrightarrow 2\ HCl + O_2).$$

Uses of chlorine

The largest consumer of chlorine is the chemical industry. The gas is used for preparation of organic and inorganic agents such as trichlorethylene, carbontetrachloride, vinyl chloride plastics, and vinylidene chloride, of pesticides and herbicides such as DDT, of refrigerants and propellants such as freons, for manufacturing of glycerine, tetraethyl lead additives, pharmaceuticals, and detergents.[62] In the pulp and paper industry, chlorine is used in bleaching operations and to oxidize odorous sulfur compounds present in the black liquor. Approximately 4% of the production of chlorine is used for water and sewage treatment (Tables 7-4 and 7-5).

In addition, a variety of inorganic chemicals are prepared with chlorine, namely the chlorine salts, metals and other compounds, paint coating, silicates, phosphates. Hydrochloric acid is emitted mainly from

Table 7-4. Uses of chlorine and hydrochloric acid in 1969 in the United States*

CHLORINE	PERCENT	HYDROCHLORIC ACID	PERCENT
Organic chlorinations	78.5	Organic chlorinations	50.0
Pulp, paper bleaching	15.0	Treatment of oil wells	17.0
Water, sewage treatment	3.5	Metallurgical processes	17.0
Manufacturing bleaches	2.0	Metal pickling	7.0
Metallurgical processes	1.0	Food processing	4.0
		Miscellaneous inorganic chemicals	5.0

*Adapted from Gerstle, R. W., and Devitt, T. W.: Chlorine and hydrogen chloride emissions and their control. Presented at the Sixty-fourth Annual Meeting of the Air Pollution Control Association, Atlantic City, New Jersey, 1971.

Table 7-5. Estimated United States emissions of chlorine and hydrochloric acid in 1969 (tons/year)*

SOURCE	ESTIMATED EMISSIONS	
	CHLORINE	HYDROCHLORIC ACID
Chlorine manufacture	47,000	0
Hydrochloric acid manufacture	800	5,700
Chemical and industrial processes	30,400	27,400
Combustion	0	874,500
Total	78,200	907,600

*Adapted from Gerstle, R. W., and Devitt, T. W.: Chlorine and hydrogen chloride emissions and their control. Presented at the Sixty-fourth Annual Meeting of the Air Pollution Control Association, Atlantic City, New Jersey, 1971.

combustion of coal and oil (Table 7-5). Domestic coal contains between 0.01% and 0.5% of chlorine by weight, 95% of which reaches the atmosphere as hydrochloric acid.[63] Near incineration dumps where vinyl plastics are burned hydrochloric acid is a major contaminant.

Chlorine is usually shipped in liquified form. During the liquification process it can become an important source of atmospheric contamination. When in contact with moisture, chlorine reacts to form hypochlorite, the active ingredient in liquid household bleaches, and hydrochloric acid, a strong corrosive, an irritant to the eyes and to the whole respiratory tract. The industrial threshold limit value (TLV) for chlorine in the United States is 3 mg/meter³ (1 ppm) for an 8-hour day. In Russia, the value is one third that adopted by our country.

Experimental data

At chlorine concentrations of 3 to 6 ppm (9 to 18 mg/meter³) a stinging and burning sensation is noted in the eyes.[64] Exposure to concentrations of 14 to 21 ppm for 30 to 60 minutes causes pulmonary edema, pneumonitis, emphysema, and bronchitis.[65] This condition is usually associated with marked bronchospasm, muscular soreness, and headache. Chlorine produces hemorrhages in the lungs more frequently than most other respiratory irritants at the same concentration.[66] After exposure, a rise in temperature and extensive tearing of eyes are not uncommon; rales remain audible in the lungs for several weeks. In long-term (up to 9 months) experiments on rabbits exposed to chlorine in concentrations of 0.7 to 1.7 ppm, loss of weight and a high incidence of respiratory disease was observed.[67]

Acute intoxication

Acute epidemics have occurred repeatedly as the result of accidents associated with handling or emptying liquid chlorine cylinders. For instance, in March 1961[68] what were supposedly empty liquid chlorine cylinders were being unloaded from a freighter in the Baltimore harbor when the main valve of a cylinder snapped off. One hundred and fifty-six persons were stricken immediately, some with hemorrhages from the lungs, others with asthmalike wheezing and pneumonialike lung infiltration, which lasted as long as 19 to 35 months and resulted in long-term impairment of pulmonary function.[68]

Two months prior to this accident on January 31, 1961, a tank car, torn open in a train wreck at LaBarre, Louisiana, a rural community, had spilled 6,000 gallons of liquid chlorine.[69] The cloud of the gas covered approximately 6 square miles and 1000 people had to be evacuated. Seven hours later the concentrations of chlorine gas in the area were still 400 ppm at a distance of 75 yards (about 70 meters) from the site of the accident and 10 ppm at the fringe of the cloud. An 11-month-old infant died as the result of the exposure and approximately 100 people were treated for varying degrees of respiratory illness. Some developed congestive heart failure. About 500 animals, namely dogs, cats, horses, mules, chickens, hogs, cows, and ducks died as the result of this accidental spillage.

Another episode that was well publicized caused a city-wide panic in New York. It occurred the first week of June, 1944.[70] A truck driver carrying a cargo of compressed chlorine detected, through the odor, that one of his tanks was leaking. He removed the tank and tried to obtain aid. He failed to realize that the truck was standing close to the ventilation intake of the Brooklyn-Manhattan transit subway station at the intersection of Myrtle and Flatbush Avenues. Chlorine not only seeped down into the subway station but was also sucked into the passing subway trains. Within a few minutes numerous people waiting for trains were unable to see or breathe. Some were lying prostrate on the street. Many fainted on the stairways and collided with others who were trying to escape from the gas above and below. The number of casualties amounted to well over 100. At one hospital all 33 patients who were admitted had tracheobronchitis, 23 had pulmonary edema, 14 developed pneumonia. Among 29 individuals who were followed up, 16 showed various anxiety reactions for periods up to 16 months. No permanent lung disease was reported.

More recently, on May 8, 1969, a leak in a liquid chlorine storage tank occurred in Cleveland.[71] Twenty-seven persons were treated in St. Luke's Hospital: eighteen of them underwent a series of studies of their pulmonary function up to 14 months following the exposure. Airway obstruction and hypoxemia (low oxygen levels in blood) cleared within 3 months. Five of the eighteen, however, had persistent reduction in air inflow at the termination of the study.

As a result of these experiences, to avoid similar incidents, health authorities have imposed strict rules including plans for evacuation of populations near threatened areas.

Chronic effects

In contrast with reports on acute poisoning by chlorine gas there is a great paucity of information on chronic effect of minute amounts. Most observations were made in factories producing the chemical. As long ago as 1909, Ronzani[72] observed that the men working with chlorine aged prematurely, suffered from bronchial trouble, and were predisposed to tuberculosis. Corrosion of teeth was widespread because of hydrochloric acid, which formed when chlorine combined with the moisture of the mouth.

Veterans of World War I, hospitalized

from gassing with chlorine, developed permanent lung damage and emphysema.[73]

I observed several individuals with advanced emphysema that was initiated by exposure to chlorine gas in World War I.* In some, it was possible to pinpoint a specific area of the lungs, which showed a localized process suggestive of a primary corrosion of bronchial and pulmonary tissue at the site of impact. This so-called asthma does not yield to the treatment that usually benefits allergic asthma.

Of particular interest is the interaction of the chlorine gas with other agents. Although the health effects of chlorine and sulfur anhydride† resemble each other closely when they are administered separately to an experimental animal, in combination their effect is considerably less serious.[74] In other words, the two gases act to neutralize each other's effect.

On the other hand, when chlorine is combined with hydrochloric acid, a higher concentration is required for detection of the odor than for each gas individually.[74]

Among other halogen compounds, hydrogen fluoride and silicon tetrafluoride are strong respiratory irritants. Since they involve many other organs they are discussed in Chapter 10.

AMMONIA

Ammonia (NH_3) is a highly irritating gas with a strong pungent odor. It forms the intensely alkaline ammonium hydroxide when it comes in contact with the moisture of the throat and bronchi.

Occurrence

Naturally. Man has contributed relatively little ammonia to global air pollution.[75] Most of it is produced and released into the air by natural biologic processes. Atmos-

pheric concentrations in the temperate zones are about 6 μg/meter³ and about 140 μg/meter³ near the equator as contrasted with average urban concentrations of about 20 μg/meter³. On the other hand, close to factories much higher concentrations (about 7.2 mg/meter³) are being recorded. The green leaves of growing plants absorb considerable quantities of ammonia from the atmosphere and thus constitute a natural sink for ammonia.[76]

Industrial uses. Ammonia serves as raw material for the production of nitric acid fertilizers and for the synthesis of many organic compounds including drugs, explosives, plastics, and dyes. Approximately 85% of ammonia is applied by farmers to the soil as anhydrous ammonia fertilizer. As a refrigerant gas, it has constituted a hazard to drivers of ice-cream trucks. Combustion fuels, incineration of wastes, and the use of internal combustion engines are man-made sources of ammonia. Chemical plants, coke ovens, and refineries also release ammonia. Around stockyards and similar installations it is produced by disintegration of biologic material.

Health effects

Despite its widespread use, ammonia does not constitute a serious threat to human health as an airpollutant. Because of its high solubility it dissolves in the moisture of the upper air passages, allowing only a small percentage of the inhaled dose to reach the lungs. Ammonia is neutralized in the upper respiratory tract, which acts as a chemical buffer.[77] At concentrations of 280 to 490 mg/meter³ the gas produces slight irritation of the eyes and throat as well as a hoarse voice. Higher concentrations of 1700 to 4500 mg/meter³ are required to induce pulmonary edema.

When seven adult males were exposed experimentally[78] to ammonia gas, at a concentration of 350 mg/meter³ difficult breathing and nasal and throat irritation ensued. In other studies in humans, the

---

*Chlorine itself was used as a war gas only for a short time. It was replaced by phosgene and mustard gas or used in combination with them.
†Compounds from which the water molecule is abstracted.

urea and ammonia content of the blood increased following inhalation of 13 mg/meter^3.[79]

Hemeon[80] has suggested that in the 1948 Donora fog disaster, zinc ammonium sulfate aerosols played an important role as an irritant to the lungs. This possibility was further explored by Amdur and Corn[81] who produced severe pulmonary irritation in guinea pigs by exposing them to inhalation of zinc sulfate, ammonium sulfate, and zinc ammonium sulfate. The double salt was the most irritating. The smaller the particles, the greater was the irritation in the lungs. The presence of sulfur dioxide further potentiated the effect.

Additional damage in humans is suggested by other animal experimentation. For instance, Dalhamn[82] observed that concentrations of ammonia as low as 2 mg/meter^3 arrested temporarily the ciliary movements of the upper respiratory tract in rats. At this concentration, however, the condition was reversible.[83]

High concentrations, caused by accidental spillage, have caused damage to the cornea, throat, and bronchi. The moist surface of these organs absorbs the highly water-soluble ammonia gas and leads to permanent injury. In concentrations of 1700 to 4500 mg/meter^3, ammonia produces asphyxiation.[75]

Following derailment of a railroad tank car on February 18, 1969, a 22-year-old white woman was exposed to anhydrous ammonia fumes for a period of 30 to 90 minutes. She fainted, became unconscious, and, following admission to a Nebraska hospital, had general convulsions. She had chemical burns on the cornea of the eyes, palate, legs, arms, and abdomen. She experienced serious respiratory distress for the first 10 of the 27 days that she was hospitalized. During this time she contracted a pneumonialike process that subsequently turned into extensive bronchiectasis, a permanent condition.[84]

The occupational threshold limit for ammonia has been set at various levels. For the Navy, for instance, the permissable limit in a submarine during a 60-day dive is 18 mg/meter^3.[85] The basic standard for long-time exposure for healthy persons[86] for an 8-hour day and a 40-hour work week is 0.1 mg/meter^3 in Czechoslovakia and 0.2 mg/meter^3 in the U.S.S.R.

REFERENCES

1. Waldbott, G. L.: Smoker's respiratory syndrome: a clinical entity, J.A.M.A. **151**:1398-1400, 1953.
2. Gaffney, E. T.: Chlorine gas inhalation: a domestic possibility, Harper Hosp. Bull. **24**: 262-69, 1966.
3. Anderson, D. O.: The effects of air contamination on health, Part I, Canad. Med. Ass. J. **97**:528-536, 1972.
4. Amdur, M. O., and Underhill, D. W.: Response of guinea pigs to a combination of sulfur dioxide and open hearth dust, J.A.P.C.A. **20**:31-34, 1970.
5. Alaire, Y., Ulrich, C. E., Busey, W. M., and others: Long-term continuous exposures to sulfur dioxide in cynomolgus monkeys, Arch. Environ. Health **24**:115-127, 1972.
6. Alaire, Y., Ulrich, C. E., Busey, W. M., and others: Long-term continuous exposure of guinea pigs to sulfur dioxide, Arch. Environ. Health **21**:769-777, 1970.
7. Kellogg, W. W., Cadle, R. D., Allen, E. R., and others: The sulfur cycle, Science **175**: 587-596, 1972.
8. Air quality criteria for sulfur oxides, Washington, D. C., 1970, United States Department of Health, Education, and Welfare, Public Service Environmental Health Service, Publication Number AP-50.
9. Amdur, M. O.: Aerosols formed by oxidation of sulfur dioxide, Arch. Environ. Health **23**: 459-468, 1971.
10. Lawther, P. J.: Climate, air pollution and chronic bronchitis,, Proc. Roy. Soc. Med., **51**: 262-264, 1958.
11. Frank, N. R.: Studies on the effects of acute exposure to sulfur dioxide in human subjects, Proc. Roy. Soc. Med. **57** (Suppl):1029-1033, 1964.
12. Nadel, J. A.: Mechanisms of airway response to inhaled substances, Arch. Environ, Health **16**:170-174, 1968.
13. Pattle, R. E., and Collumbine, H.: Toxicity of some atmospheric pollutants, Brit. Med. J. **2**:913, 1956.

14. Corn, M., Kotsko, N., Stanton, D., and others: response of cats to inhaled mixtures of So$_2$ and SO$_4$-NaCl aerosol in air. New Orleans, October 5, 1970, Air Pollution Medical Research Conference.

15. Battigelli, M. C.: Facts and opinions on the role of sulfur dioxide in causing injury, Air quality monograph, Number 69-10, New York, February, 1969. American Petroleum Institute.

16. Carnow, P. W.: Relationship of So$_2$ levels to morbidity and morality in (high risk) populations, New Orleans, October 5, 1970. Air Pollution Medical Research Conference.

17. Amdur, M. O., and Underhill, D.: The effect of various aerosols on the response of guinea pigs to sulfur dioxide, Arch. Environ. Health 16:460-468, 1968.

18. Amdur, M. O.: Physiological response of guinea pigs to atmospheric pollutants, Int. J. Air Pollut. 1:170-183, 1959.

19. Toyama, T., and Nakamura, K.: Synergistic response of hydrogen dioxide, eye aerosols and sulfur dioxide to pulmonary airway resistance, Industr. Health 2:34-45, 1964.

20. Frank, N. R., Amdur, M. O., and Whittenberger, J. L.: A comparison of the acute effects of SO$_2$ administered alone or in combination with NaCl particles on the respiratory mechanisms of healthy adults, Air Water Pollut. 8:125-133, 1966.

21. Barach, A. L.: Treatment of sulfur dioxide poisoning, J.A.M.A. 215:485, 1971.

22. Altshuller, A. P.: Thermodynamic consideration in the interactions of nitrogen oxides and oxy-acids in the atmosphere, J. Air Pollut. Contr. Ass. 6:97-100, 1956.

23. Robinson, E., and Robbins, R. C.: Gaseous atmospheric pollutants from urban natural sources, J.A.P.C.A. 20:303-306, 1970.

24. Air quality criteria for nitrogen oxides, Environmental Protection Agency, Washington, D. C., 1971, Air Pollution Control Office Publication No. AP-84, Superintendent of Documents, U. S. Government Printing Office.

25. Nationwide inventory of air pollutant emissions, 1968, Raleigh, N. C., August 1970, National Air Pollution Control Administration, Publication No. AP-73, pp. 14-16.

26. Atmospheric emissions from nitric acid manufacturing, Chemist Association and U. S. Department of Health, Education and Welfare, Cincinnati, 1966, Public Health Service Publication No. 999-AP-27.

27. Flury, F., and Zernick, F.: Schaedliche Gase, Berlin, 1931, Springer.

28. Gray, E.: Oxides of nitrogen dioxide, their oc-

currence, toxicity, hazards, Arch. Ind. Health 19:479-586, 1959.

29. Freeman, G., Stephens, R. J., Crane, S. C., and others: Lesion of the lungs in rats continuously exposed to two parts per million of nitrogen dioxide, Arch. Environ. Health 17:181-192, 1968.

30. Stephens, R. J., Freeman, G., Crane, S. C., and others: Ultrastructural changes in the terminal bronchiole of the rat during continuous low level exposure to nitrogen dioxide, Exp. Molec. Path. 14:1-9, 1971.

31. Freeman, G., and Haydon, G. B.: Emphysema after low-level exposure to NO$_2$, Arch. Environ. Health 8:125-128, 1964.

32. Henry, M. C., Ehrlich, R., and Blair, W. H.: Effect of nitrogen dioxide on resistance of squirrel monkeys to *Klebsiella pneumoniae* infection, Arch. Environ. Health 18:580-587, 1969.

33. Henschler, D., Stier, A., Beck, H., and others: Olfactory threshold of some important irritant gases and manifestations in man by low concentrations, Arch. Geverbepath. Gerverbehyg. 17:547-570, 1960.

34. Lowry, T., and Schuman, L. M.: Silo-filler's disease: a syndrome caused by nitrogen dioxide, J.A.M.A. 162:153-160, 1956.

35. United States Chemical Warfare Service: Proceedings on a board appointed for the purpose of investigating conditions incident to the disaster at the Cleveland Hospital Clinic, Cleveland, Ohio, on May 15, 1929, Washington, D. C., 1929, U. S. Government Printing Office.

36. Tse, R. L., and Bockman, A. D.: Nitrogen dioxide toxicity: report of four cases in firemen, J.A.M.A. 212:1341, 1970.

37. Vigdorschik, N. A., Andreeva, E. C., Matussevitsch, I. Z., and others: The symptomatology of chronic poisoning with oxides of nitrogen, J. Industr. Hyg. Toxicol. 19:469-473, 1937.

38. Shy, C. M., Creason, J. P., Pearlman, M. E., and others: The Chattanooga school children study: effects of community exposure to nitrogen dioxide, Parts I and II, J.A.P.C.A. 20: 539-545, and 582-588, 1970.

39. Abe, M.: Effects of mixed NO$_2$-SO$_2$ gas on human pulmonary functions, Bull. Tokyo Med. Dent. Univ. 14:415-433, 1967.

40. Stokinger, H. E.: Effects of air pollution on animals. In Stern, A. C., editor: Air pollution, vol. 1, New York, 1962, Academic Press, Inc., p. 303.

41. Henry, M. C., and Aranyi, C.: Scanning electron microscopic observations of the effects of atmospheric pollutants, Arch. Environ. Health. (In Press.)

42. Hill, E. V.: Pure ozone effect in air conditioning, Intern. Engin. **82**:101, 1942.

43. Siedlecki, J. T.: Hazard of refrigerant gases to refrigerator service man, J.A.M.A. **213**: 1044, 1970.

44. Werthamer, S., Schwarz, L. H., Carr, J. J., and others: Ozone-induced pulmonary lesions, Arch. Environ. Health **20**:16-21, 1970.

45. Goldsmith, J. R., and Nadel, J. A.: Experimental exposures to human subjects to ozone, J. Air Pollut. Contr. Ass. **19**:329-330, 1969.

46. Nasr, A. N. M.: Biochemical aspects of ozone intoxication: a review, J. Occup. Med. **9**:589-597, 1967.

47. P'an, A. Y. S., Beland, J., and Zygmunt, J.: Ozone-induced arterial lesions, Arch. Environ. Health **24**:229-232, 1972.

48. Hathaway, J. A., and Terril, R. E.: Metabolic effects of chronic ozone exposure on rats, Amer. Industr. Hyg. Ass. J. **23**:392-395, 1962.

49. Stokinger, H. E., Wagner, W. D., and Dobrogorski, O. J.: Ozone toxicity studies: Part III, Chronic injury to lungs of animals, following low level, Arch. Industr. Health **16**:514, 1957.

50. Jaffe, L. S.: Photochemical air pollutants and their effects on men and animals, Arch. Environ. Health **16**:241-255, 1968.

51. Lagerwerff, J. M.: Prolonged ozone inhalation and its effects on visual parameters, Aerospace Med. **34**:479-486, 1963.

52. Griswold, S. S., Chambers, L. A., and Motley, H. L.: Report of a case of exposure at high ozone concentrations for 2 hours, Arch. Industr. Health **15**:108-118, 1957.

53. Wilska, S.: Ozone: its physiological effects and analytical determination in laboratory air, Acta Chem. Scand. **5**:1356-1358, 1951.

54. Young, W. A., Shaw, D. B., and Bates, D. V.: Effect of low concentrations of ozone on pulmonary function in man, J. Appl. Physiol. **19**:765-768, 1964.

55. Kleinfeld, M., and Giel, C. P.: Clinical manifestations of O_3 poisoning, Amer. J. Med. Sci. **231**:638, 1956.

56. Scheel, L. D., Dobrogorski, O. J., Mountain, J. T., and others: Physiologic, biochemical, immunologic and pathologic changes following ozone exposure, J. Appl. Physiol. **14**:67-80, 1959.

57. Stokinger, H. E.: Effects of air pollution on animals. In Stern, A. C., editor: Air pollution, vol. 1, New York, 1962, Academic Press, Inc., p. 298.

58. Brinkman, R., Lamberts, H. B., and Veninga, T. S.: Radiomimetic toxicity of ozonized air, Lancet, **1**:133-136, 1964.

59. Stokinger, H. E.: Ozone toxicology: a review of research and industrial experience, 1954-1964, Arch. Environ. Health **10**:719, 1965.

60. Roehm, J. N., Hadley, J. G., and Menzel, D. B.: The influence of vitamin E on the lung fatty acids of rats exposed to ozone, Arch. Environ. Health **24**:237-242, 1972.

61. Goldstein, B. D., Levine, M. R., Cuzzi-Spada, R., and others: p-aminobenzoic acid as a protective agent in ozone toxicity, Arch. Environ. Health **24**:243-247, 1972.

62. Stahl, Q. R.: Air pollution aspects of chlorine gas, Litton Systems Inc., Bethesda, Maryland, 1969, U. S. Department of Commerce, National Bureau of Standards, Publication 188 087.

63. Gerstle, R. W., and Devitt, T. W.: Chlorine and hydrogen chloride emissions and their control, Atlantic City, New Jersey, 1971, sixty-fourth Annual Meeting of the Air Pollution Control Association.

64. Heyroth, F. F.: Chlorine, Cl_2. In Patty, F. A., editor: Industrial hygiene and toxicology, vol. II, ed. 2, New York; 1963, Interscience.

65. Kramer, C. G.: Chlorine, J. Occup. Med. **9**:193, 1967.

66. Lillie, R. J.: Air pollutants affecting the performance of domestic animals: a literature review, 1970, Agriculture Handbook No. 380, U. S. Department of Agriculture, Washington, D. C., U. S. Government Printing Office.

67. Skljanskaja, R. M., and Rappoport, J. L.: Chronic chlorine poisoning of rabbits with small doses of chlorine and the development of the fetus in chlorine-poisoned rabbits, Arch. Exp. Path. Pharmacol. **117**:276, 1935.

68. Kowitz, T. A., Reba, R. C., Parker, R. T. and others: Effects of chlorine gas upon respiratory function, Arch. Environ. Health **14**:545, 1967.

69. Joyner, R. E., and Durel, E. G.: Accidental liquid spill in a rural community, J. Occup. Med. **4**:152, 1962.

70. Chasis, H., Zott, J. A., Bannon, J. H., and others: Chlorine accident in Brooklyn, Occup. Med. **4**:152-716, 1947.

71. Kaufman, J., and Burkons, D.: Clinical, roentgenologic and physiologic effects of acute chlorine exposure, Arch. Environ. Health **23**: 29-34, 1971.

72. Ronzani, E.: Über den Einfluss der Einatmungen von reizenden Gasen der Industrien auf die Schutzkrafte des Organismus gegenüber den infektiven Krankheiten, Arch. Hyg. **70**:217, 1909.

73. Hankin, J. L., and Klotz, W. C.: Permanent pulmonary effects of gas in warfare, Amer. Rev. Tuberc. **6**:571, 1922.

74. Stayzhkin, V. M.: Hygienic determination of limits of allowable concentrations of chlorine and hydrochloride gases simultaneously present in atmospheric air. Translated by Levine, B. S., U.S.S.R. Literature on Air Pollution and Related Occupational Diseases, 9:55, 1962.

75. Miner, S.: Air pollution aspects of ammonia, Litton System, Inc., Bethesda, Maryland, 1969, U. S. Department of Commerce, National Bureau of Standards, PB 188 082.

76. Hutchinson, G. L., Millington, R. J., and Peters, D. B.: Atmospheric ammonia: absorption by plant leaves, Science 175:771-2, 1972.

77. Jacobs, M. B.: Health aspects of air pollution from incinerators, New York, 1964, Proceedings of the 1964 National Incinerator Conference, American Society of Mechanical Engineers, Incinerator Committee.

78. Silverman, L., Whittenberger, J. L., and Muller, J.: Physiological response of man to ammonia in low concentration, J. Ind. Hyg. Toxicol. 31:74-78, 1949.

79. Kustou, U. U.: Means of measuring the maximum allowable concentrations of toxic products of natural human metabolism, Washington, D. C., 1967, NASA Technical Translation, National Aeronautics and Space Administration.

80. Hemeon, W. C. L.: The estimation of health hazards from air pollution, Arch. Ind. Health 11:307, 1955.

81. Amdur, M. O., and Corn, M.: The irritant potency of zinc ammonium sulfate of different particle sizes, Amer. Ind. Hyg. Ass. J. 24:326, 1963.

82. Dalhamn, T.: Mucous flow and ciliary activity in trachea of healthy rats and rats exposed to irritant gases, Acta. Physiol. Scand. 123 (Suppl.):36, 1956.

83. Friberg, L.: Studies on absorption of and reaction to inhaled particles, Stockholm, 1963, Institute of Hygiene, Karolinska Institute.

84. Kass, I., Zamel, N., Dobry, C. A., and others: bronchiectasis following ammonia burns of the respiratory tract: a review of two cases, Chest 62:282-285, 1972.

85. Webb, P.: Bioastronautics data book, Washington, D. C., 1964, National Aeronautics and Space Administration, Washington, D. C., U. S. Government Printing Office, Special Publication.

86. Stern, A. C.: Air Pollution, vol. III, New York, 1968, Academic Press, Inc.

8

FIBROSIS-PRODUCING AGENTS: silica, iron, cobalt, and barium

When a glass slide is covered with Vaseline and exposed at a windowsill for 24 hours, a multitude of particles of all sizes and shapes collects on it (Fig. 8-1). At a roadside an assortment of solid particles interspersed with material derived from animal and plant life predominates. Inside a city the slide shows an abundance of carbon particles that range in size from 5 to 500 μ. The disease in which the principal constituents of dust are involved is pneumoconiosis, a condition characterized by fibrosis (scarring of lung tissue).

Nearly all available data on the dust diseases pertain to occupational exposures such as mining and other dust-producing operations as noted in the following list.

Dust-producing occupations

1. Mining (gold, tin, copper, mica, graphite)
2. Quarrying (granite, sandstone, slate)
3. Dressing granite, stone masonry
4. Metal grinding
5. Sand blasting
6. Cork making
7. Manufacturing pottery and ceramics
8. Abrasive manufacturing
9. Enameling, sealing, and repairing metal tanks
10. Manufacturing rubber fillers

According to a recent survey[1] the "worst" conditions currently prevail in the quartz and the construction industries.

Knowledge of damage to populations and data on safe levels has been derived from extensive studies of pneumoconiosis as an occupational disease. As an environmental problem, the agents causing the disease warrant attention for the following reasons:

1. They constitute the principal portion of flydust emitted from factories and of dust stirred up by wind, automobiles, trains, and other vehicles from fields, roads, and highways.

2. They affect the biologic action of other atmospheric pollutants.

3. They are known to damage health of persons not involved in industrial activity. For instance, a high incidence of lower ventilatory function associated with wheezing, breathlessness, cough, and phlegm[2] was found in wives of coal workers residing near Pennsylvania and West Virginia mines.

SILICOSIS

Silicosis, the chief dust disease, was recognized by Hippocrates as early as 460 B.C.

Most of the so-called inert (or harmless) dusts, such as coal, titanium oxide, hematite, and kieselguhr, are eliminated from the respiratory tract through the ciliary escalator and to a lesser extent through the lymphoid system. They have no adverse effects on health. Others remain in the lungs.

"Black lungs" caused by coal particles are an inevitable accompaniment of urban life where people are exposed to coal dust all their life (Fig. 8-1, *A* and *B*).

The principal harmful particulate responsible for pulmonary fibrosis (scarring of lungs) is silicon dioxide, usually called silica. The scar-inducing action of such dusts as asbestos, mica, talc, and kaolin depends on the presence of silica. Other agents causing pneumoconiosis are carbon, iron oxide, cobalt, and barium.

Silica exists in many natural forms as, for instance, rock crystal (quartz), sandstone, quartzite, hipoli, tridynite, opal, flint, and diatomaceous earth (kieselguhr). The crystalline forms of silica include quartz, which crystallizes below 870° C.

Formerly silica was held responsible exclusively for all respiratory disease in coal miners. Anthracite, a hard mineral, slow-burning coal causes more pneumoconiosis than bituminous coal causes. However virtually silica-free coal dust can be responsible for coal miner's pneumoconiosis, which is now recognized as a clinically distinct disease.[3]

Inhalation of particles varying in size between 0.5 and 5.0 μ is most liable to cause the disease. Large dust particles are removed from the atmosphere because they settle promptly on the ground. Should they reach the upper air passages they would be eliminated by mucus and by ciliary action.

Mechanism

Considerable research has accumulated in an attempt to explain how dust can produce fibrosis of lungs. By culturing cells from the lungs and bronchi outside of the body and by the use of the electron microscope it has been established that mineral particles that have reached the alveoli are swallowed up by the macrophages (the scavenger cells) and are removed through the lymph channels (see Chapter 6). The death of the macrophages provides the toxic proteinlike lipid (fatty) material that is needed for the products of reticulin fibril (the material that produces scarring of tis-

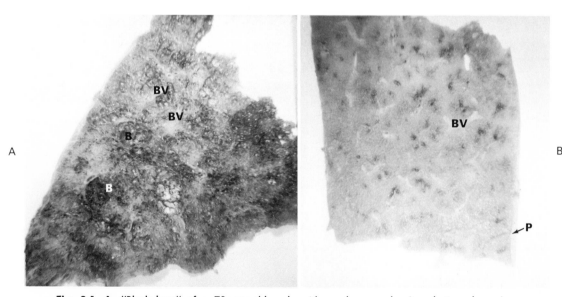

Fig. 8-1, A, "Black lung" of a 70-year-old male with emphysema showing destroyed emphysematous lung tissue (emphysematous blebs), *B,* blood vessels, *BV,* and cross section of bronchi. The dark areas contain carbon. **B,** Normal lung, natural size, of a 21-year-old male. Note uniform texture. The black spots represent carbon particles normally present. *P,* pleur, *BV,* blood vessels.

sues).[4] Even a small number of quartz particles will immobilize the macrophages and eventually tend to dissolve them.

However, certain aspects of the action of silica are not, as yet, fully understood. A sensitivity reaction has also been proposed because of formation of a silicoprotein antigen.[5]

According to Naeye and others[6] coal workers' pneumoconiosis comprises at least five distinct, but often related, disease processes:

1. The primary lesion in the lungs is the "coal dust macule," which consists of collections of coal particles surrounding the smallest ramifications of the bronchial tree and sometimes of the alveolar ducts.
2. After several years, a localized area of emphysema develops around the dust macule.
3. Crystals of silica collect within the macule, depending on the silica content of the dust, on the duration of the exposure, and, perhaps, upon other factors.
4. Eventually the macule is replaced by collagen, the material that creates scar formation.
5. Finally, general emphysema accompanied by chronic bronchitis develops. Interference with certain enzyme activities is believed to be the mediator of this process. In general, the smaller the size of dust particles the more rapid and extensive the scarring of lung tissue.

Clinical data

Clinically, pneumoconiosis can be recognized in its early stage by the roentgenographic appearance of the chest. However, a decline in pulmonary function usually precedes the development of changes visible on a roentgenogram.[7] Minute opacities are scattered throughout the lung fields. As the superimposed emphysema becomes more severe and the natural elasticity of the

lungs deteriorates, deficiency of oxygen in the alveolar air becomes more marked (Fig. 8-2). The patient cannot satisfy his demand for oxygen, especially on exertion. With increasing thinning and tearing of the alveolar walls, further loss of gas exchange between the alveoli and the blood takes place. Mucus in the bronchi becomes more abundant because of the catarrhal changes induced by the dust.

As the condition progresses further, secondary manifestations develop, which involve more widespread areas of the lungs, especially in their upper portions. In addition to the dust, such factors as infection and certain immunologic phenomena enter into the progression of the disease. Gradually the right side of the heart becomes

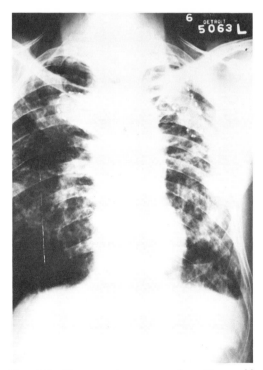

Fig. 8-2. Chest roentgenogram of a 60-year-old former coal miner with silicosis. Many small nodules throughout the lungs with two large shadows in the upper portion of each lung suggest tuberculosis. Silicosis occurs among nonmining residents near coal mines.

involved because of the heavy strain imposed upon it by the increased blood pressure in the pulmonary circulation. Silicosis predisposes the patient to tuberculosis as well as to other pulmonary infections.[8] A higher incidence of emphysema and heart disease has been observed in coal workers who smoke than in nonsmokers.[9] Lung cancer does not appear to constitute a complication of silicosis, although this question has not been resolved.[10]

In about one third of coal workers with pneumoconiosis, a more severe condition, progressive massive fibrosis, develops.[11] It is also encountered in other dust diseases such as hematite miner's lungs, kaolin pneumoconiosis, and graphite pneumoconiosis. In all of these conditions silica is present in the dusts. Because these diseases occur only after massive exposure to coal dust, those residing in the neighborhood of mines are not likely to be affected.

Another dust disease, acute silico proteinosis, which occurs in workers engaged in sand-blasting, has been identified with silica.[12] In this rapidly fatal condition a proteinlike substance fills up the alveolar spaces.

Among coal miners with rheumatoid arthritis, nodules measure 1 cm in diameter and larger. These nodules show microscopically concentric black and yellow rings that may disintegrate and turn into small cavities. This disease is called Caplan syndrome.[13] Whether or not it is of any environmental significance has not been explored.

IRON AND IRON COMPOUNDS

A comparatively harmless dust disease called siderosis occurs in mining comunities, where people are habitually exposed to inhalation of iron oxide; at autopsy the lungs show a brick red discoloration.

The health effect of airborne iron and its compounds is somewhat difficult to assess because iron oxide, the major atmospheric iron compound, rarely occurs by itself in the atmosphere. It is usually associated with other particulates, especially silicates. Damage to health, caused by persistent inhalation of iron oxide, is being attributed to its interaction with other agents rather than to the iron itself.

Sources

Iron is one of the most abundant elements in nature. The earth's crust has been calculated to contain 5.6% iron.[14] It is a constituent of water and, indeed, of all living organisms.

The major source of atmospheric contamination is the iron and steel industry. In Irontown, an Ohio steel center,[15] particulates, most of which were iron oxide, measured downwind from iron and steel plants, ranged between 190 and 212 μg/meter^3 during the interval between September 1965 and August 1967. During steel strikes, 44% to 170% fewer particulates were found in the air.[16]

Other processes emitting iron are electric arc furnaces, welding, incineration, and burning of fuel oil.[17] The National Air Sampling Network in 1964 showed an average concentration of 1.58 μg/meter^3 with a maximum of 22 μg/meter^3.[18]

Physiologic action

Iron is an essential element that is needed for formation of hemoglobin in transporting oxygen from the lungs to tissue cells. It also plays a role in the oxidation mechanism of body processes. A human adult absorbs less than 5 mg of iron per day.[19] Excess iron is stored in the liver and spleen as ferritin. Certain forms of anemia are caused by iron deficiency.

Iron as a respiratory pollutant

Besides benign siderosis, iron oxide can be responsible for sudden episodes of fever known as metal fever.[20] Furthermore, Kleinfeld and others[21] reported nodal x-ray densities in iron miners and sinterers, which were attributed largely to iron oxide, silicates, and free silica. The symptoms were cough and shortness of breath.

The role of iron oxide as a cancer-inciting agent has been well established.[10] It seems that iron oxide may by synergistic with silica in converting scarred lung tissue into a cancerous process.[22] Saffiotti and others[23] produced a variety of malignant tumors in the lungs of hamsters by using iron oxide as a carrier to transport absorbed benzo[a]pyrene, the noted cancer-producing hydrocarbon, deep into the lung. The fact that iron oxide penetrates the walls of bronchi and alveoli and enters into the lung tissue without damaging the ciliary and mucous barrier is held responsible for its ability to produce cancer.[24]

This synergistic action with other chemicals of the otherwise inert iron compounds is even more important in considering some of the irritant gases. According to Amdur and Underhill[24] iron oxide fumes produce no changes in the pulmonary flow resistance of guinea pigs. However, soluble iron compounds such as ferrous sulfate enhance the irritating effect of sulfur dioxide. The latter compound catalyzes the oxidation of sulfur dioxide to sulfur trioxide, which in turn forms the irritating sulfuric acid.

Therefore, iron, an essential nutrient can have serious damaging effects under certain conditions.

COBALT

Cobalt (Co) is another metal the inhalation of which causes changes in the lungs typical of pneumoconiosis. Among the Babylonians and Egyptians, cobalt salt, especially cobalt blue, has been employed as a constituent of pottery and glass since 1450 B.C. It accounts for their brilliant colors, which range from deep blue to green. Only during the twentieth century has cobalt been utilized in the metallurgical industry, particularly in jet engines, rocket nozzles, and gas turbines because of its high melting point and its great strength

and resistance to oxidation at elevated temperatures. Its superior magnetic properties make it desirable for high-fidelity loudspeakers. It is used in the manufacture of high-speed tools, paint, dryers, and pigments.[25] It tends to form a large number of chelates.[26] Cobalt also serves as a catalyst in many chemical processes including the synthesis of gasoline from coal. Thus, cobalt has recently become an important environmental pollutant.

In nature

Cobalt is present in soils at concentrations of 1 to 200 ppm depending on the composition of the underlying rocks.[27] In sea water its concentration is only 0.1 ppb; in fresh water it is more concentrated (0.9 ppb).[28] In ambient air the concentration of cobalt is 0.003 $\mu g/meter^3$.[29] The major source of atmospheric contamination by cobalt is burning of coal and oil.

Essentiality to life

Many species of bacteria, protozoa, fungi, and insects require cobalt to sustain life. It probably accounts for the bluegreen and red color of algae.[28] Cobalt deficiency in animals is characterized by poor growth, emaciation, and anemia,[30] a condition that can be promptly cured by administration of vitamin B_{12}. One microgram of this vitamin, the vital agent that prevents pernicious anemia, contains 0.0434 μg of cobalt.

Body burden in humans

The daily dietary intake of cobalt is approximately 300 μg,[25] about 70% to 80% of which is eliminated through the urine. Fish, cocoa beans, and molasses are among the foods containing more than 1 $\mu g/gm$ (1 ppm) of cobalt. In general, green leafy vegetables are richest in cobalt; cereals, especially refined cereals, contain the least amount.

In the blood, cobalt is carried largely by the red cells in concentrations of 0.07 to 0.36 μg in one liter of blood.[31] Normal

Table 8-1. Normal cobalt levels in human biologic material (one subject)*

	μG OF COBALT AVERAGE VALUE
Blood	0.0 per 100 gm
Urine	3.6 per liter
Feces	12.8 per 24 hour
Food	15.2 per 24 hour

*Adapted from Hubbard, D. M., Creech, F. M., and Cholak, J.: Determination of cobalt in air and biological material, Arch. Environ. Health 13:190-194, 1966.

levels of cobalt in human biologic material are presented in Table 8-1.[32]

Yamagata and others[33] estimated the whole body burden of cobalt to be 1.1 mg, about 43% of which is found in muscle, 14% in bone, and the rest in soft tissue. With increasing age cobalt is no longer stored in the system.

Cobalt intoxication

In humans, the level of cobalt toxicity is low, about equivalent to a daily dietary intake of 150 ppm. Cobalt has been administered in the treatment of nephritis, in infections, and in anemias during pregnancy.[30] However, its use has led to serious toxic manifestations, including thyroid enlargement, myxedema (a disease caused by thyroid deficiency), and congestive heart failure in infants.[34] Excessive doses have caused polycythemia (excess formation of red blood cells) in mice, rabbits, and domestic animals, which overtaxes the heart and is associated with high blood pressure.[30]

Little is known about the effect of cobalt as a constituent of ambient air. In certain industries, particularly in hard metal manufacturing, it has been a source of pulmonary fibrosis. Powdered cobalt is used as a bonding material in the manufacture of cutting tools that contain tungsten and tungsten carbide.[35] In such factories fine particulate cobalt dust measuring less than 2.0 μ in diameter is generated[36] and spreads into areas where it is not in use.[37] Whereas powdered tungsten carbide has little or no irritant effect on the lungs, powdered cobalt produces chronic lung changes leading to pulmonary fibrosis, with chronic cough and shortness of breath. This disease is usually fatal if not diagnosed early.[37]

One of my patients, Mr. J. W., age 56, had severe asthmatic attacks during the hours he was working in a hard metal factory, although he was at no time in direct contact with the metal. The attacks did not occur outside the factory. His pulmonary function was considerably impaired in the evenings compared with the values obtained when he started his work in the morning. His vital capacity was 52% of the predicted normal. Forced expiratory volume in one second was 84%. According to the factory's physician, air quality data in the plant indicated that cobalt was responsible for the asthmatic attacks and J. W.'s "asthma" cleared at first when he was transferred into an area of the plant far distant from his former location where no cobalt dust was found.

Epidemics of cobalt intoxication

When ingested with food, cobalt affects the heart and the thyroid gland. In 1965 and 1966 an epidemic of a serious heart disease occurred in Quebec, Canada. The rapidly fatal course of this disease distinguished it from other heart ailments. Of 48 persons so afflicted, 20 died in shock.[38] The essential symptoms were shortness of breath, pain in the heart and stomach area, cough, swelling of ankles, and general weakness. After numerous agents had been ruled out as the possible cause, it became apparent that the only individuals who had contracted the disease were those who had imbibed large amounts of beer. Changes in the thyroid gland of one of the diseased persons showed features characteristic of cobalt intoxication. The disease was promptly eliminated upon discontinuance of the use of cobalt in processing beer. Its use had just been introduced in the brewing industry from Denmark to stabilize foam in beer.

Subsequently, similar epidemics of primary heart disease among alcoholics were discovered in Omaha, Nebraska[39] and in Lowen, Belgium.[40] Eleven of 28 patients died in Omaha, 17 in Belgium. In a few individuals, the disease lingered for several years. In the Belgian group pericardial effusions (fluid surrounding the heart) were noted. Ulcerations in the lining of the stomach and in the thyroid tissue showed certain changes by which it was established that this disease was not the effect of alcoholism. A protein deficiency seemed to have contributed to its development.

Although the doses of ingested cobalt compounds in these cases were much greater than those of atmospheric contamination, these findings are of interest in view of the lack of data concerned with long-term cobalt ingestion and inhalation in minute concentrations in which they occur in the air.

BARIUM

Although barium (Ba) salts can affect various organs in the system, especially when taken up in large doses,[41] barium is classified here as a pneumoconiosis-producing agent: as an air pollutant, it involves primarily the respiratory tract where it leads to what is termed "baritosis" a relatively harmless "dust" disease. Considerable information exists on the toxicity of barium sulfate, the opaque agent that is administered orally in conjunction with x-ray examinations of the gastrointestinal tract, but the medical literature on the health effects of other barium compounds and on barium itself is sparse.

Occurrence

Barium is a soft silvery metallic element that occurs in nature in lead and zinc ore deposits mainly as barite, or barium sulfate ($BaSO_4$), and as witherite, or barium carbonate ($BaCO_3$). In the United States it is mined in Missouri, Arkansas, Georgia, and Nevada.[41] Trace quantities of barium are also found in coal. In the atmosphere, barium metal is highly reactive and combines rapidly with other elements, forming barium salts.

Barium is present in most soils in amounts varying from a few thousandths of a percent to 1%. In the vicinity of barite mines, soil contains as much as 3.68% barium.[42] It is poisonous to most plants in the minute quantities in which it occurs. Brazil nuts, which contain several thousand ppm, constitute an exception.[42]

In industry, metallic barium is used to remove residual gases in radio tubes, as an alloy with lead and calcium, and in the production of barium-nickel alloys. Certain fluxes used in the refining of magnesium contain from 2% to 10% barium chloride.[43] A ground baride is extensively employed in oil drilling, as a filler in paper, rubber, cloth, linoleum[44] and as a white pigment in paint. Barium is also employed in the manufacturing of glass and of ceramic enamels. In recent years, barium has been added to diesel fuels to suppress black smoke emissions.

Health effects

Metabolism. After barium has entered the digestive system, it is rapidly transmitted to and from the bloodstream, since the mucous lining of the bowels is extremely permeable to the metal. During the first 30 hours after absorption barium is retained, especially by the muscles, after which about 20% is eliminated by the bowels, only about 7% through the urine. Barium also accumulates in bones and lungs. On the other hand, liver, kidneys, brain, heart, and hair do not retain barium.

Acute barium intoxication. Poisoning was encountered frequently during the early years of gastrointestinal x-ray technique when soluble barium salts were employed as a contrast medium rather than the non-poisonous and insoluble barium sulfate. Acute poisoning occurs when either of the two barium salts, barium chloride ($BaCl_2$) or barium carbonate ($BaCO_3$), is mistaken for some other nonpoisonous powder or when taken deliberately for suicidal purposes. A strong stimulating effect on all muscles of the body, including the heart muscle, is an outstanding feature of acute barium poisoning. This effect on muscles is accompanied by pains and spasms of arms and legs, pain in the pharynx and in the stomach. A marked reduction of potassium in the bloodstream can be used as a diagnostic test. Roza and Berman[45] showed that the potassium loss is not caused by excess potassium excretion through the bowels or through the urine but that potassium enters the inner compartments of the cells from the surrounding (extracellular) fluid.[45] The low potassium level in blood is closely related to irregularities of the heart action and to paralysis of musculature.[46] Excess excretion of saliva, diarrhea, and high blood pressure are other symptoms of acute poisoning. Although the barium metal itself can be tolerated in large doses, the toxic dose of barium chloride ranges between 0.2 to 0.5 gm and the lethal dose up to 2.4 gm.[47]

Chronic intoxication. Little information is available concerning the effects of ambient air pollution by barium. The chronic phase of poisoning is an occupational disease that occurs following prolonged inhalation of barium dust.

The benign dust disease "baritosis" has been encountered in barite miners in the United States, Germany, and Czechoslovakia.[48] In a French barium smelter, Drif and others[49] observed this disease in 51 workers who experienced considerable shortness of breath and cough with expectoration of bloody sputum. In the younger individuals, who had been employed for only a short time, the lungs were studded with multiple nodes; whereas in older workers of long-standing employment the lesions were more pronounced. They resembled snow-flakes in the x-ray films. When exposure to barium ceased, the lesions cleared up, but, occasionally, chronic cough and expectoration of mucus persisted.

In addition to iron, carbon, silica, cobalt, and barium other agents contained in dust can cause scarring of lung tissue. Under certain conditions their dominant effect on the lungs is an acute fever-producing inflammatory process or in some instances so-called granuloma of lungs, which are discussed in the following chapters.

REFERENCES

1. Ahlmark, A.: Silicosis dust conditions and dust control in Sweden, Staub **29**:1-5, 1969.
2. Lanehart, W. S., Boyle, H. M., Enterline, P. E., and others: Pneumoconiosis in Appalachian bituminous coal workers, Cincinnati, 1968, Public Health Service, Bureau of Occupational Safety and Health.
3. Boren, H. G.: Pulmonary response to inhaled carbon: a model of lung injury, Yale J. Biol. Med. **40**:364-388, 1968.
4. Allison, A. C., Harington, J. S., Bierbeck, M., and others: Observation on the cytotoxic action of silica on macrophages, inhaled particles and vapors. In Davies, C. N., editor: Inhaled particles and vapours, Oxford, 1967, Pergamon Press, Ltd., pp. 121-131.
5. Crofton, J., and Douglas, A.: Respiratory diseases, Oxford, 1969, Blackwell Scientific Publications, p. 480.
6. Naeye, R. L., and Dellinger, W. S.: Lung disease in Appalachian soft coal miners, Amer. J. Pathol. **58**:557-564, 1970.
7. Hyatt, R. E., Kistin, A. D., and Mahan, T. K.: Respiratory disease in southern West Virginia coal miners, Amer. Rev. Resp. Dis. **89**:389-401, 1964.
8. Schepers, G. W. H.: Silicosis and tuberculosis, Industr. Med. Surg. **33**:381, 1964.
9. Naeye, R. L., Mahon, J. K., and Dellinger, W. S.: Effects of smoking on lung structure of Appalachian coal miners, Arch. Environ. Health **22**:190-193, 1971.
10. Spencer, H.: Pathology of the lung, Oxford, 1968, Pergamon Press, Ltd.
11. Report by committee on diagnostic criteria and disability assessment for pneumoconiosis, American Conference of Governmental Indus-

trial Hygienists, Arch. Environ. Health **21:** 221-223, 1970.

12. Buechner, H. A., and Ansari, A.: Acute silico-proteinosis disease, Chest **55:**274-284, 1969.

13. Caplan, A.: Rheumatoid pneumoconiosis syndrome, Med. Lavoro **56:**494-499, 1965.

14. Mineral facts and problems, Bureau of Mines, Bulletin 630, Washington, D. C., 1965, U. S. Government Printing Office.

15. Ironton, Ohio; Ashland, Kentucky; Huntington, West Virginia; Air pollution abatement activity, Preconference Investigations, Cincinnati, 1968, U. S. Department of Health, Education, and Welfare National Center for Air Pollution Control, Cincinnati, Ohio, Publication APTD-68-2.

16. Schueneman, J. J., High, M. D., and Bye, W. E.: Air pollution aspects of the iron and steel industry, U. S. Department of Health, Education, and Welfare, Public Health Service, Cincinnati, 1963, Division of Air Pollution, Publication No. 999-Ap-1.

17. Sullivan, R. J.: Air pollution aspects of iron and its compounds, Litton Industries, Inc., Bethesda, Maryland, 1969, U. S. Department of Commerce, National Bureau of Standards, PB 188 088.

18. Air quality data from the National Air Sampling Networks and contributing state and local networks, 1964-65, Cincinnati, 1966, U. S. Department of Health, Education, and Welfare, Public Health Service.

19. Hampel, C. A.: Iron: the encyclopedia of the chemical elements, New York, 1968, Van Nostrand Reinhold Co.

20. Akashi, S.: The mechanism producing metal fever in the process of welding with low hydrogen-type electrodes, Japan J. Industr. Health **3:**237, 1967.

21. Kleinfeld, M., Messite, J., Shapiro, J., and others: A clinical roentgenological and physiological study of magnetite workers, Arch. Environ. Health **16:**392, 1968.

22. Bonser, G. M., Faulds, J. S., and Stewart, M. J.: Occupational cancer of the urinary bladder in dyestuffs operative and of the lung in asbestos textile workers and iron-ore miners, Amer. J. Clin. Pathol. **25:**126, 1955.

23. Saffiotti, U., Cefis, F., and Kolb, L. H.: A method for the experimental induction of bronchogenic carcinoma, Cancer Res. **28:** 104, 1968.

24. Amdur, M. O., and Underhill, D.: The effect of various aerosols on the response of guinea pigs to sulfur dioxide, Arch. Environ. Health, **16:**461, 1968.

25. Schroeder, H. A., Nason, A. P., and Tipton, I. H.: Essential trace metals in man: cobalt, J. Chronic Dis. **20:**369-890, 1967.

26. Stability constants of metal-ion complexes, The Chemical Society, London, 1964, Burlington House.

27. Vinogradov, A. P.: The geochemistry of rare and dispersed chemical elements in soils, ed. 2, (Translated from Russian) New York, 1959, Consultant's Bureau.

28. Bowen, H. J. M.: Trace elements in biochemistry, New York, 1966, Academic Press, Inc.

29. Tabor, E. C., and Warren, W. V.: Distribution of certain metals in the atmosphere of some American cities, Arch. Industr. Health **17:**145, 1958.

30. Underwood, E. J.: Trace elements in human and animal nutrition, ed. 2, New York, 1962, Academic Press, Inc.

31. Aston, B. C.: The bush sickness investigation, laboratory work and results, New Zeal. J. Agric. **28:**301; **29:**14; **29:**84, 1924.

32. Hubbard, D. M., Creech, F. M., and Cholak, J.: Determination of cobalt in air and biological material, Arch. Environ. Health **13:**190-194, 1966.

33. Yamagata, N., Murata, S., and Torri, T.: The cobalt content of the human body, J. Radiat. Res. **3:**4, 1962.

34. Kriss, J. P., Carnes, W. H., and Gross, R. T.: Hypothyroidism and thyroid hyperplasia in patients treated with cobalt, J.A.M.A. **157:** 117-121, 1955.

35. Shepers, G. W. H.: The biological action of tungsten carbide and cobalt, Arch. Industr. Health **12:**140-146, 1955.

36. McDermott, F. T.: Dust in the cemented carbide industry, J. Amer. Industr. Hyg. Ass. **32:**188-193, 1971.

37. Coates, E. O., Jr., and Watson, J. H. L.: Diffuse interstitial lung disease in tungsten carbide workers, Ann. Intern. Med. **75:**709-716, 1971.

38. Morin, Y.: Quebec's medical mystery, J.A.M.A. **197:**592, 1966.

39. McDermott, P. H., Delanoy, R. L., Egon, J. D., and others: Myocardiosis and cardiac failure in men, J.A.M.A. **198:**253-256, 1966.

40. Kestelloot, H. R., Terryn, R., Bosmans, P., and others: Alcoholic perimyocardiopathy, Acta Cardiol. (Brux) **21:**341, 1966.

41. Miner, S.: Air pollution aspects of barium and its compounds. Litton Systems, Inc., Bethesda, Maryland, 1969, U. S. Department of Commerce, National Bureau of Standards, PB 188 083.

42. Browning, E.: Toxicity of industrial metals, London, 1969, Butterworth and Co., Ltd.

43. Iverson, R. E.: Environmental protection agency, Personal communication, April, 1972.
44. Ladoo, R. B., and Meyers, W. M.: Non-metallic minerals, New York, 1951, McGraw-Hill Book Co.
45. Roza, O., and Berman, L. B.: The pathophysiology of barium: hypokalemic and cardiovascular effects, J. Pharmacol. Exp. Ther. 177:433-439, 1971.
46. Habicht, W. V., Smekal, P., and Etzrodt, H.: Course and treatment of barium poisoning, Med. Welt, 28:1292-1295, 1970.
47. Lydtin, H., Kusus, T., Dietze, G., and others: Effect of an adrenergic beta-receptor blocking agent on the cardiac rhythm through experimental barium poisoning, Arzneimittelforschung 17:1456-1459, 1967.
48. Sax, N. I.: Dangerous properties of industrial materials, New York, 1968, Van Nostrand Reinhold Co.
49. Drif, M., Chaulet, P., Larbaoui, D., and others: Baritosis, initial results of a survey in two Algerian factories, Ann. Radiol. 2:67-74, 1968.

9

GRANULOMA-PRODUCING AGENTS

Sarcoidosis is a disease of the lungs that has baffled the medical profession since the turn of the century. It is a so-called granulomatous disease characterized by multiple accumulations of cells that are distributed in nodules throughout the lungs (Fig. 9-1). These lesions are often associated with raised, dusky-red patches on the skin, which do not become inflamed or form ulcers. Enlargement of lymph glands

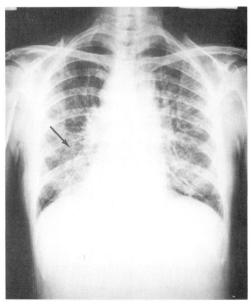

Fig. 9-1. Roentgenogram of a 36-year-old woman with sarcoidosis. Note multiple nodules (arrow) in both lungs.

is another feature of sarcoidosis. The biopsy of a lymph gland taken from an area above a clavicle (collarbone) may serve to confirm the diagnosis in a suspected case. In addition other organs, especially the liver and spleen, may be involved. A skin test, called Kveim test (consisting of an injection of spleen extract from a person with sarcoidosis), if positive, and a high calcium level of the blood are important diagnostic criteria of the disease.

Tuberculosis, fungous diseases, leprosy, syphilis, and parasitic infections of the lungs, berylliosis (a condition caused by inhalation of beryllium), and chronic zirconium poisoning are among the many diseases that simulate sarcoidosis because they exhibit granulomatous lesions in the lungs.

Numerous theories have been advanced concerning the cause of sarcoidosis. Inhalation of pine pollen has been suspected, but the weight of recent opinion points to other air contaminants as a cause. The nodules encountered in the lungs in chronic beryllium poisoning are similar to those of sarcoidosis, a fact that further points to an environmental cause or causes in sarcoidosis.

BERYLLIUM

Characteristic granulomatous changes of the lungs are brought about by long-term exposure to beryllium (Be).

Properties and uses of beryllium

Its unique combination of resistance to heat and stress, its lightness and hardness make beryllium almost indispensable for a wide range of industrial processes. Its low atomic weight and its transparency to x-ray films renders it the most suitable of all metals as a shield for roentgen rays in roentgen tubes. Since it is nonmagnetic, has a high electric conductivity, and is not liable to spark, it is used in aircraft engines and electrical devices, especially electric heaters. In the nuclear energy field it is a source of neutrons, which it emits when bombarded by alpha rays. Small amounts of beryllium are added to copper, aluminum, nickel, cobalt, and steel in order to increase their hardness and resistance to corrosion and high temperatures. Finely powdered pure beryllium is used as an additive to solid fuels for missiles. Among the many beryllium compounds, beryl ore, a beryllium aluminum silicate, is the only innocuous substance. Burning coal that contains from 1.5 to 2.5 ppm beryllium may be a significant contributor to air pollution[1] in view of the quantity of coal consumed.

Health effects

Neighborhood berylliosis. Beryllium has received much attention as an industrial pollutant, mainly because of its extreme toxicity: it also gives rise to symptoms, in individuals not exposed directly through their occupation. Cases of chronic beryllium poisoning were reported in 1946 by Hardy and Tabershaw[2] and in 1949 Eisenbud and others[3] described so-called neighborhood berylliosis in the United States. Eleven persons, residing within ¼ to 2 miles of a beryllium-producing plant, developed typical chronic pulmonary granulomatosis and other evidence of beryllium poisoning. Beryllium was found in the clothes of the husband of one of the patients. Because he worked in a beryllium plant coveralls worn for one day by 100 employees at the plant

were shaken out. The dust, analyzed for beryllium, yielded an average of 500 μg/meter[3]. It was estimated that an individual in contact with the clothes inhaled 17 μg daily.

Another instance of neighborhood poisoning involving 26 persons occurred in the vicinity of a Pennsylvania refinery and alloy fabricating plant. Most of the patients resided within 0.7 to 6 miles in the downwind sectors from the plant. Sampling of the air revealed a mean concentration of 0.015 μg/meter[3]. Beryllium levels in other parts of the state averaged 0.0002 μg/meter[3].[4]

Acute poisoning. In acute poisoning, beryllium gives rise to a chemical inflammation of the lung tissue. When exposed to concentrations of beryllium of 20 to 60 μg for about 50 days,[5] workers in beryllium-producing plants develop transient inflammation of the upper air passages, nose, pharynx, trachea, and upper bronchi, which is followed by a pneumonialike process with fever, chills, cough, sputum, and shortness of breath.[5] If not fatal, the disease can last up to 3 months. Even without further exposure,[6] in about 6.3% of the cases it is followed by the chronic form of the disease.

Chronic berylliosis. After World War II, an explosive increase of chronic berylliosis in the United States occurred in persons employed in the manufacture of fluorescent lamps.[7] The metal was used along with zinc, magnesium, and manganese silicates to coat the inside of fluorescent light tubes.

A group of researchers who examined routine chest films 20 to 25 years after workers had first been exposed to beryllium noted the granulomatous lesions in the lungs indicative of the disease.[2]

The roentgenograms of persons suspected of having berylliosis show an enlargement of lymph glands in conjunction with the typical lesions: first to appear are diffuse, finely granulated lesions that are distributed throughout the lungs. Later, when the nodules have grown to between 0.5 to 1 cm in diameter, the shadows at the roots of the lungs become enlarged.

The disease starts insidiously with progressive shortness of breath, weight loss, cough, and slight production of phlegm. Occasionally, the patients have a low-grade fever and nausea.

If much time elapses between exposure and the development of the disease[8] progressive shortness of breath is practically the sole symptom. However, if the interval between exposure and the disease is short or nonexistent, patients often develop a profound progressive emaciation. They may die within a few months.

As the disease develops, granulomatous inflammation, the typical feature of beryllium poisoning, is often followed by fibrosis (scarring) of lung tissue and by damage to the heart.

In some workers, who had been subjected to massive prolonged exposure, no clinical or roentgenographic evidence of the disease was found. Other individuals had contracted it merely by residing in the neighborhood of a beryllium factory or extraction plant.

Beryllium is believed to interfere with the passage of oxygen from the alveoli to the arterial blood, a condition called "alveolar capillary block."

An immune mechanism is indicated by the fact that beryllium ions have been found attached to protein molecules.[5] Patch tests, which consist of applying a minute amount of 1% Na_2BeF_4 to the skin by means of adhesive tape, are usually positive when the disease is present. Another valuable test for the diagnosis of the disease is a biopsy of lungs, lymph glands, or skin lesions to determine whether or not typical granulomas are present. In the granulomatous tissue, shell-like, concentrically laminated inclusions, called Schaumann's bodies, are found.

Although the pulmonary effects dominate the clinical picture of berylliosis, other organs are also involved, such as the liver, spleen, kidneys, and lymph glands. The skin, especially, is subject to eruptions, ulcers, and granulomas.[9] Serum proteins, calcium, and uric acid metabolism are frequently abnormal. About 40% of patients with chronic beryllium poisoning show a high uric acid level in the blood.[10]

Beryllium compounds have the capacity to cause malignant tumors in laboratory animals, namely osteosarcoma in rabbits and carcinoma of the lungs in rats and monkeys.[11] Whether or not patients with berylliosis are prone to the development of lung cancer has not been determined.

Large doses of adrenal steroids (cortisone preparations) constitute a useful treatment for the disease.

THESAUROSIS

In 1958 Bergman and associates[12] described a granulomatous lung disease called pulmonary thesaurosis, which they presumed was caused by exposure to hair spray. The main disability of the afflicted persons was shortness of breath on exertion and cough productive of a thin, white sputum. In 1962 they added twelve more cases to their series, including three autopsies.[13] They concluded that a chemical called polyvinylpyrrolidone (PVP), a major constituent of hair sprays, was the toxic material. However there is considerable disagreement on this question. Schepers could not reproduce the disease in animal experiments[14]; some spray deodorants and hair sprays that produced the disease did not contain PVP.[15] Other constituents of the sprays are now implicated, particularly zinc compounds, hexachlorophene, and dichlorodifluoromethane (Freon), a gas widely used as a refrigerant and spray propellant. This propellant has been considered nontoxic, but recent evidence indicates that it might be a cause of the lesion.

Gowdy and Wagstaff described the case of an 18-year-old girl with fever up to 104° F (40° C) but with a normal white blood count.* A granulomatous area in the right lung was found. Results of a tuberculin test and tests for histoplasmosis (a fungus disease) were negative. For approximately 1 month prior to the acute illness, the child had had cough and general malaise. She had been using a hairspray several times daily. When this practice was stopped, her temperature returned to normal and the condition cleared up.

Ward[16] observed granulomatous lesions simulating sarcoidosis in two women and ten young men who had been using underarm deodorants habitually for periods of approximately 2 years. These patients were essentially symptom-free but showed an impaired pulmonary function. Some experienced shortness of breath temporarily and a slight cough at the time of the use of the deodorant.

Other agents occasionally responsible for granulomas in the lungs are tungsten carbide, zinc, and manganese.

A somewhat different kind of granulomatosis was related to the use of a tooth powder as reported by Reiman and associates.[17]

In a 48-year-old housewife who died of lung cancer, granulomatous areas in the lungs and in the abdomen were studded with tricalcium phosphate crystals of less than 5 μ in size. These lesions were distributed throughout the lymph nodes, particularly in the abdomen. The patient had used a popular denture cleanser as an abrasive for more than 3 years. The powder, which contained tricalcium phosphate, was sprinkled generously into a glass of water and, occasionally, directly on the dentures. They were then immersed into the suspension, rinsed, and inserted into the mouth 8 or 10 times a day. During insertion the patient habitually inhaled deeply to avoid the gag reflex.

Reiman and associates proposed the the-

ory that the crystals had been entrapped in the mucus of the upper air passages, ejected from the lungs, and were swallowed. They had penetrated the lining of the bowels and thus entered the lymph glands of the abdomen. The patient's smoking habit was believed to be a contributing factor in the production of cancer.

Nam and Gracey[18] reported the death of a 39-year-old male newspaper truck driver who had used talcum powder liberally for 20 years at least twice daily. For 4 years prior to his death he dusted himself at least 3 times a day following frequent baths. He also dusted his bed sheets with talcum powder. At autopsy the lungs showed small firm yellowish nodules distributed around the terminal bronchioles; the alveolar spaces in the periphery of the lungs were overexpanded. They contained numerous needle-shaped particles that were identified as talc, a finely powdered hydrous magnesium silicate [$3 \text{ MgO} \cdot 4 \text{ SiO}_2 \cdot \text{H}_2\text{O}$].[18]

Another group of diseases characterized by granulomatous lesions, fibrosis, and functional impairment of the lungs is farmer's lungs, bagassosis, and byssinosis. Although they are described as occupational diseases, minor degrees of nonoccupational exposure may conceivably contribute to, or even give rise to, this type of respiratory illness.

1. *Farmer's lungs.* So-called farmer's lungs is encountered among agricultural workers 6 to 9 hours after exposure to moldy hay. They develop shortness of breath, fever, and cough and occasionally expectorate blood.[19,20] Impaired diffusion of gas, decreased compliance of the lungs, and minimal ventilatory disturbances occur.[21] This condition constitutes an allergic type of reaction and has been reproduced in animals that were previously sensitized to the hay. A fungus called *thermopolyspora* has been identified with the disease.[21]

2. *Bagassosis.* A similar disease localized mostly in the upper lobes of the lungs is

---

*A normal or low white blood count associated with fever is often indicative of a chemical inflammation.

bagassosis (sugar cane lung[22]) caused by inhalation of moldy dust of the bagasse fiber, the cane residue after removal of sugar. This fiber contains 1% protein, 1% to 2% silica, and 0.1% to 0.2% quartz. It is used in the manufacture of insulating board, paper, explosives, and poultry feed. When the material is exposed to rain during storage, a variety of fungus spores develop, estimated to be of a magnitude of 240 million/gm.[23] The disease, characterized by asthmatic wheezing and emphysema, is considered to be caused by hypersensitivity and is mediated by certain antibodies.

3. *Byssinosis.* Byssinosis occurs in those who work with cotton, hemp, and flax, both during harvesting and manufacturing of these products. Specific rounded dust bodies up to 10 μ in diameter, consisting of a center core of black dust surrounded by yellowish material, are found in the lungs.

REFERENCES

1. Abernethy, R. F., and Gibson, F. H.: Rare elements in coal, Pittsburgh Coal Research Center, Pittsburgh, 1963, U. S. Bureau of Mines Information Circular 1c 8163.
2. Hardy, H. L., and Tabershaw, I. R.: Delayed chemical pneumonitis occurring in workers exposed to beryllium compounds, J. Industr. Hyg. Toxicol. **28**:197-211, 1946.
3. Eisenbud, M., Wanta, B. S., Duston, C., and others: Nonoccupational berylliosis, J. Industr. Hyg. Toxicol. **31**:282, 1949.
4. Sussman, V. H., Lieben, J., and Cleland, J. G.: An air pollution study of a community surrounding a beryllium plant, Amer. Industr. Hyg. Ass. J. **20**:504, 1959.
5. Nishimura, M.: Clinical and experimental studies on acute beryllium disease, Nagoya J. Med. Sci. **28**:17-44, 1966.
6. Hardy, H. L.: Beryllium poisoning: lessons in control of man-made disease, New Eng. J. Med. **273**:1188, 1965.
7. Durocher, N. L.: Air pollution aspects of beryllium and its compounds, Litton System, Inc., Bethesda, Maryland, 1969, U. S. Department of Commerce, National Bureau of Standards, PB 188 078, p. 38.
8. Hardy, H. L., Rabe, E. W., and Lorch, S.: United States beryllium registry (1952-1966):

review of its methods and utility, J. Occup. Med. **9**:271-276, 1967.
9. Jones-Williams, W., and Lawrie, J. H.: Skin granulomata from beryllium oxide, Brit. J. Surg. **54**:292, 1967.
10. Kelley, W. N., Goldfinger, S. E., and Hardy, H. L.: Hyperuricemia in chronic beryllium disease, Ann. Intern. Med. **70**:977-983, 1969.
11. Vorwald, A. J., Reeves, A. L., and Urban, E. C.: Experimental beryllium toxicology. In Stokinger, H. E., editor: Beryllium: its industrial hygiene aspects, New York, 1966, Academic Press, Inc.
12. Bergmann, M., Flance, I. J., and Blumenthal, H. T.: Thesaurosis following inhalation of hair spray, New Eng. J. Med. **258**:471-476, 1958.
13. Bergmann, M., Flance, I. J., Cruz, P. T., and others: Thesaurosis due to inhalation of hair spray: report of twelve new cases, including three autopsies, New Eng. J. Med. **266**:750-755, 1962.
14. Schepers, G. W. H.: Thesaurosis versus sarcoidosis, J.A.M.A. **184**:851-857, 1963.
15. Nevins, M. A., Stechel, G. H., Fishman, I., and others: Pulmonary granulomatosis: two cases associated with inhalation of cosmetic aerosols, J.A.M.A. **193**:266-271, 1965.
16. Ward, G. W., Jr.: Lung changes secondary to inhalation of underarm aerosol deodorants, Presented at the Meeting of the American Thoracic Society in Los Angeles, 1971.
17. Reiman, H. A., Ducarves, T., and Supple, L. K.: Tricalcium phosphate crystallosis, J.A.M.A. **189**:195-198, 1964.
18. Nam, K., and Gracey, D. R.: Pulmonary talcosis from cosmetic talcum powder, J.A.M.A. **221**:492-493, 1972.
19. Fuller, C. J.: Farmer's lung: a review of present knowledge, Thorax **8**:59, 1953.
20. Dickie, H. A., and Rankin, J.: Farmer's lung: an acute granulomatous interstitial pneumonitis occurring in agricultural workers, J.A.M.A. **167**:1069, 1958.
21. Pepys, J., and Jenkins, P. A.: Precipitin (F.L.H.) test in farmer's lung, Thorax **20**:21, 1965.
22. Slavaggio, J. E., Buechner, H. A., Seabury, J. H., and others: Bagassosis: precipitins against extracts of crude bagasse in the serum of patients with bagassosis, J. Allerg. **37**:107, 1966.
23. Spencer, H.: Pathology of the lungs, ed. 2, Oxford, 1968, Pergamon Press, Ltd.

10
FEVER-PRODUCING AGENTS

METAL-FUME FEVER

So-called metal-fume fever follows inhalation of finely dispersed particulate matter, which is formed when certain metals are heated and become volatile. Since the particle size of metal fumes is very small (usually about 1 μ or less) they can be dispersed widely and affect populations in the environment of industrial establishments.[1] The oxides of the following metals are capable of causing the disease: antimony, arsenic, cadmium, cobalt, copper, iron, lead, magnesium, manganese, mercury, nickel, tin, and zinc.

The disease starts with dryness, irritation of the throat, and a sweetish taste in the mouth, which is followed within a few hours by tightness, constriction in the chest, and dry cough. The condition is accompanied by general lassitude, fatigue, frontal headaches, low back pains, and, occasionally, blurred vision. A malarialike chill and high fever develop, with considerable muscular pain, nausea, and occasional vomiting. These episodes last from 6 to 12 hours and, in rare instances, as long as 24 hours. The patients experience general weakness and prostration before complete recovery.

The two metals with which this disease is most often identified are manganese and zinc. Although both agents produce systemic effects in addition to their action on the lungs, they are presented here because the pulmonary symptoms dominate the clinical picture.

Manganese

Sauda, a small town on the western shore of Norway, had been a tourist center up to the early 1930s when a newly built plant in the town began manufacturing manganese (Mn) alloys. The town soon became known as an area of high morbidity, where eight times more people died of pneumonia than elsewhere in Norway.[2] Inside the plant the ventilation system of the electric smelting furnaces was adequate, but the smoke, containing manganese compounds, was discharged into the surrounding area. Particles of the size of 5 μ or greater were found 3 km from the plant.

Near another factory in Aosta, Italy, among residents and miners[3] a high incidence of so-called croupous pneumonia was attributed to the presence of manganese dust. Of 1200 residents within a 500-meter zone of the plant, an epidemic of ear, nose, and throat problems associated with neurologic disorders, especially in children, occurred in 1962. However, workers in the plant had no such disease. In 62% of 700 children, mostly of preschool age, the mucus from the nose contained up to 95 μg of manganese and about 40% suffered from ear, nose, and throat diseases. Sixteen out of 204 children complained of dizziness and severe general asthenia (weakness).

Properties and uses of manganese. Manganese, a gray-white metal that resembles iron, is an element essential to human life. Its presence in the body is required for the action of many enzymes. However, it is also a source of environmental disease.

It occurs in many minerals widely scattered over the earth.[4] Montana, Minnesota, and New Mexico have manganese mines.[5] Its main commercial source, manganese dioxide, or pyrolusite (MnO_2), is used in steel making to reduce oxygen and sulfur. It is an ingredient of special alloy steels. Manufacturing of dry-cell batteries, welding, and coloring and bleaching of glass release manganese. In the chemical industry it serves as an oxidizing agent for the production of potassium permanganate and other manganese chemicals. Organic manganese compounds added to gasoline and fuel oil for internal combustion and turbine engines account for environmental pollution. Basic slag contains about 10% manganese.

Atmospheric manganese. In 1964, the National Air Sampling Network found an average of 0.1 μg/meter^3 of manganese in urban areas. The highest values of 10 μg were recorded in Charleston, West Virginia.[6] The official threshold limit value for manganese in Pennsylvania is 5 μg/meter^3 for an exposure up to 30 minutes.[7]

Manganese occurs in the atmosphere mainly as manganese oxide, which interacts rapidly with other pollutants, as for example sulfur dioxide and nitrogen dioxide, to form water-soluble manganese compounds.

Body burden. The daily average intake in humans is between 3 to 9 mg.[8] Manganese salts are absorbed slowly by the gastrointestinal tract. Blood contains between 12 and 15 μg% and urine from 1 to 10 μg%.[9] Most manganese taken into the body appears in the feces, but some[10] is retained, especially in liver and lymph nodes.

Manganese deficiency. In animals manganese deficiency causes retardation of growth, bone abnormalities, disturbance of reproduction, and disease of the central nervous system. These conditions have been associated with a low level of liver aldol-ase, an enzyme involved in carbohydrate metabolism, and of bone alkaline phosphatase activity, a condition that can be rectified by administering manganese. The metabolism of choline is linked with that of manganese; both decrease liver fat in rats and in birds.

Manganese intoxication. Manganese poisoning has been recognized for more than 100 years, but little is known about the long-term effects of minute amounts present in the atmosphere. Data on its toxicity must, therefore, be gleaned from the experience of occupational poisoning.

Acute intoxication. Manganese pneumonia differs from an infectious pneumonia inasmuch as the white blood cells present in the lungs are lymphocytes (round cells) in distinction to the usual kind of pus cells, the so-called neutrophiles.[11] Nasal congestion and nosebleed are often associated with the disease. Before pneumonia develops, the chest symptoms are usually mistakenly diagnosed as "influenza." Administration of antibiotics, the customary treatment for febrile diseases, does not change their course, but adrenal steroids (cortisone preparations) are valuable as treatment.

Chronic intoxication. Whereas acute intoxication involves the respiratory system, chronic manganese poisoning affects the central nervous system, mainly the midbrain between the cerebellum and the cerebral cortex, and the large ganglion cells of the brain cortex. The disease causes disorders in mentation, disorientation, impairment of memory and judgment, acute anxiety, even hallucinations and delusions.[12] Compulsive behavior including singing, dancing, fighting, a tendency to weeping, and purposeless laughter and running about, is frequently reported.

The following case, reported by Tanaka and Lieben[13] illustrates the course of this illness. In 1962, a 47-year-old Negro who had worked in a manganese ore processing plant for 16 years experienced low back pain, pain in the left flank, and difficulty in maintaining his balance. Various aches and pains in the extremities had persisted for many months. His gait was disturbed and he stumbled frequently. In one hospital, physicians suspected lead poisoning; in another, posterolateral sclerosis (a spinal cord disease); in a third, tabes dorsalis (a spinal disease caused by advanced syphilis). Laboratory and physical findings were essentially negative; the electromyogram, the recording of electric potentials developed in muscle, revealed an abnormal pattern only in the area of the lower spine.

Six years later he was again admitted to a hospital. This time his principal complaints were nervousness, drowsiness, inability to concentrate, muscle cramps, and sexual impotency. Examination revealed tremor of the hands, stiffness of extremities, and an impediment in his speech. He had a slightly positive Romberg test, which is indicative of inability to control one's equilibrium. His urine contained 71.0 μg/liter manganese (normal 1 to 8 μg/liter).

Tanaka and Lieben related the details of a second patient who was unable to control his bladder action. He had a weak voice and a "frozen" facial expression suggestive of Parkinson's disease. This patient was unable to rise from a prone to an erect position without assistance. The dust of the plant where this patient had been working contained from 2.6 mg/meter^3 manganese to a maximum of 6.4 mg/meter^3.

Laboratory tests that aid in the diagnosis of manganese poisoning are a reduction in the urinary excretion of 17 ketosteroids (an adrenal gland hormone), an increase of lymphocytes (round white cells) of the blood, and a rise in the basal metabolic rate.[8]

Examination of the hair for manganese assists in the diagnosis. Elevated levels ranging from 4.7 to 29 ppm manganese have been reported.[12] The chest hair may contain more than threefold the content of scalp hair. The symptoms of manganese poisoning are usually reversible at least temporarily when a medication called Levodopa, a chelating agent, is given in daily doses up to 8 gm.[14]

Zinc and zinc compounds

Zinc (Zn) is another common metal that evokes "metal-fume fever."

Zinc as essential trace element. Zinc occurs in the earth naturally, in relatively small quantities, as zinc blende (ZnS) associated with lead and iron sulfides.[15] It is an important essential trace element that is required for the function of many enzymes. It plays a part in the normal development of the skin and of the skeleton.[16] It also limits the normal synthesis of proteins and of deoxyribonucleic acid (DNA), the principal constituent of genes, which plays an important role in the genetic action of chromosomes. An adult man stores between 1.2 and 3 gm. The average daily dietary intake is 10 to 15 mg. Normal blood levels are remarkably constant, namely from 0.8 to 1.6 ppm. Their day-to-day variations are smaller than those of plasma copper and plasma magnesium.[17] However, plasma zinc levels are below normal in patients with certain liver diseases and, especially, in cancer of the bronchi.[17]

Zinc deficiency causes stunted growth, lack of sexual development in young males, and poor wound healing in older persons.[18]

Zinc as air pollutant. Its role as an air pollutant is difficult to assess because zinc is commonly associated with other toxic contaminants, especially cadmium and lead. It is emitted, mainly, as zinc oxide fumes from industrial factories that produce copper, lead, and steel and from secondary processing operations that recover zinc from scrap brass alloy, from galvanizing processes, and from incineration of zinc-bearing materials.

Measurements of 24-hour atmospheric concentrations of zinc in United States cities revealed annual values averaging 0.67 μg/meter^3 between 1960 and 1964. The highest value was recorded in East St. Louis in 1963, namely 58 μg/meter[3]. These concentrations in the air are generally considered nontoxic to humans, animals, and plants. The maximum allowable concentration for zinc oxide fumes for an 8-hour work day in the United States, Federal Republic of Germany, and U.S.S.R. is 5 mg/meter[3].

Toxicity. In animal experiments, the toxic dose varies with the kind of animal and with the kind of zinc compound. For instance, in rats, inhalation of zinc oxide in concentrations of 400 to 600 μg/meter[3] for 10 to 120 minutes produces damage to lungs and liver, which is fatal in approximately 10%.[19] Dogs and cats, on the other hand, tolerate concentrations up to 1 gm a day of zinc oxide with only slight damage, involving mainly the pancreas.[15]

To humans zinc is usually nontoxic in open atmospheres, but inside factories inhalation of zinc or zinc compounds at a magnitude of 48 and 74 mg/meter[3] for 10.5 and 12 minutes, respectively, has given rise to metal-fume fever.[20]

Symptoms of zinc intoxication. Just as in manganese fever, this malarialike illness lasts approximately 24 hours, causing chills, high fever, malaise, depression, nausea, and vomiting, as well as aching of head and muscles.[1] After the temperature has reached 103° to 104°, it drops to normal within 12 to 24 hours. Recovery is rapid and complete. It is postulated that inhaled zinc fume particles induce a release of protein into the body, which causes this characteristic foreign protein response.[15]

Another pulmonary disease that appears to be a distinct variation of metal-fume fever is encountered following massive inhalation of zinc chloride as, for instance, in welders[20] or in military personnel[21] employing smoke screen zinc compounds. Fever and chills are accompanied by throat irritation, bronchitis, joint muscle pains, vomiting, diarrhea, nasal catarrh, and vertigo. Matsui[20] induced this disease in rats

following a 12-minute exposure to 48 mg/meter[3] of zinc. Zinc sulfate and zinc ammonium sulfate are believed to have played a role in the development of pulmonary symptoms during the Donora disaster.[22] It is possible that the sulfate in these compounds could have been the determinant factor.

The particle size of zinc oxide and zinc chloride is largely responsible for the type and degree of respiratory symptoms and for their differing toxic effects.[23]

When excessive amounts of the metal are ingested with food and drinks, especially when acid foods are prepared in galvanized containers, another form of zinc poisoning occurs.[8,24] It is largely confined to the gastrointestinal tract with vomiting, bowel disorders, and diarrhea.[25] In an episode of mass poisoning,[26] for instance, 44 out of 51 persons who drank punch stored in a galvanized container became ill. The punch contained 3.7% zinc (3675 ppm). It is possible, however, that cadmium and fluoride, which are also present in galvanized material, contribute to this kind of poisoning. The zinc ion ordinarily is not absorbed in sufficient quantities to cause systemic effects. Another local manifestation of zinc salts is their caustic effect on the skin, leading to ulcerations.

POLYMER-FUME FEVER

A condition similar to, if not identical with, metal-fume fever but not caused by metal, is encountered when the widely used plastic teflon (polytetrafluorethylene, PTFE) is heated above 400° C.[26,27] The close interrelation of this disease with cigarette smoking is illustrated by a report on two workers in the laboratory of an airplane factory.[28]

On their way home from work, they experienced an influenzalike chill, aching arms and chest, followed by high fever. The condition came on shortly after one of the men had started to smoke a cigarette that had a bad taste and made him cough.

The other person, a pipe smoker, had been complaining of chronic fatigue and aching in arms and chest since he began to work in the area. A third man, working in the same area, who did not smoke, had no symptoms.

When other employees, who were also smokers, investigated the condition in the laboratory, they had the same unpleasant reactions. Shortly after entering the laboratory they developed tightness in the chest, cough, and bad taste. Within ½ hour they began to shake and experienced chills and fever, which lasted for 2 to 3 hours.

It was determined that the polytetrafluoroethylene covering of the cables that were wired to a small electric furnace had become overheated and had emitted toxic fumes.* When the cables were removed, they had shrunk in size as a result of the heat. More than half of the original weight had been burned up within 50 to 100 hours. It was calculated that the workers developed their first chills upon exposure to a small fraction of the fumes, less than 1 mg/meter^3 for 4 hours. The exact nature of the breakdown product was not revealed. Carbonyl-fluoride, hydrogen fluoride, and carbon monoxide were among them. Chills, fever, severe chest pains, and a rise in white blood cells rarely last more than 1 day.[26]

A more recent report[29] described the case of a 50-year-old woman who had about 40 febrile episodes during a period of 9 months. In her work at an electronic equipment factory she used a fluorocarbon spray, which contaminated her fingers with a white sticky powder deposit. Minute amounts of this material were transferred to cigarettes that she smoked without first washing her hands.

Cavagna, Finulli, and Vigliana[27] believe that the fever results from accumulation of granulocytes (white blood cells) in the lungs and subsequent release of a fever-producing protein from the cells. Tobacco smoke is thought to accelerate the accumulation of breakdown products of the plastic in the lungs.

That extensive exposure to the overheated plastic can have more serious effects than a temporary rise in temperature was indicated in a *Canadian Medical Association Journal* report of 1961. An individual developed pulmonary edema, cough, and died after he had laid a lighted cigarette on the edge of a sheet of teflon and later picked it up and resumed smoking.[30]

OTHER FEVER-INDUCING POLLUTANTS

In distinction to these suddenly appearing and quickly clearing lung diseases, there is an entirely different group of fever-producing diseases caused by air pollutants, which closely follow the usual pattern of pneumonia. They occur among persons handling parrots, parakeets (psittacosis) and other birds, especially pigeons (pigeon breeder's disease).

In 1945, I described the case of a pigeon fancier who collapsed suddenly while feeding his pigeons.[31] He was taken in shock into the hospital where after several hours he developed chills, fever up to 104° F and cough, which were diagnosed as pneumonia. Skin tests with an extract of pigeon feathers *during the acute phase* of the illness were unrevealing; however, 6 weeks later, the disease gradually developed into asthma and a strongly positive reaction to pigeon feathers was obtained. The patient recovered completely after he had abandoned pigeon raising.

Within recent years, considerable interest has revolved around this kind of disease. Some investigators believe the precipitating cause to be a fungus rather than an allergic response to the pigeon feathers. Antibodies for fungi have been found in patients' blood serum.

A rather unique case has come to my attention, which demonstrates the manner

---

*The toxic gas contained perfluoroisobutene, a highly toxic agent.[29]

in which this disease can occur without occupational exposure. Furthermore the case combines two unusually rare pulmonary diseases, both caused by environmental sources.

A 49-year-old woman was admitted to a midwestern hospital on July 21, 1969, because of chills, fever, and severe chest pains of 4 days' duration. At first she had little cough but after 2 days she coughed and expectorated heavy mucus. Examination revealed a low-grade pneumonialike process, but the culture of the expectorated material showed no bacterial growth. Since the patient had had contact with parrots, a test for psittacosis (parrot fever) was performed but failed to produce evidence of the disease. After some sleuthing it was determined that, on a hot day 1 week prior to the onset, the patient had buried a pigeon that she had found lying dead in her yard.

Shortness of breath, cough, and expectoration of mucus persisted for several months. Pulmonary function studies showed severe airway obstruction with marked restriction of the ventilatory capacity of the lungs. Roentgenograms revealed a number of local infiltrative processes distributed throughout the lungs. A biopsy of a lymph gland at the neck showed a condition that was suggestive of berylliosis. From 1938 to 1958 the patient had been working in the fluorescent lamp division of an electric appliance company. Earmarks of chronic beryllium poisoning had been identified since the early 1940s.

After recovery from the pneumonia the patient moved into a rural area about 40 miles distant from contaminating urban sources. In spite of the two disabling lung conditions, she has made a remarkable recovery.

REFERENCES

1. Rohrs, L. C.: "Metal" fume fever from inhaling zinc oxide, Arch. Intern. Med. **100:** 44-49, 1957.
2. Elstad, D.: Manganholdig Fabrikkrvek som Medvirkende Arsak ved Peumoni-Epidermier i en Industribygd, Nord. Med. 3:2527, 1939.
3. Pancheri, G.: Industrial atmospheric pollution in Italy. In Mallette, F. S., editor: Problems and control of air pollution, New York, 1955, Van Nostrand Reinhold Co., p. 263.
4. Dokuchaev, V. F., and Skvortsova, N. N.: Atmospheric air pollution with manganese compounds and their effect on the organism. Levine, B. S., translator, U.S.S.R. literature on air pollution and related occupational disease 9:40, 1962.
5. Sullivan, R. J.: Air pollution aspects of manganese and its compounds, Litton System, Inc., Bethesda, Maryland, 1969, U. S. Department of Commerce, National Bureau of Standards.
6. Air Quality Data from the National Air Sampling Network and Contributing State and Local Networks 1964-1965, Cincinnati, 1966, U. S. Department of Health, Education, and Welfare, Public Health Service, Division of Air Pollution.
7. Regulations Establishing Threshold Limits in Places of Employment, Article 432, Pennsylvania Department of Health, Adopted October 27, 1961.
8. Patty, F. A., editor: Industrial hygiene and toxicology, vol. 2, ed. 2, New York, 1963, Interscience Publishers, Inc.
9. Cholak, J., and Hubbard, D. M.: Determination of manganese in air and biological material, Amer. Industr. Hyg. Ass. J. **21:**356-360, 1960.
10. Hygienic Guide Series: Manganese and its inorganic compounds, Amer. Industr. Hyg. Ass. J. **24:**284, 1963.
11. Davies, T. A. L.: Manganese pneumonitis. Brit. J. Industr. Med. 3:111-135, 1946.
12. Rosenstock, H. A., Simons, D. G., and Meyer, J. S.: Chronic manganism, neurologic and laboratory studies during treatment with levadopa, J.A.M.A. **217:**1354-1356, 1971.
13. Tanaka, S., and Lieben, J.: Manganese poisoning and exposure in Pennsylvania, Arch. Environ. Health **19:**674-684, 1969.
14. Mana, I., Court, J., Fuenzalida, S., and others: Modification of chronic manganese poisoning, treatment with L-Dopa and 5-OH tryptophane, New Eng. J. Med. **282:**5-10, 1970.
15. Athanassiadis, Y. C.: Air pollution aspects of zinc and its compounds, National Technical Information Service, Litton Industries, Inc., Bethesda, Maryland, 1969, U. S. Department of Commerce, National Bureau of Standards, PB 188 072.
16. Zinc: editorial, Lancet 2:268, 1968.
17. Davies, I. J. T., Musa, M., and Dormandy,

T. L.: Measurements of plasma zinc, J. Clin. Pathol. 21:359-365, 1968.

18. Prasad, A. S.: Zinc: human nutrition and metabolic effects, Ann. Intern. Med. 73:631-635, 1970.

19. Beeckmaus, J. M., and Brown, J. R.: Toxicity of catalytically active zinc oxides, Arch. Environ. Health 7:346-50, 1963.

20. Matsui, K., and others: Studies on the metal fume fever and pneumoconiosis due to welding work in the holds, Japan J. Industr. Health 7:3-7, 1965.

21. Gafafer, W. M., editor: Occupational diseases, U. S. Department of Health, Education and Welfare, Public Health Service Publication No. 1097, Washington, D. C., 1964, U. S. Government Printing Office.

22. Amdur, M. O.: Aerosols formed by oxidation of sulfur dioxide, Arch Environ. Health 23:459-468, 1971.

23. Handbook of Air Pollution, 1968, U. S. Department of Health, Education, and Welfare, Public Health Service.

24. Prasad, A. S., editor: Zinc metabolism, Springfield, Ill., 1966, Charles C Thomas, Publisher, p. 429.

25. Brown, M. A., Thom, J. V., Orth, G. L., and others: Food poisoning involving zinc contamination, Arch. Environ. Health 8:657-660, 1964.

26. Lewis, C. E., and Kerby, G. R.: An epidemic of polymer fume fever, J.A.M.A. 191:103-106, 1965.

27. Cavagna, G., Finulli, M., and Vigliana, E. C.: Experimental study on the pathogenesis of teflon fume fever, Med. Lavoro 52:251, 1961.

28. Welti, D. W., and Hipp, M. J.: Polymer fume fever, J. Occup. Med. 10:667-671, 1968.

29. Waritz, R. S., and Kwon, B. K.: The inhalation toxicity of pyrolysis products of PTFE heated below 500°, Amer. Industr. Hyg. Ass. J. 29:19-26, 1968.

30. Mach, G. J.: Letter to the Editor, Canad. Med. Ass. J. 85:955, 1961.

31. Waldbott, G. L.: Problems in the diagnosis of bronchial asthma, Ann. Allerg. 3:12-20, 1945.

11
ASPHYXIATING POLLUTANTS

When a person becomes asphyxiated, his blood is deprived of its oxygen supply and and he can no longer eliminate carbon dioxide. This condition leads to certain changes throughout his system. Most organs become waterlogged. Tiny hemorrhages are widely distributed throughout the organism and incapacitate the vital organs.

Numerous agents that obstruct the main air passages can produce this kind of condition, such as strangulation, general anesthesia, or tumors of the throat and bronchi. Most irritating gases, when inhaled in very high concentrations, flood the lungs with fluid; this as well as spasm of the bronchi prevent exchange of oxygen and carbon dioxide.

Carbon monoxide (CO), which deprives the hemoglobin of its oxygen-carrying ability, is the asphyxiant most often encountered. Another asphyxiating gas, hydrogen sulfide (H_2S), does not act on hemoglobin like carbon monoxide but paralyzes the brain center that controls the respiratory movements of the chest.* It impedes exchange of oxygen and carbon dioxide in the alveoli.

Whereas complete cessation of breathing occurs only after exposure to relatively

---

*Although carbon monoxide and hydrogen sulfide also induce systemic effects, they are classified here as respiratory pollutants, since they involve principally respiration and enter the system through the respiratory tract.

high concentrations of these gases, long-term impairment of oxygenation of blood by lesser amounts of the pollutant leads to systemic damage involving mainly heart, brain, and blood vessels.

CARBON MONOXIDE
Shinshu myocardosis

In 1955 a Japanese physician, Dr. Fumio Komatsu,[1] observed an unusual disease called Shinshu myocardosis in the Japanese village of Kinasa, Nagano Prefecture, situated a thousand meters above sea level and surrounded by mountains. Because of the cold climate and the limited arable land, the 6000 inhabitants depended for their livelihood on silkworm raising and lumber cutting in the summer and on manufacturing tatami mats during the winter. The indoor work in winter was carried out in so-called kakoi (closed rooms), the windows and crevices of the walls of which were tightly sealed. The crowded rooms, heated by an open charcoal fire, provided approximately 5 meters^3 of air volume per person, about as much as a boy scout tent.

In the beginning stage of the disease the patients complained of stiffness in the shoulders, backache, fatigue, and dizziness. As the disease progressed, they became short of breath on exertion, experienced tightness and pain below the breastbone, numbness in arms and hands, and swelling of the face. The attacks of shortness of breath came on mostly at night; whereas the episodes of pain and tightness around the heart, a condition known as angina pectoris, followed light work during the day.

Of the 1022 inhabitants investigated by Dr. Komatsu, 35.5% were afflicted with a disease involving the heart valves, an incidence far above the national average. Eighteen percent of the heart patients, mostly middle-aged women, had a specific kind of heart involvement designated as Shinshu myocardosis. Even young people had arteriosclerotic heart disease.

Investigation at Shinshu University established that the disease was caused by carbon monoxide inhaled at high levels over long periods of time. The carbon monoxide concentration in the rooms ranged between 0.2% and 0.3% (2000 to 3000 ppm) in the morning and the carboxyhemoglobin (COHb), the part of hemoglobin altered by carbon monoxide, reached 20% to 30%. Anything above 10% to 15% is considered dangerous.

After the cause of the illness was detected and the rooms in the village were remodelled, the incidence of heart disease decreased to one half. Subsequently, the disease cleared up entirely[2] when a change in agricultural procedures in the area made work in the small rooms unnecessary.

Properties of carbon monoxide

Carbon monoxide, a poisonous gas, is a product of incomplete combustion. The fact that it can neither be seen, smelled, nor tasted prevents its recognition in the atmosphere by its prospective victims. Unlike many other pollutants, carbon monoxide is quite stable and undergoes only slight changes in the atmosphere. A minimal amount of it is slowly converted into carbon dioxide. Inhalation of carbon monoxide from an automobile parked in a closed garage[3] with its engine running or from an open unlighted gas burner in a home has become a favorite method of suicide.[4] In fact, carbon monoxide is responsible for half of all fatal poisoning in the United States.

Table 11-1. Estimated emissions of carbon monoxide in the United States during 1968 in million metric tons per year*

Stationary fuel combustion	1.7
Mobile fuel combustion	57.9
Combustion of refuse	7.1
Industrial processes	8.8
Total	75.5

*Compiled from Morgan, G. B., Ozolins, G., and Tabor, E. C.: Air pollution surveillance systems, Science 170:289-296, 1970.

Sources of carbon monoxide

Formerly the ocean was thought to be a sink, that is, a place for *disposal* of carbon monoxide, not a source. Recently, however, carbon monoxide was shown to *originate* in the ocean, which is likely to be its largest natural source.[5]

On land, the automobile is the most significant source of contamination of the air by carbon monoxide; cigarette smoking occupies second place. In 1963 the Los Angeles County Air Pollution District[6] estimated that exhaust from automobiles contained 8000 tons of carbon monoxide per day or about 5 pounds per vehicle; as of January 1971, it amounted to about 9000 tons.[7] The yearly emission of carbon monoxide from automobiles in the United States is calculated to be 57.9 million tons[8] (Table 11-1). Other operations that release carbon monoxide are heating with gas and coal, distillation of coal and wood, furnaces, stoves, forges, and kilns. Inhalation of certain chemicals used in household and industry also lead to substantial formation of carbon monoxide and to temporary rise in carboxyhemoglobin of the blood. Dichloromethane (CH_2Cl_2), for instance, a paint remover, forms between 500 and 1000 ppm[9] carbon monoxide in human beings following exposure for 1 to 2 hours.* In domestic

---

*At approximately 1000 ppm a volunteer develops lightheadedness, thick tongue, and an inability to enunciate words clearly.[9a]

Table 11-2. Important sources of carbon monoxide*

SOURCE	PERCENT
Domestic coal	2 to 15
Coke oven gas	15 to 20
Water gas	30 to 40
Fires	0.5 to 1

*Adapted from Simpson, K.: Forensic medicine, ed. 5, London, 1964, The Williams & Wilkins Co.

and industrial gases the carbon monoxide content varies from as little as 0.5% to as much as 40%[10] (Table 11-2).

The current high rate of carbon monoxide production throughout the world of about 200 million metric tons a year has given rise to fears of accumulation of gas to dangerous levels. Inman and Ingersoll,[11] however, recently demonstrated that fungi (molds) present in soil constitute an efficient "sink" by which carbon monoxide is being removed at the rate of about 500 million tons a year.

Carboxyhemoglobin

When carbon monoxide is inhaled, it enters the capillary blood vessels through the alveoli. Its principal damage to health lies in the fact that it has an affinity for the hemoglobin of blood, the carrier of oxygen, 300 times greater than that of oxygen. Therefore, even a small concentration of carbon monoxide in the inhaled air will displace life-sustaining oxygen in the blood. After a 2-hour exposure to 250 ppm at sea level, about 16% of the blood's hemoglobin is converted into carboxyhemoglobin.[12] Since the portion of hemoglobin with which carbon monoxide has combined is no longer available for transporting oxygen, such inactivation of hemoglobin is equivalent to withdrawing a corresponding amount of blood.

The carboxyhemoglobin content of blood varies widely with a city's automobile traffic, the time of day, atmospheric conditions and many other factors. On the streets of the French city of Bordeaux[13] the average carboxyhemoglobin content of blood of traffic policemen on duty was found to be 1.2% in the morning and 2.7% in the evening. Policemen who smoked had higher values in their blood, with an average 2.35% in the morning and 4.7% in the evening. Among officers involved in desk work away from traffic, the mean level was 1.6% in the morning and 1.14% in the evening.

In contrast with these values, Gordon and Rogers[2] reported carboxyhemoglobin levels up to 44% in Denver firefighters exposed to smoke for more than 5 minutes. About half of the exposed individuals showed minor abnormal changes in the heart as indicated by the electrocardiogram.

Atmospheric carbon monoxide concentrations

In cities. In urban air the concentration of carbon monoxide is higher than that of any other gaseous pollutant. Approximately 97% of the air pollution in New York City is currently attributed to exhaust gases from vehicles.[14] The carbon monoxide levels in the atmosphere are very sensitive to variations of traffic. They rise at an intersection when vehicles are stopped for a traffic light and when cars idle near the monitoring station. In 1960 Clayton and collaborators[15] measured the concentrations of carbon monoxide in Detroit throughout several months. Some of their findings are shown in Table 11-3. A sampling made in a parked police car with its motor idling averaged 17 ppm with a peak value of 120 ppm. The maximum concentration in a Detroit residential site was 29 ppm compared with that at the Oxford Circus in London, which on frequent occasions exceeded 100 ppm. In Los Angeles, where the air contains between 10 to 12 ppm carbon monoxide, the level along the

Table 11-3. Average carbon monoxide concentration in Detroit in 1960

	PPM	WEEKS
Residential area	2	18
Shopping district	10	58
Downtown street	9	21
Expressway	8	21

route of heavy traffic was 37 ppm with peaks as high as 120 ppm.[16] Eight-hour exposures to levels greater than 30 ppm are considered hazardous. According to a Japanese study[17] the carbon monoxide pollution range extended 20 meters (65.5 feet) distant from the edge of a street.

In the streets of large cities carbon monoxide levels have declined in recent years. The average hourly concentration in New York streets in 1922 was 32 ppm compared with 8 ppm in 1967.[14]

In tunnels and garages. In garages, tunnels, and behind automobiles the above concentrations are often exceeded. In toll takers at the floating bridge across Lake Washington near Seattle, Breysse[18] noted levels up to 300 ppm during rush hours. In employees of a parking garage, carbon monoxide concentrations averaged 59 ppm during weekdays.[19] The annual average in a United States city is about 4 ppm.

Threshold limits. In 1970, an international committee[20] proposed that the threshold limit value for carbon monoxide in industry should be less than 50 ppm, which was thought to be a safe day-to-day level for a 40-hour week for healthy workmen. Such exposures cause carboxyhemoglobin levels from 8% to 10% in nonsmokers. Critical factors that account for wide variations are the duration of exposure and an individual's susceptibility. Persons under physical strain and particularly arteriosclerotic individuals are vulnerable at such levels.

Smoking. Cigarette smoke as inhaled contains 200 to 800 ppm carbon monoxide; smoke from cigar or pipe tobacco contains considerably more.[21] The highest concentration of carbon monoxide is emitted when the last portion of a cigarette is smoked.[22] Addition of cigarette smoke to the daily exposure from vehicle exhaust, even though only temporary, can take an unforseen toll. Smokers with arteriosclerosis, especially in the 30 to 39 age group, show a carboxyhemoglobin level two to three times higher than nonarteriosclerotic smokers.[23] On the other hand, habitual, "healthy," one-pack-a-day smokers show a concentration of 5% to more than 7% of carboxyhemoglobin. This compares with 0.4% to 0.5% in a typical nonsmoker[24] without apparent adverse manifestations. The fact that smokers have no overt symptoms of poisoning has led to the belief that they acquire some kind of tolerance through constant exposure to carbon monoxide.[25] This might also be true among nonsmoking urban dwellers exposed to carbon monoxide day after day.

Adverse effects

The deficiency of oxygen in blood caused by carbon monoxide affects mainly respiration and function of the brain and heart, the two organs most sensitive to oxygen deprivation. Persons with a chronic heart and lung disease or with anemia, whose hemoglobin supply is limited, as well as individuals residing in high altitudes, are particularly prone to poisoning. Carbon monoxide can also harm pregnant women and account for small-sized babies.[26,27] In Los Angeles[28] an increase in death rates occurred on days of highest atmospheric carbon monoxide concentrations.

The initial symptoms of carbon monoxide poisoning occur when carboxyhemoglobin levels range between 10% and 20%. They consist of dizziness, headaches, nausea and general fatigue, impairment of memory, and loss of muscular control. Because carbon monoxide accumulates in muscle tissue, muscular weakness may persist for days after the pollution has stopped. Short-term exposure to between 15 and 50 ppm, which produces 2% to 8% carboxyhemoglobin, causes impaired ability to detect a flashing light against a dim background.[29] At a concentration of 250 ppm, a person's mental acuity deteriorates to the extent that perception of light is reduced by 60%. Auditory vigilance and comprehension are likewise markedly inhibited during exposures to carbon monoxide concentrations of 50 to 250 ppm for ½ to 2½ hours.[30] It is conceivable that, at a concentration of carbon monoxide that a car may pour out,* the perception of the driver of the following vehicle could be impaired to such an extent that he could not apply the brakes in time.

Acute intoxication. Abundant data are available on acute carbon monoxide poisoning caused by exposure to large doses. A pertinent illustration of the clinical picture of acute carbon monoxide poisoning is presented in a paper by Anderson and others[31] of the University of Texas, which points up the variations in symptoms from person to person.

In one incident a family of four was found unconscious in a tightly sealed house where one unvented natural gas heater and a pilot light were burning; in another incident three women were stricken while riding in a closed ambulance.

In the first incident, an infant boy was dead on arrival at the hospital. The carboxyhemoglobin saturation of his venous blood was 55%. The father, age 33, was unconscious, his blood pressure was elevated, and spastic reflexes indicated brain damage. Two hours after admission to the hospital his blood contained 10% carboxyhemoglobin. Forty-six hours later, he regained consciousness and on the fifth day he was able to attend the funeral of his infant son after which he developed sudden pain in the heart region and died. The postmortem examination revealed marked degenerative changes in the heart muscle.

*On rare occasions automobile drivers in California have been subjected to such concentrations.[12]

His wife, age 27, was disoriented and unconscious upon admission to the hospital but soon began to speak coherently. On the sixth day of hospitalization, an electrocardiogram showed marked changes indicative of heart damage. The description of her chest pains agrees with Dr. Komatsu's account of the Japanese cases. One month after the exposure, the electrocardiogram was normal, and the patient had fully recovered.

Unlike the other members of the family, a 7-year-old daughter was awake and talking coherently on admission to the hospital. She had right-sided palsy of the face and hemorrhages in the retina; her heart, however, showed no electrocardiographic abnormality.

The three patients in the second incident described by the Texas physicians were all exposed to the same concentration of carbon monoxide while riding in the ambulance together for the same amount of time, approximately 6 hours. One female, age 29, who had always been in good health, developed significant damage to the heart, whereas two elderly women aged 68 and 52 with diabetes experienced relatively little harm. In general, there was a lack of resemblance of symptoms from one person to the other.

Chronic intoxication. In contrast with acute carbon monoxide poisoning the medical literature contains much less information on the chronic phase of intoxication. In a survey on residents in gas-equipped apartments in Leningrad, Sorokina[32] found that 65 of the 80 residents had headaches, chest pain, dizziness, nausea, vomiting, general weakness, and rapid fatigability. Blood carboxyhemoglobin values were above 9% in 62 of the persons investigated; 33.5% of the housewives had a low blood pressure and low temperatures. In approximately 10% of the patients, both the hemoglobin and red blood counts were higher than normal, a condition often encountered in carbon monoxide poisoning. Carbon monoxide determinations were made on 895 air samples in the center of each apartment at a level of 1.5 meters above the floor under normal gas-burning conditions. The values, 1.5% to 35.5%, exceeded the maximum allowable carbon monoxide concentration in Russia. Carbon monoxide was emitted primarily from gas-burning heaters and stoves.

Fainting spells in persons working in street traffic or in a garage can be the result of carbon monoxide inhalation, especially when sudden bursts of carbon monoxide are emitted. Mr. J. L., a 57-year-old worker, was constantly exposed to exhaust from trucks in a poorly ventilated machine shop. For months he had been complaining about muscular weakness, headaches, and dizziness. While at work, he suddenly collapsed and fractured his skull and a cervical (neck) vertebra. Although during hospitalization the above symptoms cleared up completely within a few days, he was unable to recollect the events leading to the accident. The possibility that something, perhaps a part of a machine, had hit him on the head while he was working was ruled out by the available evidence.

After he returned to work, the former symptoms gradually recurred. Because carbon monoxide had not been suspected as the cause of his illness at the time of admission to the hospital, neither tests for carboxyhemoglobin were performed nor were determinations made of the carbon monoxide levels of the polluted air where the accident had occurred. Subsequent samplings of the air showed 72 and 45 ppm carbon monoxide. After retiring from work, the patient gradually recovered and had no further discomfort.

Although it could not be established with certainty that this illness actually represented carbon monoxide intoxication, the case is presented here because its course and its clinical features are typical of chronic poisoning. Furthermore, it illustrates the difficulties for attending physicians, who are unaware of a pollutant's effect, in establishing a diagnosis in such cases and in presenting final proof of the causal relationship to a certain pollutant.

Glowing charcoal brick in a grill or makeshift burner used for outdoor cooking can cause fatal poisoning when placed for heating purposes in an enclosed, unventilated space such as a sealed room or in a locked vehicle, station wagon, cabin cruiser, or other area. Five such cases were reported by Wilson and associates.[33] At autopsy carbon monoxide concentrations in the blood of the heart ranged as high as 71% as determined by gas chromatography.

Principal organs involved in poisoning

Heart. Dr. Komatsu's observations underline the effect of protracted carbon monoxide poisoning upon the heart. In rabbits 200 to 350 ppm of carbon monoxide in the air for 8 to 10 weeks produces changes in the blood vessels and enhances cholesterol uptake in vessel walls.[34] The damage to the heart may not necessarily be caused by the lack of oxygen but could be related to the toxic effect of carbon monoxide.[20] Just how much the habitual inhalation of carbon monoxide at low concentrations, especially in large cities, contributes to the incidence of heart disease or to coronary thrombosis is a subject in need of further exploration.

Brain. It has long been recognized that acute carbon monoxide intoxication affects the central nervous system. The following case report from a hospital in the British town of Leeds focused attention on this phase of poisoning.

Four workers were admitted to a hospital September 29, 1965, in an unconscious state following their attempt to repair a gas leak in a closed basement.[35] After a brief period of unconsciousness, a diversity of neurologic and psychiatric symptoms ensued, which resembled those of severe head injury—namely, difficulty in speech, inability to carry out simple activities such as buttoning their clothes or tying a knot, visual failure, disorientation, and lack of memory. Weeks and months passed before the individuals could recall the incident. The clinical picture differed in each patient. The patient exposed to carbon monoxide for only a few minutes showed signs no less severe than the other three who were exposed to the gas for about 3 hours at what appeared to be the same magnitude.

Skin. Dermatologists have recently become interested in carbon monoxide poisoning. They have long recognized that a cherry red color of the skin is a characteristic sign of carbon monoxide intoxication. Victims of carbon monoxide poisoning develop erythema, a bright red skin eruption[36] that tends to blister and usually clears up after 2 to 3 weeks. Prolonged inhalation of carbon monoxide is featured by white discoloration of the fingernails, a condition that indicates that the blood supply to the fingertips has been temporarily impeded.

Whereas most physicians are familiar with the clinical picture of acute carbon monoxide intoxication, only little is known about the effects of low-level exposures of the kind that is encountered in a large city with much automobile traffic or in a poorly ventilated dwelling. It is therefore necessary to study acute intoxication in order to recognize adverse effects from low-grade intoxication, which is bound to take its toll in those exposed over long periods of time. Because of its inconspicuous manifestations low-grade chronic carbon monoxide intoxication has not received the attention that it deserves.

HYDROGEN SULFIDE

Although hydrogen sulfide (H_2S) is a strong irritant to the respiratory organs, it is presented among asphyxiants because its major effect is its paralyzing action on the respiratory center that controls the respiratory movements.

Hydrogen sulfide is the gas with the "rotten-egg" odor. It occurs naturally near volcanoes and in mines when sulfur-containing organic matter decomposes without complete oxidation. It is also emitted by many chemical industries, especially oil wells and oil refineries and particularly in the production of gas for fuel. Large quantities originate when sulfur and protein-containing material undergo putrification.[37]

Hydrogen sulfide is corrosive to many metals and blackens numerous materials. Because of its high density (specific gravity) of 1.92g/liter it accumulates and remains in underground locations such as sewers and wells where it is formed. Here it is usually associated with other asphyxiant irritants and toxic gases, especially ammonia, methane, carbon monoxide and dioxide, ethylene, sulfur dioxide, phosphine.

Acute intoxication

Air pollution by hydrogen sulfide is usually localized to the vicinity of the emission. In the concentrations of 1000 mg/meter[3],[38] in which it occurs in underground passages, hydrogen sulfide is extremely toxic and as rapidly fatal as hydrogen cyanide. By immediately paralyzing the olfactory (smell perceiving) nerve, it deprives the potential victim of a warning of its presence.[39] Nor can it be seen, since it is colorless. Even in severe poisoning, rapid recovery[36] can be anticipated upon prompt removal of a victim into uncontaminated air.

Such acute intoxication, caused by H_2S formation in underground locations, is not rare. The following is a typical example:

In fall 1965 a 36-year-old employee of the Ohio State Highway Department collapsed and died within "a minute or two" after having descended on a ladder into a 15-foot deep sewer.[40] Two would-be rescuers, who tried to tie a rope around the victim, dropped dead in their tracks within a few seconds of one another.

At the autopsies of the three bodies, a characteristic rotten-egg odor and a striking grayish-green color of the skin, brain, internal organs, and blood were indicative of hydrogen sulfide poisoning. Death was attributed to hemorrhages and to edema (waterlogging) of the lungs. Coins and keys in the clothing of the victims were deeply blackened. When the coins were bathed in diluted sulfuric acid, hydrogen sulfide evolved.

The gas had been emitted into the sewer at the rate of approximately 500 pounds of hydrogen sulfide every 36 hours by a factory that converted fish oil and crude petroleum oil into a gear lubricant. Customarily, it was metered into the sewer at the safe ratio of 1 part of hydrogen sulfide to 2,000 parts of water. But on the day before the fatal exposures something had gone amiss: a defective fire hydrant had reduced the water pressure to the factory and to the neighborhood. The water had been shut off completely for about 2½ hours, which had permitted the extremely high hydrogen sulfide concentration to occur. In addition, the discharge of acid into the same sewer from another industrial plant contributed to the release of the gas.

The hydrogen sulfide concentration that caused the three fatalities was estimated to be between 1,000 and 2,000 mg/meter³. Between 400 and 700 mg/meter³ is considered dangerous.[41] Ambient urban concentrations range from 1 to 92 μg/meter³, but near industrial establishments, they may reach up to 1,400 μg/meter³.[37]

High hydrogen sulfide concentrations cause almost instantaneous paralysis of the entire central nervous system. The heart usually continues to beat for several minutes after breathing has stopped. Unlike carbon monoxide, hydrogen sulfide does not combine with hemoglobin. The formation of so-called sulfhemoglobin takes place after death as a result of decomposition of tissue. The sulfur-containing hemoglobin complexes are responsible for the green and greenish-blue discoloration of body tissue, which are observed at autopsy. The classical mass poisoning by hydrogen sulfide that occurred in Poza Poca, Mexico in 1950 is described in Chapter 5.

Nonfatal exposures

In low concentrations hydrogen sulfide, although extremely unpleasant in odor, is relatively harmless. The odor perception level varies among individuals between 1 and 45 μg/meter³. In smokers and in persons who have been exposed to the gas repeatedly, the odor threshold is higher.

In the bloodstream hydrogen sulfide promptly combines with oxygen derived from hemoglobin and is converted into inactive compounds such as sulfates and thiosulfate. Because of this rapid oxidation it does not accumulate in the body. However, nonfatal exposures to hydrogen sulfide may leave permanent aftereffects such as chronic kidney and liver disease, as well as injury to the brain.[42]

The following illustrates the events of a nonfatal exposure to hydrogen sulfide:

Mr. B. was pouring 1 gallon of an industrial grade of hydrochloric acid into a well, located in the 5 × 6 feet well room of his basement, in the presence of his wife.[43] Immediately a blue smoke was emitted from the well, which caused both to collapse. Their 12-year-old son who tried to be of assistance also became unconscious. After the concentration of fumes had somewhat diminished an 8-year-old neighbor came to their aid. He became nauseated and suffered severe back and chest pains.

The 35-year-old Mrs. B. who had received the full dose remained in deep coma for several hours with pupils dilated. Rales were present in both lungs; feet and hands were in a spasm and her blood pressure was unobtainable. Subsequently, she became extremely excited and her white blood count rose to 17,350 (normal, up to 9000) an indication of a secondary infection. An acute kidney disease with pus and red blood cells in the urine developed. Eventually the patient recovered and the sole after-effect was an impaired memory.

The 44-year-old Mr. B. was extremely "hyperirritable." He vomited profusely and showed extensive moisture in the lungs indicative of pulmonary edema. Prompt improvement followed withdrawal of blood from the vein to relieve the congestion of the waterlogged organs. He and the three other persons recovered completely.

The addition of hydrochloric acid to sulfur-containing organic materials in the well was responsible for production of hydrogen sulfide.

An example of much less disabling effects from emission of a relatively low-level concentration of hydrogen sulfide in a population occurred in May and June 1964 in Terre Haute, Indiana. Residents complained of shortness of breath, nausea, and loss of sleep. They also noted damage to property, mainly blackening of paints. The hydrogen sulfide odor was traced to a 36-acre lagoon into which organic industrial wastes had been dumped. Atmospheric concentrations of hydrogen sulfide during the episode ranged from 34 to 450 μg/meter[3].[44]

Other symptoms described in nonfatal hydrogen sulfide poisoning are metallic taste, fatigue, diarrhea, blurred vision, intense aching of eyes, and dizziness.[45]

Hydrogen sulfide can have synergistic effects with other pollutants: a mixture of hydrogen sulfide and naptha gas for instance and the combination of hydrogen sulfide with carbon monoxide potentiate each other's action.[39]

REFERENCES

1. Komatsu, F.: Digest of science of labour, **10**:315-318, 1955.
2. Quoted by Goldsmith, J. R.: Carbon monoxide research: recent and remote, Arch Environ. Health **21**:118-120, 1970.
3. Larsen, R. I.: Air pollution from motor vehicles, Ann. N. Y. Acad. Sci. **136**:275-301, 1966.
4. McBay, A. J.: Carbon monoxide poisoning, New Eng. J. Med. **272**:252, 1965.
5. Coburn, R. F.: Biologic effects of carbon monoxide, Ann. N.Y. Acad. Sci. **174**:1-430, 1970.
6. Summary of Air Pollution Statistics for Los Angeles County. Los Angeles County Air Pollution Control District, Los Angeles, 1963.
7. Profile of Air Pollution Control. Los Angeles County Air Pollution Control District, Los Angeles, 1971.
8. Morgan, G. B., Ozolins, G., and Tabor, E. C.: Air pollution surveillance systems, Science **170**:289-296, 1970.
9. Fisher, T. N., Hosko, M. J., Peterson, J. E., and others: Carboxyhemoglobin elevation after exposure to dichloromethane, Science **172**:295-296, 1972.
9a. Stewart, R. D., Fisher, T. N., Hosko, M. J., and others: Experimental human exposure to methylene chloride, Arch. Environ. Health **25**:342-348, 1972.
10. Simpson, K.: Forensic medicine, ed. 5, London, 1964, The Williams & Wilkins Co.
11. Inman, R. E., and Ingersoll, R. B.: Uptake of carbon monoxide by soil fungi, J.A.P.C.A. **21**:646-647, 1971.
12. Goldsmith, J. R., and Rogers, L. H.: Health hazards of automobile exhaust, Public Health Rep., **74**:551-558, 1959.
13. Coudray, P., and Mear, J.: Étude de l'imprégnation oxcarbonée des gardiens de la paix assurant la circulation des vehicles automobiles à Bordeaux, Pollution Atm. **11**:20-22, 1969.
14. Eisenbud, M., and Ehrlich, L. R.: Carbon monoxide concentration in urban atmospheres, Science **176**:193-194, 1972.
15. Clayton, G. D., Cook, W. A., and Fredrick, W. G.: a study of the relationship of street level carbon monoxide concentration to traffic accidents, Amer. Industr. Hyg. Ass. **21**:46-54, Feb. 1960.
16. Haagen-Smith, A. J.: Carbon monoxide levels in city driving, Arch. Environ Health **12**:548-551, 1966.
17. Kobayashi, Y., and Takamatsu, K.: carbon monoxide pollution in urban atmospheres by automobile exhaust gases, J. Jap. Soc. Safety Eng. **9**:29-36, 1970.
18. Breysse, P. A.: Use of expired air for evaluating carbon monoxide exposures. Ninth Conference on Methods in Air Pollution and Industrial Hygiene Studies, Pasadena California, Feb. 7-9, 1968.
19. Ramsey, J. M.: Carboxyhemoglobinemia in parking garage employees, Arch. Environ. Health **15**:580-583, 1967.
20. Grut, A., Astrup, P., Challen, P. J. R., and Gerhardsson, M. S.: Threshold limit value for

carbon monoxide, Arch. Environ. Health **21:** 542-544, 1970.

21. Patty, F. A.: Industrial hygiene and toxicology, vol. II, New York, 1962, Interscience Publishers, p. 932.

22. Effect of chronic exposure to low levels of carbon monoxide on human health, behavior and performance, Washington, D. C., 1969, National Academy of Science, National Academy of Engineering, p. 5.

23. Kjeldsen, D.: Smoking and atherosclerosis, Copenhagen, 1969, Munksgarr.

24. Air Quality Data for Carbon Monoxide, 1970, U. S. Department of Health, Education, and Welfare, National Air Pollution Control Administration, No. AP-62.

25. Lilienthal, J. L., Jr.: Carbon monoxide, Pharmacol. Rev. **2:**324-354, 1950.

26. Abramowicz, M., and Kass, E. H.: Pathogenesis and prognosis of prematurity, New Eng. J. Med. **275:**938-943, 1966.

27. Haddon, W., Jr., Nesbitt, R. E. L., and Garcia, R.: Smoking and pregnancy: carbon monoxide in the blood during gestation and at term, Obstet. and Gynec. **18:**262-267, 1961.

28. Hexter, A. C., and Goldsmith, J. R.: Carbon monoxide: association of community air pollution and mortality, Science **172:**265-267, 1971.

29. McFarland, R. A., Roughton, F. J. W., Halperin, M. H., and others: The effects of carbon monoxide and altitude on visual thresholds, J. Aviation Med. **15:**381-384, 1944.

30. Beard, R. R., and Wertheim, G. A.: Behavioral impairment associated with small doses of carbon monoxide, Amer. J. Publ. Health **57:**2012-22, 1967.

31. Anderson, R. F., Allensworth, D. C., and DeGroot, W. J.: Myocardial toxicity from carbon monoxide poisoning, Ann. Intern. Med. **67:**1172-1182, 1967.

32. Sorokina, S. T.: A study of carbon monoxide concentrations in the air of living dwellings and its effect on the organism, U.S.S.R. Literature **8:**207-213, 1963.

33. Wilson, E. F., Rich, T. H., and Messman, H. C.: The Hazardous hibachi: carbon monoxide poisoning following use of charcoal, J.A.M.A. **221:**405-406, 1972.

34. Astrup, P. Kjeldsen, K., and Wanstrup, J.: Enhancing influence of carbon monoxide on the development of atheromatosis in cholesterol-fed rabbits, J. Atheroscler. Res. **7:**343, 1967.

35. Garland, H., and Pearce, J.: Neurological complications of carbon monoxide poisoning, Quart. J. Med. **36:**445-454, 1967.

36. Leavell, U. W., Farley, C. H., and McIntyre, J. S.: Cutaneous changes in a patient with carbon monoxide poisoning, Arch. Derm. **99:**429-433, 1969.

37. Miner, S.: Air pollution aspects of hydrogen sulfide, Litton Systems, Inc., Bethesda, Maryland, 1969, U. S. Department of Commerce, National Bureau of Standards, PB 188 068.

38. Permissible emission concentrations of hydrogen sulfide, Subcommittee of effects of hydrogen sulfide of the Committee on Effects of Dust and Gas of the Verein Deutscher Ingenieure Committee of Air Purification, VDI Verlag G.M.B.H. Düsseldorf 2107, 1960.

39. Petri, H.: The effects of hydrogen sulfide and carbon disulfide, Staub **21:**64, 1961.

40. Adelson, L., and Sunshine, I.: Fatal hydrogen sulfide intoxication, Arch. Path. **81:**375-380, 1966.

41. Threshold limit values for 1966, Cincinnati, Ohio, 1966, American Conference of Governmental Industrial Hygienists, p. 10.

42. Hurwitz, L. J., and Taylor, G. I.: Poisoning by sewer gas with unusual sequellae, Lancet **1:**1110-1112, 1954.

43. Thoman, M.: Sewer gas: hydrogen sulfide intoxication, Clin. Tox. **2:**383-386, 1969.

44. The air pollution situation in Terre Haute, Indiana, with special reference to the hydrogen sulfide incident May-June 1964. A Joint Report to the City of Terre Haute by U. S. Public Health Service, Division of Air Pollution, and Indiana Air Pollution Control Board, Division of Sanitary Engineering, June 1964.

45. Halley, P. D.: Hazards of hydrogen sulfide, Med. Bull. **27:**219, 1967.

12
SYSTEMIC POISONS: lead and mercury

In contrast to the agents that mainly involve the lungs, the following chapters deal with systemic atmospheric poisons that affect numerous organs. Among them, lead, mercury, fluoride, and cadmium warrant foremost attention as atmospheric pollutants. They are emitted from both moving and stationary sources. They constitute the greatest threat to our environment at the present time because they accumulate in the system and produce illnesses that develop slowly and insidiously.

Ill effects from lead have been recognized for centuries; damage to human health by mercury has come to the fore during the last decade. Cadmium has only recently emerged as a significant atmospheric pollutant. On the other hand, damage by fluorides to plant and animal life was established years ago, but its deleterious effect upon human health has been underrated and is only now attracting the attention it warrants.

Systemic poisons that rival the above-mentioned ones in significance, the chlorinated hydrocarbons and organophosphates, are discussed in Chapter 18.

LEAD

On June 11, 1967, two sisters, age 2 and 3, were admitted to the Bradford (England) Children's Hospital. They died in convulsions within a few days.[1] At the same time several domestic animals in the neighborhood where the two sisters lived had convulsions and died. Prompted by this coincidence, local health officials investigated the area, particularly the homes of the pet owners. An initial survey on 60 persons revealed 5 additional children and 2 adults with lead (Pb) poisoning caused by inhaling fumes of lead-containing storage batteries that were being burned in the area. Blood tests revealed the characteristic stippling of red blood cells; and roentgenograms showed the typical "lead lines" in long bones, that is, dense horizontal zones indicative of lead poisoning. Substantial quantities of lead had adhered to the plastic cases of the batteries and had been emitted into the air during burning. The plastic cases themselves appeared to be harmless. Both the inhalation of airborne lead particles and food contaminated by airborne lead had poisoned the children.

Sources

The hazard of lead as a powerful poison has been recognized since early civilization. Water pipes and primitive tools were made of lead; vessels used for cooking, eating, and wine storage contained the metal.

Lead is produced in larger quantities than any other poisonous heavy metal. The current world production per year is estimated to be 3.5 million tons, 3.1 of which are produced in the northern hemisphere.[2] In modern times lead has played a role in occupational disease among miners and smelters, automobile finishers, foundry and storage battery workers, typesetters, sheet metal workers and spray painters. In the southeastern United States lead in equipment used for the illegal distillation of whiskey took its toll of illness and death during the prohibition era. Lead-containing paints, especially white lead, chrome green, and chrome yellow,* and lead in solder used to seal food cans have contributed materially to the incidence of plumbism (chronic poisoning) in recent years. In 1918, 40% of all painters showed evidence of lead poisoning.[2] Less common sources of the disease are inorganic and organic lead salts, which are added as stabilizers to plastics, to ceramic glaze, and to enamel jewelry.[3]

New interest in lead as an environmental hazard was stimulated by the discovery in 1952 by members of the staff of John Hopkins Hospital in Baltimore that, in children between the ages of 1 and 3, chronic lead poisoning is common and, indeed, frequently fatal. In Philadelphia, for instance, over a 14-year period, 804 cases of plumbism with 76 deaths were discovered.[4] Eighty-two percent of the deaths occurred between the ages of 12 to 36 months.

According to the U. S. Public Health Service, in 400,000 American children lead blood levels are elevated and 16,000 require treatment for lead poisoning. Approximately 3200 will suffer moderate to severe brain damage and will require years of special care.[5]

Lead poisoning in children is caused in part by their habit, referred to as "pica," of consuming strange and unnatural material such as soil, flaking paint from cribs, or plaster from walls (Fig. 12-1). Habitual chewing on toothpaste tubes[6] and on the painted surface of lead pencils has caused

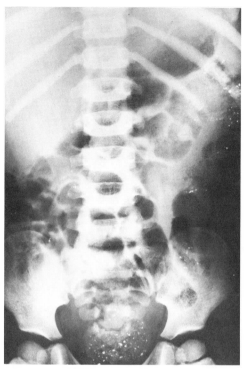

Fig. 12-1. This roentgenogram shows lead particles in a 3-year-old girl with pica (chewing on painted plaster). The small dots throughout the abdomen represent lead particles inside the bowels. (Courtesy X-ray Department of Children's Hospital of Michigan, Detroit.)

lead poisoning in children. Residing and playing near highway construction areas or where old buildings containing lead paint are being torn down* is a significant cause of poisoning in children, who are much more susceptible to it than adults (Table 12-1).

During the past four decades the development of the lead alkyls—namely, tetraethyl and tetramethyl lead as an antiknock gasoline—has created one of the most hazardous sources of environmental pollution. One gallon of gasoline contains up to 4 gm of lead (Table 12-2). About 300,000

---

*Recently suggestions have been made that famous painters such as Goya and Van Gogh may have died of poisoning as the result of chronic inhalation and ingestion of toxic lead-based paints. (Niederland, W. C., N. Y. J. Med. **72:**413-418, 1972.)

---

*Lead based paint is still being used today for the exteriors of buildings and remains a potential source of exposure.

Table 12-1. Nonfood items ingested by 58 children with an increased body burden of lead*

Crayons and toys	43
Paper and clothes	38
Dirt and sand	37
Lead paint-impregnated plaster	34
Paint flakes	20
Furniture	15
Window sills	14
Wallpaper	7

*Adapted from Pueschel, S. M., Kopito, L., and Schwachman, H.: Children with an increased lead burden, J.A.M.A. **222**:462-66, 1972.

Table 12-2. Average lead content of gasoline 1970-1971*

	GM PER GALLON	
	1970	1971
Regular gasoline	2.43	2.22
Premium gasoline	2.81	2.67
Low-lead and no lead gasoline		0.75

*Adapted from Use of lead in gasoline declining, Chemical and Engineering News, **50**:4, 1972.

tons of lead were used in gasoline additives in 1968. This amount constitutes about 25% of the total lead used in the United States.[3]

Ubiquity of lead

In soil. Lead is present in soil, water, food, and air and in numerous industrial products. The average lead content of soil is about 16 ppm.[8] In agricultural soils the levels range somewhat higher, namely from 14 to 95 ppm, because of the use of lead-containing sprays. Lead in antiknock gasoline has contributed materially to existing lead levels of soil.[9] In city dust the lead content is about 1% (10,000 ppm). Figures approaching 5% have been reported from Germany.[10] Such concentrations are similar to those of many lead ores.

At the Staten Island Zoo where animals suffered from lead poisoning, soils and leaves contained 3900 ppm (dry weight) an amount equal to or exceeding the levels alongside heavily travelled expressways.[11] Although lead arsenate sprays are no longer used in the United States, the contamination of soils where tobacco is grown is still responsible for traces of lead in tobacco. In filtered cigarettes, 24.1 ppm has been reported.[12] In 1961 Schroeder and associates[13] reported that smokers inhaled from 1.0 to 3.3 μg of lead per cigarette or 20 to 66μg per pack, which is believed to be derived from lead arsenate sprays.

In water. Since in most plumbing lead pipes have been replaced by copper and galvanized piping, water now contributes little to the total lead intake in humans. In ground and surface water, concentrations of lead range from 6 to 50 μg/liter.[14] This concentration, however, may be considerably exceeded when the water is conducted into storm drain outlets.[15] Furthermore, drinking water that remains for a prolonged period in lead-containing pipes or inside water storage tanks that have been painted with lead chromate may show higher lead values than those encountered ordinarily in water. Soft and acid waters dissolve more lead from pipes and plumbing joints than do hard waters.

In air. In ambient air, the greatest sources of lead are leaded gasoline, production and processing of lead, natural lead fallout, and, to a lesser extent, coal that contains approximately 54 ppm lead. Over 180,000 tons of lead annually spew into the air in the United States from tail pipes of automobiles, trucks, and busses.[16] In large cities such as Cincinnati and Los Angeles, 1860 kg and 14,000 kg, respectively, of lead is being burned per day with gasoline,[8] one quarter to one half of which reaches the air as bromide, chloride, and ammonium complexes. Lead levels in ambient air range from 1.6 μg/meter[3] in Cincinnati[17] to 9.8 μg/meter[3] in Paris, France.[8] During a peak traffic period in Los Angeles county, 71.3 μg/meter^3 was recorded.[18] In the Great Plains and Rocky Mountain areas, Schroeder and others[13] found 0.2 μg/meter^3; in New England and at the Pacific coast, 0.7 μg/meter^3 of lead in air was found. Some of the lead particles tend to fall out on the street.

Lesser amounts in ambient air are derived from radon decay, from the surfaces of the earth, from evaporation of sea salts, and from forest fires. About 1% of lava exuded from a volcano is lead.

In food. The major source of environmental lead intake in humans is food. An average daily diet is estimated to provide about 0.3 mg.[19] Plants take up lead mainly from leaves and relatively little from soil, to which lead is tightly bound in insoluble compounds. Plants growing on soils containing 1 ppm of lead have shown 20 to 25 ppm lead per gram in their ash.[20] Samples taken from different portions of a plant vary considerably in their lead content. Therefore, a lead assay of a leaf or of the total plant does not necessarily disclose the amount of lead contained in fruit or grain.

Along heavily traveled highways, fruit and vegetables nearest to the traffic show the highest lead load. Levels up to 3000 ppm have been recorded.[21] In an extensive survey of lead in food, Schroeder and others[13] found the highest lead levels in lettuce (1.04 ppm), kale (1.26 ppm), Swiss chard (0.75 ppm), puffed rice (7.49 ppm), and lobster (2.5 ppm).

Body burden of lead

Uptake. In modern United States communities, the daily intake of lead has been estimated by Kehoe[19] to be about 0.35 mg, 0.31 mg of which is derived from food, 0.02 mg from water, and 0.02 mg from air.* However, only about 5% to 10% of ingested lead reaches the bloodstream with food

from the intestinal tract,[19] in contrast to 30% to 50% of inhaled lead. The small size of airborne lead ($<$ than 1 μ) facilitates its absorption through the alveoli.[22] In comparing the daily absorption of inhaled with that of ingested lead it appears that in a contaminated area lead that reaches the bloodstream through inhalation is of greater significance than lead consumed with food and water. Table 12-3 presents the daily amounts of inhaled lead in a person breathing 20 meter^3/day of air, the normal amount.

The last two figures in Table 12-3 are much higher than the "normal" amount of lead absorbed from food and water, namely 15 to 30 μg, based on 5% to 10% of the 300 μg average consumed daily with food and water.

Thus a person breathing congested traffic air containing 5 to 10 μg/meter^3 of lead is already absorbing lead at or close to the toxic level (100 to 300 μg/day), excluding the amount ingested from food and water.

Transport. Blood levels range from 0.05 to 0.4 ppm with much more lead in red blood cells than in blood plasma—namely, 0.24 ppm and 0.015 ppm, respectively.[23] The threshold for acute intoxication is believed to be in the range of 0.5 to 0.8 ppm.[24]* Blood values for lead in persons exposed persistently to automobile exhaust as, for instance, traffic policemen and those residing adjacent to busy highways are decidedly higher than normal.[25] The lead level in the blood of those working in downtown Philadelphia was found to be almost twice as high as the level found in those living in Philadelphia suburbs.[25]

---

*Kehoe's figure of inhaled lead is considered by some investigators to be too low.[8,17,18]

*Inmates of two Swiss prisons, one in open country, the other near a highway, have recently been found to have the abnormally high mean lead blood levels of 0.406 and 0.433 ppm, respectively. Yet the corresponding mean urinary levels were only 0.0288 and 0.0355 ppm. Such high blood levels are usually associated with much higher urinary values, perhaps twice those found in the Swiss prisons.[26a]

Storage. Lead accumulates in bones, where it replaces calcium. Bones store almost one half of the total body pool,[23] with long bones (arms and legs) accumulating about 3 times more than flat bones (breast bone, vertebrae). Becker and coworkers[26] found 5 ppm lead in ancient bones 500 years old in comparison to 50 ppm, which is present in bones today. They implicated contemporary air pollution as the primary cause of this increase.

With advancing age, some of the metabolized lead accumulates in soft tissues (Table 12-4). Newly absorbed lead is retained in the body as lead triphosphate, especially in liver, kidneys, pancreas, and aorta.

Table 12-3. Lead absorbed into the bloodstream from inhalation

LEAD CONTENT OF AIR μg per meter^3	ESTIMATE OF LEAD ABSORBED BY A PERSON BREATHING 20 METER^3/DAY (BASED ON 30% TO 50% OF LEAD INHALED) μg
0.5	3 to 5
1.0	6 to 10
2.0	12 to 20
5.0	30 to 50
10.0	60 to 100

Table 12-4. Mean tissue lead concentrations (ppm wet weight)*

TISSUE	NONOCCUPATIONAL EXPOSURE		HEAVY EXPOSURE
	MALES	FEMALES	FOUR MALES
Bone			
Tibia	21.03	16.05	221.00
Rib	8.66	6.43	61.00
Hair	18.44	19.07	——
Nails	9.40	——	——
Adrenal glands	0.16	0.18	0.11
Aorta (atheroma)	2.39	0.85	9.95
Blood	0.22	0.14	0.20
Brain cortex	0.12	0.15	4.17
Feces†	0.21	0.21	——
Fat	0.15	0.08	——
Gastrointestinal tract	0.10	0.14	0.11
Heart	0.07	0.08	0.35
Kidney	0.58	0.42	0.53
Liver	0.98	0.63	1.36
Lung	0.20	0.22	0.16
Lymph glands (lungs)	0.42	0.44	0.33
Muscle	0.06	0.05	——
Ovary	——	0.34	——
Pancreas	0.42	0.26	0.33
Prostate gland	0.32	——	0.38
Skin	0.11	0.09	——
Spleen	0.25	0.18	——
Testis	0.09	——	——
Thyroid	0.17	0.25	0.19
Urine	0.05	0.03	——

*Adapted from Barry, P. S. I., and Mossman, D. B.: Lead concentrations in human tissues, Brit. J. Industr. Med. 27:339-351, 1970.

†As ppm ash weight.

Table 12-5. Approximate daily lead balance in a normal individual*

From food	0.22 mg	Feces	0.30 mg
From water	0.10	Urine	0.50
From inhaled dust	0.08	Stored in bones	0.05
Totals	0.40 mg		0.40 mg

*Adapted from Durum, W. H., Hem, J. D., and Heidel, S. G.: Reconnaissance of selected minor elements in surface waters in the United States, Washington, D. C., 1971, Geological Survey Circular 643, Department of Interior.

Excretion. The principal routes of elimination of lead are the feces and, to a lesser extent, urine and sweat. In febrile diseases and disturbances of the calcium-phosphorus metabolism, lead that had been stored in the body may be mobilized and cause recurrences of poisoning years after exposure.

Biochemical aspect

Lead affects the formation of blood in two important ways: (1) by retarding the normal maturation of red blood cells in the bone marrow, it produces stippling of red blood cells and anemia; and (2) it inhibits the synthesis of hemoglobin by interfering with two important substances necessary for formation of hemoglobin—namely, delta-aminolevulinic acid and coproporphyrin III. In lead poisoning both substances are excreted in the urine in excess. Normal daily coproporphyrin values in urine vary between 0.5 to 1.5 μg/liter as compared with levels of 9.8 μg/liter in lead intoxication. The inhibition of the activity of delta-aminolevulinic acid dehydrogenase in red blood cells, an enzyme involved in the synthesis of hemoglobin, serves as a diagnostic criterion in the early stage of lead intoxication before symptoms are pronounced. This enzyme is inhibited when inorganic lead levels in the blood are between 0.2 and 0.4 ppm, those now prevalent in the general population.[28] The concentration of delta-aminolevulinic acid in plasma rises in lead poisoning from about 30 to 125 μg/100 liter.

Symptoms of poisoning

Lead gives rise to a wide variety of symptoms that involve mainly the blood-forming mechanism, the gastrointestinal tract and, in the advanced stage, the nervous system. Kidneys and heart can also be affected in lead poisoning.

The early stage. In the beginning stage of the disease the patients are anemic. They feel weak and tired. They complain of headaches and pains in muscles. They become clumsy and irritable. They are restless, easily distracted, and impulsive. Children develop pain in the stomach and lower abdomen; they are constipated, often nauseated, and complain of heartburn. In adults the abdominal pains can become so severe as to suggest bowel obstruction.

When the anemia fails to improve with the usual medications, physicians become suspicious of lead poisoning. They look for stippling of red blood cells and check the urine for coproporphyrin III and delta-aminolevulinic acid; they also analyze the urine and blood: lead levels in the blood higher than 0.6 ppm are indicative of lead poisoning. Roentgenograms reveal an increased density of the bones, horizontal lines at the epiphyses (the terminal portions of long bones) (Fig. 12-2, A and B), and condensation of the inner table of the skull, especially at the forehead. Occasionally, opacities of lead itself can be visualized in the bowels (Fig. 12-1). Black stools caused by occult bleeding from the bowels and the so-called lead line, a pigmentation on gums, which have been em-

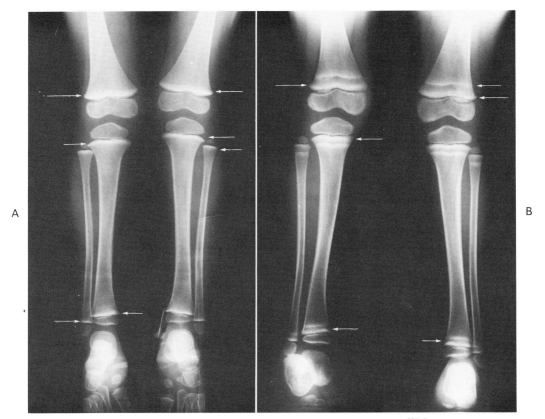

Fig. 12-2. A, Roentgenogram of legs of a 3-year-old girl showing typical lead lines (arrows). **B,** Second episode of poisoning 6 months later produced a second line in the same area as before. The former line had moved farther into the bone substance.

phasized in the literature as characteristic signs of lead poisoning, in reality occur infrequently, especially in adults.

Kidney diseases, particularly damage to the arteries of the kidneys[29] and involvement of the proximal tubules, occur in connection with lead poisoning with crippling atrophy (shrinkage) of the organ. Jaundice and gout have also been encountered in individuals with chronic kidney disease caused by lead poisoning.

Advanced intoxication—brain damage. The most serious manifestation of the disease is the involvement of the nervous system. A strong affinity of lead to nerve tissue accounts for a wide variety of neurologic symptoms ranging from drowsiness to coma and epileptic convulsions. Children lose their balance, become clumsy and lethargic. After prolonged, grossly excessive lead absorption, paralysis of the eye muscles and of the extensor muscles of legs and feet occurs.

A classic sign of advanced plumbism is the wristdrop caused by palsy of the medianus nerve, which supplies the extensor muscles of the hand. Damage to the optic nerve leading to blindness has also been reported in lead poisoning. The cerebrospinal fluid is under pressure and contains a high concentration of protein and of white blood cells.

Course of the disease. The disease can lead to early death or result in permanent injury. In a Chicago survey[30] 257 of 405 children with chronic lead poisoning recovered completely, the remaining ones had permanent neurologic symptoms, mainly mental retardation and recurrent epileptic seizures; 9 had contracted cerebral palsy with spasticity in the extremities; 5 had optic nerve atrophy (blindness).

In women, lead causes sterility and cessation of menstruation.[7] A pregnant woman and her fetus seem to be particularly vulnerable to lead. Abortions and stillbirths, as well as premature births have been encountered in women exposed to excessive amounts of lead.[31]

Diseases with which lead poisoning is often confused are vitamin B deficiency, diabetes, and arsenic poisoning.

Case reports

Lead poisoning involving a physician's family was described in November 1969 in a popular magazine.[32] The following account of the illness illustrates the enigma with which the diagnostician is confronted.

Five of the six members of the family experienced fatigue, poor appetite, vague pains in the stomach, and vomiting. Unexplained changes in personality in three of the four children as well as in the parents took place. They left most of their meals unfinished. They became increasingly irritable to the point of quarreling with each other. Only the infant who was still on formula experienced no ill effect. A slight trauma of the head of one of the boys, which precipitated vomiting and paralysis of the left extremities, prompted an exploratory opening of the skull. This procedure showed that the spinal fluid was under pressure. The blood count disclosed marked anemia, suggestive of severe malnutrition. Tests on the other four members of the family revealed that they too had a serious anemia indicative of some kind of poisoning. Eventually the diagnosis was established on the basis of typical stippling of red blood cells.

Considerable detective work was required to identify the source of the lead poisoning: an earthenware pitcher had contaminated the orange juice that all members of the family, with the exception of the infant, had been drinking daily. Because the pitcher had not been fired long enough at a high temperature, lead had leached from the pitcher's glaze into the acid juice. The local health department determined that enough lead chromate came out of the juice pitcher in one washing with acid to kill two people. Lead in the orange juice, after 24 hours in the pitcher, was estimated at 15 mg in 100 ml of juice.

Table 12-6. Laboratory data on the McDevitt family*

Blood		Normal
Lead: on admission	194 μg% (1.94 ppm)	0–60 μg%
after recovery	6 μg% (0.06 ppm)	
Uroporphyrin	161 μg/liter	0–30 μg/liter
Coproporphyrin III	1.008 μg/liter	none
Stippled red blood cells	10 to 15 per oil power field	none
Blood platelets	302,000–650,000	300,000
Urine (24 hour)		
Lead: before recovery	14 mg/liter	0.1 mg/liter
after recovery	6.5 mg/liter	
Delta-aminolevulinic acid	3.3 mg/liter	1.3–7.0 mg/liter
Coproporphyrin III	5.4 μg/liter	0–60 μg/liter

*Courtesy Dr. T. J. McDevitt, Pocatello, Idaho.

The child who had undergone surgery and the other members of the family recovered after discovery and removal of the cause.

Tetraethyl and tetramethyl lead poisoning

Poisoning with tetraethyl and tetramethyl lead, the two contaminants from automobile exhaust, differs from inorganic lead intoxication because of their predominant effect on the central nervous system. Heat in the combustion chamber, in the crankcase, or in the carburetor of an automobile tends to decompose most organic lead to inorganic lead, which constitutes an additional hazard to human health. About 75% of particulate lead from automobile combustion is less than 0.9 μ in mean diameter, a size that easily reaches the alveoli.[33]

In its acute phase, caused by massive doses,* this kind of poisoning which has occurred only in workers engaged in the production of leaded gasoline, constitutes a classic example of how a serious mental disease can originate from a poisonous agent. Patients exposed to these compounds, even for short periods, show nervous irritability, sleeplessness, terrifying dreams, emotional instability, and gastrointestinal symptoms with vomiting and diarrhea. With more intensive exposure the victims of the disease become irrational and develop delusions and hallucinations with dramatic suddenness. They may have to be restrained even when under the influence of sedatives. The disease resembles acute alcoholic hallucinations or a catatonic schizophrenia, a common mental disease.

Because of the rapid elimination of organic lead compounds through the urine, anemia and elevation of lead levels in blood and urine do not occur as they do in inorganic lead poisoning. In contrast with in-

*A concentration of alkyllead (0.1 to 2 μg/meter[3]) observed in central Stockholm is considered too small to cause acute toxic effects in a city population.[34]

organic lead poisoning, the patients show a marked tremor. Some develop impaired vision and optic nerve degeneration associated with high tension of the eyeball of the kind encountered in glaucoma. Others experience disturbances of the inner ear.

There are indications that chronic lead poisoning from automobile exhaust fumes may either contribute to or cause low-grade lead encephalitis (inflammation of the brain) among urban populations, the symptoms of which are depression, headache, and undue fatigue. Treatment with the lead chelating agent calcium-EDTA rapidly leads to improvement or complete cure in 85% of the cases.[35]

With the awareness of physicians, especially health authorities, of the seriousness of the three kinds—namely, pediatric, adult inorganic, and organic lead poisoning—measures to restrict the use of lead and to assure safe handling of the metal are likely to reduce the incidence of lead intoxication.

MERCURY

In March 1968 Swedish health officials warned their citizens not to eat fish from most fresh and coastal waters more than once a week because of the hazard of methyl mercury poisoning.

For the same reason on April 14, 1970 Michigan's governor issued a decree that stopped fishing in Lakes St. Clair and Erie. On March 31 of that year the Canadian fishing authorities had taken a similar step. Subsequently, Ohio's governor followed suit. Along the St. Clair River, Lake St. Clair, the Detroit River, and Lake Erie, large chloralkali plants had been discharging daily approximately 200 pounds of waste metallic mercury (Hg) into the waters. About one half pound of mercury is emitted for each ton of chlorine produced. Other contaminating sources were pulp and paper factories and the electrical industry. Pickerel caught in Lake St. Clair contained 5 ppm mercury. The economic impact of this measure was particularly painful to Ontario's fishing industry; about 95% of the pickerel caught in Lake Erie is sold to the United States.

Less than a year prior to these events, the magazine *Environment* pointed to the "new pollution problem" that had arisen as the result of mercury poisoning.[36] Actually the problem of mercury pollution has been cropping up repeatedly in the United States during the last two decades, ever since mercury poisoning was reported in 1935 by Neal and Jones[37] in a detailed study of 529 workers in the fur-cutting industry, where pelts were treated with a solution containing inorganic mercury. Eight percent of these workers were afflicted with chronic poisoning. One-tenth milligram of mercury per cubic meter of air has been set as the safe 8-hour limit for industrial workers.

Properties of mercury

Mercury compounds are divided chemically into inorganic salts—namely elemental mercury, mercuric and mercurous salts, and organic compounds. The latter contain a carbon atom covalently bound to mercury.

Inorganic mercury is insoluble in water, in alkalies, and in dilute hydrochloric acid. It vaporizes at room temperature. With every degree of rise in temperature its volatility rises by 10 degrees. When spilled on floors and dirty tables, evaporation is further increased by dust and grease with which it combines to form minute globules, thus exposing larger surface areas to air.

Three groups of *organic* mercury compounds are important toxicologically—aryl mercury (phenyl mercury), alkyl mercury (methyl and ethyl mercury), alkoxyalkyl mercury (methoxy ethyl mercury).

Uses of mercury

In medicine. As early as the year 1500, mercury was used in treatment of syphilis. Undoubtedly it has contributed to the death of many patients. Similarly calomel (mercurous chloride) was a popular ca-

thartic until a few decades ago, when physicians became aware of its toxic action. Even today, certain organic mercury compounds serve as effective diuretics to induce elimination of excess fluids from the kidneys. Amalgams (an alloy of mercury with other metal) are still extensively used in dentistry today. For instance, in Sweden, dentists use between 15 and 20 tons of mercury a year.[38]

In agriculture. In agriculture, mercury compounds have had widespread uses, principally because of their ability to counteract the growth of fungi (Table 12-7). Fungi tend to grow wherever moisture is combined with a proper growth medium, especially sugars and starches in grain. To prevent spoilage of grain by fungous growth, a method of treating seed grain with mercury compounds was introduced in Germany in 1914. In the 1930s, the dry spray was supplemented by a liquid solution of alkylmercury (a powerful poison) for spraying, particularly, apple trees, tomato and potato plants, and rice fields in Japan. In the United States 16.5% of some 6 million pounds of mercury marketed yearly are thus added to agricultural soils. Much of the metal leaches from soil into waterways.

The pesticide accumulates in a growing plant. It is transmitted from the leaves throughout the branches and stalks and thus contaminates the food that is marketed. For some reason, the fruit of an apple tree accumulates more mercury than any other portion.

The U. S. Food and Drug Administration prohibits the sale of food containing mercury. Nevertheless, grain, apples, eggs, milk, and other products show levels in the range of 0.01 to 0.1 ppm as compared to 0.05 ppm, the highest allowable concentration suggested by the World Health Organization. In Germany the sale of food contaminated by mercury pesticides is forbidden. Czechoslovakia permits concentrations up to 0.03 ppm.[39]

Table 12-7. Quantities of mercury compounds used in agriculture, 1965 to 1966*

COUNTRY	METRIC TONS OF MERCURY COMPOUNDS
Japan	1,600 (approx.)†
United States	400
Germany	41
Italy	26
Turkey	22.5
Great Britain	20
Poland	9
Spain	7.1
Bulgaria	5
Austria	4
Denmark	3.5
Sweden	2
Finland	1
Morocco	1
New Zealand	0.5
Norway	0.4
Israel	0.2
Portugal	0.2

*Adapted from Novick, S.: A new pollution problem; Löfroth, G., Duffy, M. E.: Birds gave warning; Grant, N.: Legacy of the mad hatter, Environment, 11:2-23, 1969.
†During the past few years public pressure has led to almost complete abandonment of spraying rice fields with mercury.

In industry. The two principal industries in which mildew must be prevented are paint and paper manufacturing. The laundry industry, also, particularly the diaper services, must prevent fungous growth. In nuclear research, fungi tend to attack plastic portions of research reactors, especially in tropical, moist climates that favor the production of molds. The favorite compound used for this purpose is phenylmercury acetate (PMA). This compound added to paints has become one of the largest uses of mercury in the United States. As the paint dries, mercury evaporates and reaches the air in toxic concentrations.

In the paper industry mercury protects wood pulp stored for processing from becoming moldy. It is also employed in cleansing the paper-making machinery of the slimy fungous material that adheres to it. Mercury thus finds its way into the paper itself. When paper is burned, mercury becomes airborne. In recent years, its use in the paper industry is being restricted and replaced by chlorine.

Municipal incinerators and coal-burning power and industrial plants are emitting from 100 to 5400 pounds of mercury vapor per year at individual sites. The total yearly amount released by coal, petroleum, and asphalt constitutes the largest contribution of mercury to air pollution.[40]

Other applications of mercury are in the electrolytic production of chlorine and caustic soda. In chlorine factories, mercury electrodes release mercury into the air and into the water. In many other chemical manufacturing processes mercury serves as a catalyst, especially in the manufacture of vinyl chloride, the important building stone of many plastics. In manufacturing of scientific instruments, thermometers,* barometers, gauges and mercury-vapor lamps, and in laboratories and hospitals where they are used, mercury vapor has led to poisoning.

Ubiquity of mercury

Mercury is widely distributed in nature.

In *soil* it is present at levels of 0.05 ppm, but certain volcanic rocks consisting largely of cinnabar (HgS) may contain from 1 to 30 ppm.[41] According to Joensuu[42] coal contains from 0.09 to 33 ppm. About 3000 tons are released annually throughout the world from this source.

Atmospheric concentrations may reach up to 16 ppb near mercury mines. Since it is carried considerable distances by the wind, both as a particulate and in vaporized form, food can become contaminated by mercury from the air without direct application. This possibility was driven home when fish from a lake called Joe's Pond in Vermont far distant from industry,

*It is estimated that 1.8 million mercury-containing thermometers are broken yearly in Canadian hospitals and 1.2 million in Canadian homes.[40]

Table 12-8. Mercury in blood and hair*

	WHOLE BLOOD (PPB)	RED BLOOD CELLS (PPB)	HAIR (PPB)
Normal levels	5	10	10
Estimated maximum "safe" level	50	100	—
Estimated level for overt symptoms	500	1,000	150
Fatal level of Niigata case	1,300	2,400	500

*Adapted from Eyl, T. B., Wilcox, K. R., and Reizen, M. S.: Fish and human health, Mich. Med. 69:873-880, 1970.

contained four times the United States allowable content of mercury.[43]

Rainwater contains an average of 0.2 ppb according to Swedish reports. In ocean water mercury varies widely with a range of 0.03 to 5.0 ppb. Near mercury deposits, waters contain from 5 to 100 ppb. Inorganic mercury from industrial wastes settles at the bottom of lakes and rivers because of its heavy specific gravity. Concentrations as high as 692 ppm have been found in Lake Ontario mud and up to 1800 ppm near a Saskatoon chloralkali plant.[44] In the absence of oxygen, the inorganic mercury is converted into the very toxic methyl mercury $(CH_3)_2$ Hg by the bacterium *Methanobacterium amelanskis.*

Through the *food chain* mercury becomes more concentrated as it is taken up by its various links: mercury penetrates the surface of plankton by passive absorption. In contrast, fish take up methyl mercury both through consumption of food, mainly plankton, and through their gills. Fish that breathe faster and eat more than other species, such as tuna, concentrate more mercury in their bodies during their lifetime than other fish. The older the fish, the greater is the mercury concentration in its body. The metal accumulates in its body fats. A long retention time in some fish (mercury's half-life is 200 days)* accounts for added accumulation.[40] Birds that eat fish concentrate even more mercury in their

body. Whales and seals have been found to contain very high levels of mercury.[45]

Body burden of mercury

The kind of symptoms produced by mercury, its distribution, accumulation, and excretion from the body, depend on whether elemental mercury or a mercury compound is involved, as well as upon the kind of chemical transformation of the mercury compound that takes place inside the human body.

Inorganic mercury is absorbed through inhalation of its vapors and through prolonged contact of the skin with the metal. Normal blood levels range from 1 to 3 $\mu g/100$ mg (0.030 ppm).

Table 12-8 shows a comparison of levels in blood and hair at various stages of toxicity.[46]

Amounts of methyl mercury of 0.2 ppm have been identified with symptoms of poisoning.[47] Urinary mercury levels in poisoning are below 20 $\mu g/100$ ml. However, such values cannot always be utilized in the diagnosis of mercury poisoning, since mercury disappears rapidly from blood. Individuals with signs of poisoning may have less mercury in their blood and urine than those without evidence of poisoning.[48]

Mercury levels in body tissue were presented in a study by Howie and Smith[49] on routine autopsies in the Glasgow area of persons who had died as the result of violence. The kidneys, hair, and thymus gland showed the highest mercury concentrations (Table 12-9).

_____
*Time required for half of the mercury to be eliminated.

Table 12-9. Mean mercury values in dry tissue*

TISSUE	PPM	TISSUE	PPM
Adrenal gland	0.80	Nail (finger)	2.27
Aorta	1.39	Nail (toe)	2.40
Blood (whole)	0.09	Ovary	2.14
Bone	0.45	Pancreas	1.14
Brain	2.94	Prostate	0.65
Breast	1.79	Skin	3.34
Hair (head)	5.52	Spleen	1.50
Hair (in groins)	1.62	Stomach	2.27
Heart	1.76	Teeth	3.22
Kidney	9.03	Thymus	4.75
Liver	3.66	Thyroid	3.38
Lung	2.55	Uterus	1.43
Muscle (breast)	0.71		

*Adapted from Howie, R. A., and Smith, H.: Mercury in human tissue, Forensic Sci. 7:90-96, 1967.

Mass poisoning

In Japan. Between 1953 and 1960, a strange illness disabled 111 persons severely and killed 43 of them. They were mostly members of the families of fishermen in the Japanese coastal town of Minamata on the island of Kyushu (Minamata Bay). The illness began with vague symptoms. People became tired and irritable; they complained of headaches, numbness in arms and legs, and difficulty in swallowing. Their vision became blurred and their visual fields restricted. They became hard of hearing and lost muscular coordination. Some were constantly aware of a metallic taste in their mouth. Their gums were inflamed and diarrhea was widespread. Death resulted from a supervening infection or from gradual inanition.[50]

A factory producing plastics from vinyl chloride and acetaldehyde had discharged its mercury waste into the Minamata Bay and subsequently (1958) into the Minamata River. Fish in these waters contained between 27 and 102 ppm (dry weight) mercury.

In addition to the 111 cases, nineteen babies born in that area had congenital defects. Significantly, the symptoms of mercury poisoning in the mothers were min-imal or completely absent. For instance, in an infant girl who died at age 2½, the mother's only complaint was slight numbness of the fingers during pregnancy; otherwise, she had been perfectly healthy. The child had been nursed by the mother for 1 month and had not eaten enough fish to be harmful. At 3 months of age, the first convulsions occurred; arms and legs became spastic and the parents noted that the baby was mentally retarded. At postmortem, an unusually high level of mercury in the hair and other features of poisoning were found. The evidence strongly suggested that alkyl mercury was transferred from the mother to the fetus through the placenta.

Another epidemic of the same disease, caused by mercury emitted from an industrial plant, occurred in 1965 in Niigata on the Japanese island of Hon Shu.[51] Of 26 persons thus poisoned, 5 died. One hundred and twenty additional cases of illness were not classified as mercury poisoning because health authorities had stipulated that each individual must manifest every specific symptom in order to establish the diagnosis. The families had consumed fish containing 5 to 20 ppm mercury up to three times each day.

In Sweden. In the Japanese incidents the

Table 12-10. Mercury in Scandinavian meat products*

PRODUCT (RAW)	MERCURY (PPM)		
	SWEDISH (1965-1966)	DANISH	SWEDISH 1968 (MARCH-MAY)†
Pork chops	0.030	0.003	0.008
Beef	0.012	0.003	0.003
Bacon	0.018	0.004	—
Pig's liver	0.060	0.009	0.021
Ox liver	0.016	0.005	0.005

*Adapted from Westöö, G.: Mercury compounds in animal foods, Nordic Conference on Mercury, Norfcrsk, October 11-12, 1968; Prof. Gunnel Westöö of the Staten Institute Fôr Folkhälsan has carried out an enormous amount of work on methyl mercury assays from which most available data on mercury in food in Sweden have been obtained.

†After methyl mercury was banned in Sweden.

mercury compound constituted industrial waste discharged into water and consumed by fish. In Sweden poisoning developed in the early 1960s in a different manner: a drastic decrease of the bird population drew the attention of the health authorities to the mercury problem. The birds had been feeding on grain that had been treated with Panogen, a methyl mercury fungicide used to prevent mildew. Mercury had entered the food chain from grain to hen, to egg, to meat, and, finally, to man.[52] Because of the Japanese experience the Swedish authorities recognized the ability of mercury to damage human health.

Swedish eggs (Table 12-10) contained four times as much mercury as those from continental European countries, that is, an average of 0.029 ppm compared with 0.007. Revocation of the license to sell methyl mercury compounds for agricultural uses on February 1, 1966, produced a drastic reduction in mercury contamination of meat and eggs.

In addition to eggs, meat products were also contaminated by methyl mercury. Swedish and Norwegian meat contained considerably more mercury than the Danish products, where use of the poison had been restricted. Meat from wild life, especially from pheasant, was another signifi-

cant source of mercury intake in Sweden. Mercury emissions were also discovered in northern Sweden near Sundswall where a vinyl chloride factory discharged its mercury waste into the gulf of Bothnia.

Extensive investigations began in Sweden to survey the mercury distribution in other parts of the environment. Fish in midoceans were found to be relatively free of mercury, but fish caught in fresh and coastal waters of Sweden showed concentrations from 0.2 to 1 ppm. A pike caught in southern Sweden contained 9.8 ppm in wet muscle tissue.*

Middle East. Another mode of mass poisoning from agricultural organic mercury has been reported from the Middle East. In 1956 more than 100 patients including 14 who eventually died were admitted to Mosul Hospital in Iraq.[54] A subsequent outbreak in 1960 affected 221 farmers, at least 22 of whom died. They had consumed bread baked with wheat that had been dressed with Granosan M, a fungicide containing 7.7% ethyl mercury-toluene sulfonanilide with a total mercury content of 3.2%. Organ tissues at autopsy

_____

*In fish caught in coastal waters of the Irish Sea the concentration of mercury ranged from 0.10 to 0.5 mg/kg wet weight.[55a]

contained high levels of mercury. In one instance, the liver showed 65.8 ppm.

Pakistan. In Pakistan in 1961, 4 of 34 hospitalized patients died[55] of the same disease. Because of scarcity of wheat in Pakistan at that time, mercury dressed seed wheat was being consumed. The typical symptoms were burning sensation in the mouth, nausea, vomiting, weakness in arms and legs, mental confusion, slurred speech, and inability to stand and walk. Several patients had degenerative changes of the optic nerve. The organic mercury compound was Argrosan GN, a mixture of phenyl mercury acetate with ethyl mercury chloride, the mercury content of which was 1%. Autopsies showed ulcers in the stomach, damage to liver cells, and evidence of kidney involvement (pyelonephritis).

Inorganic vs. organic mercury compounds

Inorganic mercury. The action of inorganic mercury differs considerably from that of organic methyl mercury. Inorganic mercury usually settles in and damages the liver and kidneys, especially the kidney tubules, the portion of the nephron involved in reabsorption of vital agents from the urine. In the small intestines, it accounts for diarrhea. Mercury vapor diffuses readily through the alveolar membrane and reaches the brain, where it interferes with coordination.[56]

An example of the hazard of airborne inorganic mercury is the following acute case of poisoning reported by Howie and Smith.[49] A school boy took about 200 gm of mercury to his home where he played with it. The metal spilled over the living room carpet, from which it was further dispersed by means of an electric vacuum cleaner. Every member of the household contracted mercury poisoning.

All had a generalized tremor, a skin eruption, and one member experienced hallucinations. After father and son had received adequate treatment and the home had been thoroughly cleaned they returned home,

apparently cured. Two months later, however, the disease recurred possibly because of incomplete cleaning of the house.*

Organic mercury. In distinction to inorganic mercury the much more soluble methyl mercury and other compounds of the alkyl mercury group mainly affect the brain (Fig. 12-3). They penetrate easily through biologic membranes, which accounts for their wide distribution through the human body. They circulate in the bloodstream unchanged, bound to red blood cells, and then diffuse slowly into and destroy brain cells that control coordination. For unexplained reasons, the onset of these symptoms rarely occurs prior to 3 weeks following exposure; in some cases, no symptoms become manifest before 2 months have elapsed.

Whereas inorganic mercury compounds are excreted through the kidneys, methyl mercury is eliminated mainly through the bowels. Only 10% of it leaves the body through the kidneys.

Methyl mercury poisoning is characterized by atrophy (shrinkage) of brain cells in both the cerebellum and the brain cortex. The first symptoms are numbness in the fingers, lips, and tongue; the patient's speech becomes blurred, his gait atactic (incoordination of voluntary muscular movements) and he has difficulties in swallowing. Subsequently the patient develops deafness, blurred vision, and constriction of the visual fields. If mercury uptake ceases, the symptoms may gradually disappear.[52]

In the advanced stage the speech becomes loud, explosive, and unmoderated. Hearing is impaired inasmuch as the patient has difficulty in comprehending the meaning of what other persons say. Since those around him cannot understand his inarticulate speech, the patient is likely to lose contact with his surroundings. Some of these individuals have been classified

---

*The usual method of cleaning with a vacuum sweeper tends to spread the contamination further.

as neurotics, others have spent years in mental hospitals, their condition diagnosed as an unidentified mental disorder.

Alkyl mercury also penetrates the placental barrier as indicated by the fact that, in the Minamata episode, infants had been poisoned prior to birth. Engleson and Herner[57] described the case of a woman who had eaten food prepared from methyl mercury-treated seeds. Her infant girl was born with congenital cerebral palsy. Two other members of the family showed evidence of methyl mercury poisoning but the mother herself was free of symptoms. It is generally acknowledged that the fetus is more sensitive to poisoning than the mother. In newborn children, the average mercury concentration in the blood corpuscles is considerably higher than in the mother's blood corpuscles.[58] It is likely that methyl mercury has a strong affinity for the placenta and fetal tissue, thus protecting the mother from being poisoned.

Sometimes advanced organic mercury poisoning takes on the clinical features of amyotrophic lateral sclerosis, a disease of the spinal chord characterized by muscular wasting. In 1954 Brown[59] reported such a case in a 39-year-old farmer who developed weakness and progressive wasting of muscles in arms and legs, which, after 6 months, terminated fatally. In 24 hours he excreted 340 μg of mercury through his urine. When treatment to eliminate mercury was instituted, the daily excretion rose to 740 μg. For six to seven seasons, the farmer had been dusting his oat seeds with ethyl phenyl mercury, which contains as much as 7.7% mercury in inorganic form.

A 5-year-old boy had frequent pains in the abdomen and muscles.[60] He became weak and irritable, sensitive to light, and lost the muscular tone in arms and legs. His skin was dry and scaly and his hands had a peculiar pink color, a condition called

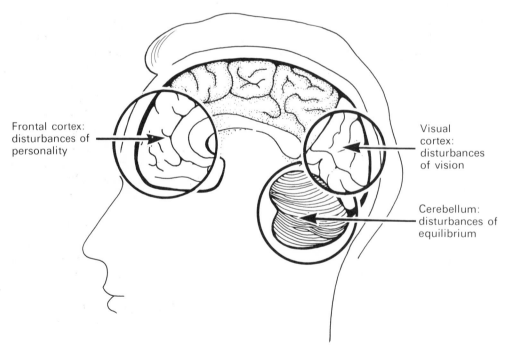

Frontal cortex: disturbances of personality

Visual cortex: disturbances of vision

Cerebellum: disturbances of equilibrium

Fig. 12-3. Methyl mercury attacks the cerebellum (small brain), which regulates balance, the visual cortex—the organ of visual perception—and, to a lesser extent, the frontal lobe, which produces disturbances of personality.

acrodynia. The urine showed from 0.1 to 0.5 ppm mercury. The child had helped paint the room in which he had been sleeping. The paint contained 0.036% phenylmercuric propionate or 0.02% metallic mercury on a weight basis. Mercury vapors had emanated from the painted wall in sufficient amounts to poison the child.

In December 1969, in Alamogordo, New Mexico, three children became permanently disabled after eating meat from hogs that had been fed, accidentally, grain treated with an organic mercury. It contained 27 ppm mercury. The mother, who was pregnant at the time although symptom-free herself, bore a fourth child who had convulsions.

That methyl mercury can cause abnormal breakage and faulty division of chromosomes[61] (carriers of genetic material) is indicated by experiments on fruitflies that consumed food containing 0.25 ppm methyl mercury. In their offspring, one extra chromosome was identified. In humans exposed to methyl mercury through fish consumption, chromosome breakage was reported at relatively low levels[61] of airborne mercury.

Treatment for mercury poisoning is based on withdrawal of mercury from the system by such chelating agents as BAL (British antilewisite), CaEDTA (calcium ethylene diamine tetra-acetate) and NAP (N-acetyl-D,L-penicillamine). The last-mentioned drug, which has recently been introduced, seems to produce the best results[62]; but further data are needed concerning any possible untoward side effects.

The recent recognition of the many modes of exposure to mercury and its entry into the food chain through soil, water, and air has brought to the fore the significance of this metal as one of the major environmental pollutants. Further exploration of its action will undoubtedly reveal additional medical phenomena that have baffled physicians in the past.

REFERENCES

1. Turner, W., Banford, F. N., and Dodge, J. S.: Lead poisoning at Bradford, Brit. Med. J. **3:**56, 1967.
2. Dyrssen, D.: The changing chemistry of the oceans, Ambio **1:**24, 1972.
3. Craig, P. P., and Berlin, E.: The air of poverty. Environment **13:**2-9, 1971.
4. Miano, S.: The problem of lead poisoning in children, J. Environ. Health **27:**510, 1964.
5. Barnako, D.: Childhood lead poisoning, J.A.M.A. **220:**1737-1738, 1972.
6. Berman, E., and McKiel, K.: Is that toothpaste safe? Arch. Environ. Health **25:**64-66, 1972.
7. Use of lead in gasoline declining, Chemical and Engineering News, **50:**4, 1972.
8. Haley, T. J.: Air quality monographs 69-7: a review of toxicology of lead, New York, 1969, American Petroleum Institute.
9. Chow, T. J., and Johnstone, M. S.: Lead isotopes in gasoline and aerosols of Los Angeles basin, Calif. Sci. **147:**502-503, 1965.
10. Von Lahmann, E., and Möller, M.: Luftverunreinigung in Städten durch bleihaltige Stäube, Bundesgesundheitsblatt **10:**261-264, 1967.
11. Bazell, R.: Lead poisoning: zoo animals may be the first victims, Science **173:**130-1, 1971.
12. Cogbill, E. C., and Hobbs, M. E.: Transfer of metallic constituents of cigarettes to mainstream smoke, Tobacco Sci. **1:**68, 1957.
13. Schroeder, H. A., Balassa, J. J., Gibson, F. S., and others: Abnormal trace metals in man: lead, J. Chron. Dis. **14:**408-525, 1961.
14. Durum, W. H., Hem, J. D., and Heidel, S. G.: Reconnaissance of selected minor elements in surface waters in the United States, Washington, D. C., 1971, Geological Survey Circular 643, Department of Interior.
15. Ettinger, M. B.: Lead in fishing water, Symposium on environmental lead contamination, March 1966, Public Health Service Publication No. 1440, pp. 21-27.
16. Bazell, R. J.: Lead poisoning: combating the threat from the air, Science **174:**574-576, 1971.
17. Survey of Lead in the Atmosphere of Three Urban Communities. U. S. Public Health Service Publication No. 999-AP-12, Washington, D. C., 1965, U. S. Government Printing Office, p. 94.
18. Bove, J. L., and Siedenberg, S.: Airborne lead and carbon monoxide, Science **167:**986, 1970.
19. Kehoe, R. A.: Metabolism of lead under ab-

normal conditions, Arch. Environ. Health 8:225-243, 1964.

20. Warren, H. V.: Some aspects of the relationship between health and geology, Canad. J. Public Health 52:157-164, 1961.

21. President's Science Advisory Committee, Restoring the quality of our environment. Report on Environmental Pollution Panel, P.S.A.C., Washington, D. C., 1965, Executive office of the President, The White House.

22. Lee, R. E., Jr., Patterson, R. K., and Wagman, J.: Particle size distribution of metal components in urban air, Environ. Sci. Tech. 2:288-290, 1968.

23. Kehoe, R. A.: The metabolism of lead in man in health and disease, The Normal Metabolism of Lead, The Harben Lectures, J. Roy. Inst. Public Health, 28:81, 1961.

24. Patterson, C. C.: Contaminated and natural lead environments of man, Arch. Environ. Health 8:235, 1964.

25. Goldsmith, J. R., and Hexter, A. C.: Respiratory exposure to lead: epidemiological and experimental dose-response relationships, Science 158:132-134, 1967.

26. Becker, R. O., Spadaro, J. A., and Berg, E. W.: The trace elements of human bone, J. Bone Joint Dis. 50:326-334, 1968.

26a. Lob, M., and Desbaumes, P.: Etude de la plombomie et de la plomburie chez deux groupes de detenus, les uns internés à la compagne, les autres à proximité immediate d'une autoroute, Schweiz med. Wschr. 101: 357-361, 1971.

27. Barry, P. S. I., and Mossman, D. B.: Lead concentrations in human tissues, Brit. J. Industr. Med. 27:339-351, 1970.

28. Millar, J. A., Battistini, V., Cumming, R. L. C., and others: Lead and aminolevulinic acid dehydratase levels in mentally retarded children and in lead-poisoned suckling rats, Lancet 2:695-698, 1970.

29. Goldsmith, J. R.: Epidemiological basis for possible air quality criteria for lead, J. Air Pollut. Contr. Ass. 19:714, 1969.

30. Perlstein, N. A., and Attala, R.: Neurologic sequelae of plumbism in children, Clin. Pediat. 5:292-298, 1966.

31. Wilson, A. T.: Effects of abnormal lead content of water supplies on maternity patients, Scot. Med. J. 11:73-82, 1966.

32. Block, J. L.: The accident that saved five lives, Good Housekeeping, November 1969, pp. 60-70.

33. Habibi, K.: Characterization of particulate lead in a vehicle exhaust, experimental techniques, Environ. Sci. Tech. 4:55, 1970.

34. Laveskog, A.: A method for determination of tetramethyl lead (TML) and tetraethyl lead (TEL) in air. In Englund, H. M., and Barry, W. T., editors: Proceedings of the Second International Clean Air Congress, New York, 1971, Academic Press, Inc.

35. Blumer, W.: Toxische Enzephalose infolge langdauernder Einwirkung von Auto-Abgasen, Z. Praeventivmedizin, 15:389-390, 1970.

36. Novick, S.: A new pollution problem; Löfroth, G., Duffy, M. E.: Birds gave warning; Grant, N.: Legacy of the mad hatter, Environment 11:2-23, 1969.

37. Neal, P. A., and Jones, R. R.: Chronic mercurialism in the hatter's fur-cutting industry, J.A.M.A. 110:337, 1938.

38. Halldin, A.: Industrial sources, Nord. Hyg. T. 50:154-159, 1969.

39. Teisinger, J., and Krivucová, M.: Documentation of MAC in Czechoslovakia, Czechoslovak Committee of MAC, Praha, June, 1969.

40. Grant, N.: Mercury in man, Environment 13:2-15, 1971.

41. Jonasson, I. R., and Boyle, R. W.: Geochemistry of mercury. Special symposium on mercury in man's environment, Ottawa, Ontario, February 1971.

42. Joensuu, O. J.: Fossil fuels as a source of mercury pollution, Science 172:1027, 1971.

43. Cohn, W.: Lethal mercury: a warning from Sweden, Detroit News, August 1970, p. 1 E.

44. Aaronson, T.: Mercury in the environment, Environment 13:21, 1971.

45. Hammond, H. L.: Mercury in the environment: natural and human factors, Science 171:788-789, 1971.

46. Eyl, T. B., Wilcox, K. R., and Reizen, M. S.: Fish and human health, Mich. Med. 69:873-880, 1970.

47. Tejning, S.: Report No. 68 02 20 from Department of Occupational Medicine, University Hospital, Lund, Sweden.

48. Jacobs, M. B., Ladd, A. C., and Goldwater, L. J.: Absorption and excretion of mercury in man. Part VI, Significance of mercury in urine, Arch. Environ. Health 9:454-463, 1964.

49. Howie, R. A., and Smith, H.: Mercury in human tissue, Forensic Sci. 7:90-96, 1967.

50. Irukayama, K.: Third International Conference Water Pollution Research, 1966, paper No. 8. Washington, D. C., Water Pollution Control Federation.

51. Special Research Group, Japanese Ministry of Health, First report, March 1966; Second report, 1968.

52. Löfroth, G.: Methyl Mercury, ed. 2, Stockholm, 1970, Ecology Research Committee, Swedish Natural Science Research Council.

53. Westöö, G.: Mercury compounds in animal

foods, Nordic Conference on Mercury, Nordforsk, October 11-12, 1968.

54. Jalili, M. A., and Abbasi, A. H.: Poisoning by ethyl mercury toluene sulfonanilide, Brit. J. Industr. Med. **18:**303-308, 1961.

55. Haq, I. U.: Agrosan poisoning in man, Brit. Med. J. **1:**1579-1582, 1963.

55a. Grimstone, G.: Mercury in British fish, Chem. Brit. **8:**244-247, 1972.

56. Berlin, M., Nordberg, G. F., and Serenius, F.: On the site and mechanism of mercury vapor resorption in the lung, Arch. Environ. Health **18:**42-50, 1969.

57. Engleson, G., and Herner, T.: Alkyl mercury poisoning, Acta Pediat. **41:**289-294, 1952.

58. Suzuki, T., Miyama, T., and Katsunuma, H.: Comparison of mercury contents in maternal blood, umbilical cord blood and placental tissues. Bull. Environ. Contam. Toxicol. **5:**502-508, 1970.

59. Brown, I. A.: Chronic mercurialism: a cause of the clinical syndrome of amyotrophic lateral sclerosis, Arch. Neurol. Psychol. **72:** 674, 1961.

60. Hirshman, S. Z., Feingold, M., and Boylen, G.: Mercury in house paint as a cause of acrodynia, New Eng. J. Med. **369:**889, 1963.

61. Löfroth, G.: A review of health hazards and side effects associated with the emission of mercury compounds into natural systems, ed. 2, Stockholm, 1970, Swedish Natural Science Research Council, pp. 49, 50.

62. Kark, R. A. P., Poskanzer, D. C., Bullock, J. D., and others: Mercury poisoning and its treatment with N-acetyl-D,L-penicillamine, New Eng. J. Med. **285:**10-16, 1971.

13

SYSTEMIC POISONS: fluoride and cadmium

FLUORIDE

A 54-year-old Ontario farmer's wife experienced a progressive disease characterized by increasing malaise and debility, constant pain in the lower spine, and frequent migrainelike headaches. Dishes and glasses frequently dropped from her hands because of numbness and pain in fingers and hands, which prevented her from gripping objects firmly. Her abdomen was constantly bloated and painful. Diarrhea alternated with periods of constipation. Because of her gradually deteriorating health and increasing weakness she was forced, at first, to rest for 2 to 3 hours daily. Gradually she became bedridden most of the time.

Her 13-year-old son had an illness similar to her own. He had always enjoyed good health until the triple phosphate fertilizer factory, ¼ mile from his home, began operations. Pains in the shoulders and knee joints, below the ribs, and in the lower spine limited his movements and activities. His legs frequently stiffened, his big toes cramped and, on several occasions, his knees collapsed under him. He experienced involuntary, uncontrollable twitching of muscles in various parts of his body, a phenomenon known as muscular fibrillation, usually caused by a temporary deficiency of calcium or magnesium in the bloodstream. The boy's nose and eyes were frequently irritated.

The family had witnessed gradual deterioration and eventual destruction of strawberry and rhubarb plants, current bushes, and apple and pear trees on their fifty acre farm. Eighty-three of their eighty-six colonies of bees had been wiped out.

On their one-acre garden plot, burns had appeared on the tips and margins of begonia and geranium leaves. Lilac bushes wilted early in spring even before they had borne flowers. The window glass of their house was etched and the finish of their automobile damaged. The cistern water that the family was using for drinking, contained 14.3 ppm of fluoride (F).

Altogether, I interviewed 28 farmers residing in that area within a radius of 3 miles of a triple phosphate fertilizer factory. Subsequently I examined fifteen, four of whom were hospitalized. All showed evidence of the same disease, which seemed to be occurring in epidemic proportion.[1]

An Ontario government investigation[2] revealed that airborne fluoride had, indeed, damaged vegetation and livestock. The investigators however failed to carry out meaningful studies on the afflicted individuals to determine whether or not their illness was related to the fluoride emission. Subsequent investigations in three other fluoride emission areas near Bolzano, Italy, Kitimat, British Columbia, and in southern Ohio, have shown that fluoride damage to vegetation and animal life is accompanied by adverse effects to human health.

Occurrence of fluorides

Fluorine, a gas so reactive that it does not occur in nature in elemental form, has a strong tendency to combine with other elements or molecules to form new combinations and can thus account for formation of a multitude of highly complex compounds.

In nature the three most common compounds containing fluoride are the minerals fluorspar or calcium fluoride (CaF_2), the aluminum compound cryolite (Na_3AlF_6) and apatite, a calcium phosphate complex of the formula $Ca_{10}X_2(PO_4)_6$ where X represents either fluoride, chlorine, or the hydroxide (OH^-) atoms.

Fluorides in industry

Throughout the early part of the twentieth century, up to the 1930s fluoride compounds constituted useless by-products of many industrial processes, such as the manufacture of aluminum, superphosphate fertilizers, steel, magnesium, beryllium, zirconium, enamel, and bricks. The only commercial outlet was as an insecticide and a rodenticide.

During the 1940s fluorine compounds began to enter the refrigerant, aerosol, lubricant, and plastic fields. The fluorine atom was also introduced into pharmaceutical preparations for the purpose of reinforcing their action. Hydrogen fluoride (HF) began to replace sulfuric acid in the production of high octane gasoline.

Simultaneously the use of fluoride expanded rapidly into the area of nuclear energy and missile propulsion. Its uses range from automobile bearings that never need greasing to replacements of diseased or ruptured blood vessels in the human body, from clothing that resists stains to anticancer drugs and blood substitutes.

The chemical industry is one of the largest consumers of fluorspar, especially in the manufacturing of hydrofluoric acid. In steel production fluorspar functions as a fluxing agent and assists in the refining process. It is also used in opalescent glass, iron and steel enamelware, refining of lead and antimony, and as a catalyst in manufacturing high octane fuels.

Cryolite is in great demand as a flux for electrolytic production of aluminum. Fluorine is the most effective element for extracting vital uranium 235 atoms from natural uranium. Indeed, there is no end in sight to further expansion of fluorine's industrial uses (Table 13-1).

Ubiquity of fluoride

In air. Fluoride compounds are present in air, water, soil, and in all living matter. In a nationwide air survey by the National Air Pollution Control Administration (N.A.P.C.A.) based on over 7700 measurements for fluoride ion in 24-hour samples of suspended particles[3] 87% of measurements at urban stations yielded ambient air concentrations of "total water soluble

Table 13-1. Some uses of fluorine compounds

IN MANUFACTURING	IN OTHER INDUSTRIES	
Aluminum	Welding (flux)	Rust removal
Steel	Cleaning	Lubricant
Enamel	Refrigerant	Oil refining
Pottery	Preserving wood	Plastics
Glass	Reinforcing cement	Separation of
Bricks	Aerosol propellant	uranium isotopes
Phosphate fertilizer	Optical	Missile propulsion
Beryllium		
Tantalum		
Niobium		

Table 13-2. Fluoride in water (ppm)

Rainwater	
"Uncontaminated" area	0.16[7]
Near heavy industry	0.63—36.3[7]
Sea water*	1.0—1.4[8]
In Persian Gulf	8.7[8]
Lake water	
Near volcanoes; East Africa	2,800[8]
Effluent water	
From a Florida fertilizer plant	2,810—5,150[9]
Well water	
In most wells	Traces or less than 1.0[8]
In high fluoride areas	Up to 28[10]

*About 50% of total fluoride in seawater is bound as the double ion MgF+.

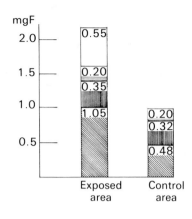

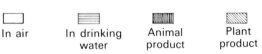

In air   In drinking water   Animal product   Plant product

Fig. 13-1. Estimated fluoride intake into the body of children through ingestion and inhalation in an air-contaminated area compared to a noncontaminated one. Food, especially plant products, constitute the bulk of fluoride uptake. Fluoride from drinking water was calculated at 0.1 to 0.3 mg/liter in exposed and control areas. (Courtesy Dr. G. Balazova, Dr. P. Macuch, and Dr. A. Rippel, C.S.S.R.)

fluoride" below 0.05 μg/meter³, 0.2% exceeded 1 μg/meter³. In rural areas, 97% showed no detectable amounts of fluoride. This is in contrast to 0.018 ppm (18 ppb) reported by Cholak in Baltimore where phosphate fertilizer factories are located.[4] Earlier determinations near an aluminum factory were 0.02 to 0.22 mg/meter³ (20 to 220 ppb).[5] Discrepancies in these values can be explained on the basis of time and place of exposure, season, mode of sampling, and method of analysis, and especially on the basis of the industrial activity in the emission area. Gasoline is estimated to contain 0.4 ppm fluoride and gasoline exhaust about 0.03 ppm. The latter value represents 0.1% of the total fluoride of the atmosphere.

In water. Fluoride values in water are also highly erratic, as shown in Table 13-2. The level called "optimum" for prevention of tooth decay, namely 1 to 1.2 ppm (somewhat less in hot climates), was selected to provide minimum caries with maximum safety.[6]

In food. Fluoride-containing foods and beverages are the most important sources of fluoride intake (Fig. 13-1). The fluoride content of our daily food varies erratically according to where it is produced, pro-

cessed, and prepared. Seasonal and climatic changes, variations in composition of soil, and the proximity of fluoride-emitting factories affect its content. Continuous exposures to fluoride-laden atmosphere increase the fluoride content of edible vegetation.

Fluoride levels in most food are below 1 ppm with the exception of tea, which contains naturally between 8 and 400 ppm in dried substance (1 mg fluoride to 2 cups), fish, and seafood. In gelatin as well as in polished rice and peas, fluoride levels run as high as 10 ppm.[11]

When food is boiled in fluoride-containing water, it takes up additional fluoride.[12] Food grown in industrial areas, particularly fruit and leafy vegetables such as lettuce, spinach and cabbage, accumulates more than the normal amounts of fluoride. Root vegetables such as beets, sugar beets, and potatoes grown in phosphate fertilized soils

Table 13-3. Fluoride assays of foods consumed by farm families near a phosphate fertilizer factory

	PPM	NORMAL VALUES
Wheat (grain)*	2.6	0.7 to 2.0*
Apples	6.6	0.8
Carrots	7.0	2.0
Beets	7.0	0.7 to 2.8
Squash	10.4	—
Corn	1.3	0.7
Sauerkraut	10.7	—
Currants	8.0	0.7
Cabbage leaves	9.6	—
Chicken vegetable soup†	4.6	—
Hamburger with onions	2.4	—
Potatoes (boiled)	7.7	0.4
Beans (cooked)	17.3	1.7
Strawberries (frozen)	4.6	—
Oatmeal (cooked)	5.1	0.2
Lettuce‡	44.0	0.1 to 0.3

*Analysis by Dr. K. Garber, State's Institute of Botany, Hamburg, Germany.
†Analysis by Dr. W. Oelschlager, Agricultural University, Hohenheim, Germany.
‡Analysis by Ontario Water Resources Commission.

remove from the soil at harvest[13] between 0.1 to 0.4% of the amount of fluoride that was added as fertilizer. Food fluoride levels at the table of a farmer residing near a fertilizer factory are presented in Table 13-3.

In 1968 Cheng and associates[14] observed that in soybeans fluoride is present in the form of organic fluoroacetate, a substance 550 times more toxic than inorganic fluoride. Fluoroacetate inhibits the action of aconitase, an enzyme essential to carbohydrate metabolism. In the mammalian organism, it is converted into the highly toxic fluorocitrate, which is also found in contaminated hay.[15]

Fluoride metabolism

Uptake. Data on total fluoride intake are very sparse. An early report by McClure[16] indicated that most common foods contain only 0.1 to 0.3 ppm fluoride. Subsequently, in Newfoundland where drinking water was practically fluoride-free, a daily fluoride uptake of 2.74 mg was recorded[17] on the basis of a traditional diet containing considerable "high fluoride" seafood and tea. According to surveys carried out in fluoridated Ottawa, Canada[18] and Hines, Illinois, Veterans Hospital[19] the average daily ingestion of fluoride was estimated to range between 2 and 5 mg from food and water. In North Vietnam[20] where fluoride in water ranged from 0.2 to 0.6 ppm, total daily dietary intake was 7.44 mg, that is, 5.64 mg from food and 1.8 mg from water. In addition to that in diets, fluoride is taken into the body through a variety of organic fluoride compounds such as aerosols, pharmaceuticals, and cosmetics. Although fluoride is readily absorbed from the respiratory tract,[21] this mode of uptake constitutes only a relatively small proportion of the total body burden of fluoride.

Fluoride reaches the bloodstream with food and water, mainly from the stomach and upper intestinal tract, as promptly as 10 minutes after ingestion.[22] When such elements as calcium, aluminum, and magnesium are present in food and water, they inhibit fluoride absorption from the digestive tract.[8] Food-borne fluoride is absorbed less rapidly than waterborne fluoride.[23]

Total fluoride concentrations in blood are 0.12 to 0.13 ppm,[24] about 85% of which is transported tightly bound to protein.[25] The remaining unbound form of fluoride, that is, the free ion, is able to enter into any number of reactions with body fluids. An equilibrium between fluoride in blood plasma and fluoride anchored to blood protein is established within minutes.[22] Fifteen minutes after an intravenous injection of radioactive fluoride (F^{18}), its concentration in the kidneys and in the parotid gland (a saliva-producing gland) is twice as high as in the blood.[22]

Excretion. When fluoride is inhaled or ingested in the form of a readily-absorbed

Table 13-4. Soft tissue storage of fluoride (ppm) in patients with kidney stones*

KIDNEY STONE	HAIR	NAILS	FAT	SKIN	OTHER TISSUES	
101			121	195	Kidney	181
188	171		30	290		
197				41	Prostate	50
380			97	104	Prostate	86
412			10	82	Bladder	116
850	124	186				
1119	162		2	100	Prostate	15
1357	65		80	24		
1575	143	77				

*Modified from Herman, J. F., Mason, B., and Light, F.: Fluorine in urinary tract calculi, J. Urol. 80:263-267, 1958.

compound, persons with healthy kidney function eliminate the largest portion of it with the urine, less through the bowels and salivary and sweat glands.[26] However, urinary fluoride excretion is highly erratic. Whereas individuals with normal kidney function can excrete in their urine from 54% to 61% of ingested fluoride,[27] those with disturbed kidney function excrete only 17% to 22%.[28] I recovered 99.5% of a given test dose in the urine of one individual, only 3.6% in that of another.[8] Children excrete less fluoride than adults.[29] During pregnancy, urinary excretion of fluoride falls progressively up to the eighth month.[30] After fluoride intake into the body has been reduced, stored fluoride is gradually released from the body and continues to be excreted in the urine in excess of the amount of fluoride consumed.[8] For instance, 11 weeks after the U. S. Public Health Service had reduced the fluoride level of Bartlett, Texas, drinking water from 8 to 1 ppm, the average fluoride concentrations in urine of residents still ranged as high as 2.2 and 2.5 ppm (3.3 to 3.7 mg) per day.[31]

Storage takes place principally in bones and teeth, especially during the early years of life. A diet high in fat, as well as continuous rather than intermittent fluoride ingestion, enhance fluoride storage.[8] Variables that affect fluoride storage in bones and teeth are age, sex, diet, the portion of

tooth or bone examined, whether the bone is cancellous or compact, and many other factors. Furthermore, procedures in different laboratories differ and have in the past accounted for variations in results.

Normal bone levels range from 44 to 490 ppm fluoride,[32] whereas in bones of habitual tea drinkers in the British town of W. Hartlepool where water contained 1.9 ppm fluoride levels from 2500 to above 6000 ppm fluoride were recorded.[33] In bones of patients with chronic fluoride intoxication, fluoride levels range from 600 to 6800 ppm.[34] In persons with advanced kidney disease undergoing long-term hemodialysis with fluoridated water, levels of fluoride from 800 to 22,100 ppm were found.[35]

In teeth, as in bones, the fluoride content varies widely. In communities where fluoride levels in water are low, average fluoride levels in enamel ranged from 54 to 299 ppm; those in dentine from 86 to 911 ppm.[36]

Under certain, thus far unexplained, conditions considerable fluoride is stored in soft tissue organs. The usual levels in most organs range below 1 ppm. In patients with kidney stones,[37] up to 290 ppm fluoride in the skin has been reported (Table 13-4). These high fluoride concentrations in soft tissue organs occurred in New York City, where, at that time, drinking water contained as little as 0.1 ppm fluoride.

Therefore, the storage must have been caused by contaminated food or by excess inhalation of contaminated air or by a combination of both.

Among other soft tissues, fluoride levels are highest in the aorta and other blood vessels, particularly if they are calcified.[38]*

Toxicity of fluoride

Biologic action of fluoride. The strong affinity of fluoride for magnesium, manganese, and other metals, which causes it to interfere with the activity of many enzymes,[8] can affect adversely the function of endocrine processes. Most thoroughly documented is an increase in the function of the parathyroid glands, which regulate the metabolism of calcium.[39] Damage to the pituitary gland,[32] the main regulator of water balance in the human organism, indicated by the occurrence of polydipsia and polyuria (excess thirst and urination), is an early sign of fluoride intoxication. The effect of fluoride on the thyroid gland is not clearly established, although a large volume of research on this subject exists. Although fluoride appears to counteract thyroid activity, many factors, especially the extent of simultaneous intake of iodine, alter its action.[40]

In large doses, fluoride interferes with the secretion of gastric juice in experimental animals.[41] Experimental and clinical data point to fluoride's adverse effect on kidneys following long-term fluoride intake in minute doses. For the mutagenic effect of fluoride see Chapter 17.

Acute intoxication. Acute fluoride poisoning occurs following excessive ingestion of fluoride compounds, usually for suicidal or homicidal purposes. Highly soluble compounds such as sodium fluoride are more toxic than the less soluble ones. Sodium silicofluoride or sodium fluoride in doses 3 to 5 gm, mistaken for flour, sugar, and bicarbonate of soda, have caused several epidemics, one with as many as 75 fatalities.[42] Severe stomach pains and cramps in the bowels, vomiting of bloody material, bloody diarrhea, marked dehydration (fluid loss), and epilepsylike seizures caused by low blood calcium are typical symptoms.[42] Rabinowitch reported a case of hypocalcemia (low blood calcium) as low as 2.6 mg% (normal 9 to 11 mg%). Convulsions may occur several hours after ingestion of the poison.

The acute phase of the disease is of significance in evaluating the chronic effects caused by air and water pollution, since acute abdominal episodes are not uncommon during the chronic stage, probably because of temporary consumption of food or water extraordinarily contaminated. Such episodes usually constitute a serious diagnostic problem to physicians and are rarely attributed to their real cause.[43]

Chronic fluoride intoxication

Dental and skeletal fluorosis. The two conspicuous and most thoroughly studied manifestations on which physicians usually depend for the diagnosis of chronic fluoride poisoning are dental and skeletal fluorosis. However, they are not obligatory features of the disease: dental fluorosis (or mottling of teeth) occurs only in individuals who have consumed or have been exposed to fluoride during childhood, up to age 10 or 12. The skeletal changes of the disease develop only after many years of low but persistent fluoride intake.

Dental fluorosis is a permanent defect of tooth enamel, characterized by white chalky patches (Fig. 13-2, *A* and *B*). It is caused by imperfect calcification as indicated by irregular development of enamel rods (rows of cells forming the enamel)

---

*As much as 2340 ppm fluoride was found in the aorta of an individual less than 20 years old who was consuming New York City water at a concentration of only 0.1 ppm prior to fluoridation of the water supply. (Geever, E. F., McCann, H. G., McClure, F. J., Lee, W. A., and Schiffmann, E.: Fluoridated water, the skeletal structure and chemistry, Health Services and Mental Health Administration Health Reports, 86:820-27, 1971.)

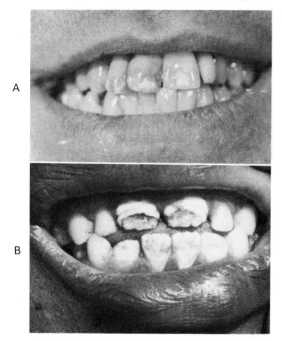

A

B

Fig. 13-2. A, Mottled teeth in a 32-year-old man who had always resided in low-fluoride (0.1 ppm) Detroit. Consumption of fluoride-contaminated food or fluoride-containing vitamins in early childhood is likely to have precipitated this condition. **B,** Advanced dental fluorosis in a high-fluoride area of India where water contains 2.5 to 11.8 ppm naturally. (Courtesy Prof. A. H. Siddiqui, Mecca, Arabia.)

and absence of cementing substance. Dental fluorosis has been recorded in communities with artificially fluoridated water (1 ppm),[44]* from natural fluoride water, and in hot climates such as India[45] and North Africa at lower levels (> 0.6).[46] In the advanced stages, the areas affected by mottling become yellow, brown, and even black.

In skeletal fluorosis, tissue and ligaments about the joints, especially in the pelvic area and spine, become calcified. Bony protrusions develop on the surface of ribs and of long bones (Fig. 13-3). The bones of arms and legs themselves show excess calcifications in some portions but can be undermineralized in others (Fig. 13-4). As this condition progresses, neurologic disturbances can develop in the spine. In India paralysis of legs, arms, bladder, and bowels ensue because of pressure of newly formed bone upon the spinal cord and the

---

*In a survey of the teeth of Grand Rapid school children during the seventeenth year of fluoridation[44] the incidence of enamel opacities caused by fluoride in those with continuous residence was 19.3% of 337 Caucasian children and 40.2% of 82 Negro children.

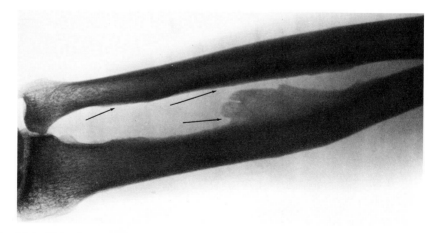

Fig. 13-3. Skeletal fluorosis caused by drinking water containing between 3 and 6 ppm fluoride naturally. Roentgenogram of the two bones of the forearm shows extensive thickening of the bone substance. The marrow in the center of the bones is hardly discernible. New grotesque bone formation is seen at the membrane connecting the two bones. At the surface (periosteum) of the bones newly developed bone substance (arrows) is visible.

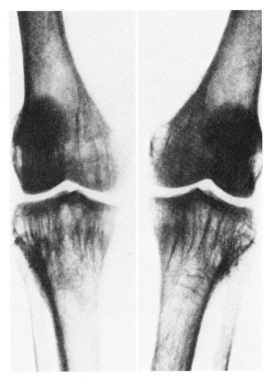

Fig. 13-4. Osteoporosis (decalcification of bones) alternating with excessive calcifications in skeletal fluorosis. The vertical lines represent increased density of trabeculae, the building blocks of bone.

nerves as they leave the vertebral column.[45] The bone changes cause rigidity of the chest cage, which interferes with breathing and, because of increased brittleness of the bones, can induce spontaneous fractures. Arthritic changes occur when the capsules surrounding the joints become calcified.[47] Calcifications of blood vessels have also been reported[38] in conjunction with skeletal fluorosis from different parts of the world.

When large doses of fluoride are ingested without concomitant calcium supplementation, osteomalacia (bone softening) ensues.[48]

Depending on the principal sources of fluoride uptake by the body, chronic intoxication can be classified into four categories:

Hydrofluorosis caused by drinking water, the most common phase of the disease

Alimentary fluorosis caused by fluoride-containing food

Industrial fluorosis, the incidence of which has been reduced materially through preventive measures

Neighborhood fluorosis, which occurs in populations residing in the vicinity of fluoride-emitting industries.

To be sure, fluoride uptake into the system is never confined to a single source. Therefore, total fluoride intake from all sources—food, water, and air—must be considered.

Alimentary and hydrofluorosis

Fluoride uptake through water is closely linked with that from food because the fluoride content of food increases when it is prepared or processed with fluoride-containing water. There are, however, instances in which contaminated food primarily accounted for fluorosis.

Soriano[47] in Barcelona reported 29 cases of advanced skeletal fluorosis caused specifically by long-term consumption of wine contaminated by 8 to 72 ppm fluoride. Chronic alcoholism in these patients might have modified and perhaps aggravated the skeletal changes. In a man from Hampshire, England[49] advanced skeletal fluorosis was confirmed by roentgenogram but no obvious source of fluoride uptake either from water or from the air was established. Excess tea consumption, a high fluoride staple of the British diet, could have been responsible. (One cup of tea contains about 0.5 mg fluoride.)

The seriousness of hydrofluorosis in hot climates is driven home by reports of widespread epidemics of this disease in India, the Middle East, and North Africa. In the Punjab province of India, Jolly and associates[45,45a] surveyed 46,000 inhabitants in 358 villages: 1320 cases of fluorosis with bone changes were detected by roentgenograms (some occurred where fluoride in water was as low as 1.2 ppm); 144 of the patients had crippling deformities, 125 had neurologic complications as a result of encroachment of newly formed bone on nerve substance, 309 had no symptoms, the remaining 742 showed bone changes but were not crippled. The extremely hot climate, excess water consumption, and poor nutrition* are conducive to the development of the disease in India.

More pertinent to air pollution in the United States are reports[50] from "natural" fluoride volcanic regions of northern Sicily, where the climate is moderate and conditions are similar to those encountered in many parts of the United States. Fradà and associates[50] reported patients with pains in stomach and bowels, nausea, vomiting, diarrhea alternating with constipation, involvement of the liver, headaches, numbness, and pain in arms and legs, arthritis in the spinal column, and muscular pains. The fluoride level in water ranged from 3 to 6 ppm.

In the United States two fatal cases with skeletal fluorosis, which occurred in the West Texas fluoride belt, have been the subject of much controversy. A 22-year-old Texas soldier[51] who sustained a kidney injury in early life had been consuming water containing 1.2 to 5.7 ppm fluoride for about 20 years; the drinking water of the other man, age 63[52] contained 2.2 to 3.5 ppm fluoride throughout his life.

The death of a newborn child with advanced calcifications of blood vessels was reported in Ames, Iowa.[53] The infant's aorta contained 59.3 ppm fluoride.[38] This case suggests that fluoride passes through the placenta from mother to child.

Industrial and neighborhood fluorosis

In 1961 an estimated 2500 tons of fluoride was released into the atmosphere of England and Wales from coal burning alone.[54]

*Recently Jolly and associates[45] found inhabitants of this area better nourished than in other regions in India.

A Swiss report[55] estimates that processing 1 ton of aluminum emits 0.56 kg of gaseous fluoride and 4.56 kg as particulate. In view of such enormous emissions, and of the well-documented fluoride contamination of vegetation and drinking water, relatively few reports of intoxication of workers in fluoride-emitting factories and of persons residing in the vicinity of such factories have appeared. Although measures to control pollution inside of industrial establishments have greatly reduced damage to employees, adverse health effects to those residing near factories has received little attention.

Neighborhood fluorosis was first described in the household of nine of a farmer residing near a fluoride-emitting ironstone works in South Lincolnshire, England.[56] Here too, the symptoms were gastric upsets, stiffness, and pains in the legs and

Table 13-5. Symptomatology in 32 cases of "neighborhood" fluorosis*

Musculoskeletal	Number of cases
Arthritis, especially in cervical and lumbar spine	30
Myalgia; myasthenia; paresthesias (muscle pains, weakness, numbness)	30
Spasticity in extremities	3
Muscular fibrillation (twitching)	8
Migrainelike headaches	20
Visual disturbances (scotomata, blurred vision)	8
Gastrointestinal	
Gastric (nausea, vomiting, epigastric pain)	18
Intestinal distention; spastic constipation, diarrhea	16
Acute condition within abdomen	9
Respiratory	
Nasal and eye irritation	28
Emphysema; asthma	4
Epistaxis (nose bleed)	7
Chizzola maculae	10

*From Waldbott, G. L.: "Neighborhood" fluorosis, Clin. Toxicol. 2:387-396, 1969.

joints. The subjects had been exposed to fluoride air pollution from 3 to 14 years with the exception of one farm worker who had been residing in the area for 1 year only. The same disease occurred in a farmer's family of three in the vicinity of a fluoride-emitting Oregon aluminum smelter.[57] In addition to the above-mentioned manifestations, the patients experienced liver and kidney damage. Neither the British nor the Oregon cases exhibited evidence of osteosclerosis. In children residing close to a Czechoslovakian aluminum factory, Balazova and assoicates[58] found anemia and significantly lower hemoglobin but higher than normal red blood cell values.

I reported additional cases of fluorosis among people residing near an Ontario fertilizer factory (Table 13-5).[43] More recently I have had occasion to observe 24 patients in Italy near fluoride-emitting factories; 36 patients near an Ohio aluminum plant; and 28 patients near a British Columbia aluminum plant. In the last-mentioned area, 18 were workers in the plant.

The preskeletal phase of fluorosis

In addition to the involvement of bones and teeth, a wide spectrum of manifestations has been described in the classical book by Roholm[32] and subsequently by Fradà[50] and Waldbott.[8] Like many other kinds of chronic intoxication, the symptoms (Table 13-5) vary from person to person,

depending on his individual susceptibility, his state of health and nutrition, food habits, age, sex, duration and extent of former and current fluoride intake, on whether fluoride is inhaled or ingested, on the simultaneous intake of other chemicals from the atmosphere and on fluoride interaction with other agents in the intestinal tract.[8]

If fluoride compounds are inhaled in conjunction with other irritant dusts and fumes, respiratory symptoms such as bronchitis, emphysema, asthma, conjunctival and nasal irritation predominate.[59]

In India, as stated above, fluorosis is associated with neurologic symptoms such as paralysis of legs and arms.[45,60] On the other hand, in the Sahara desert, only one patient among 148 with advanced skeletal changes had palsy of both arms.[46] In Sicily, where seafood predominates in the diet, paralysis is rare; instead, 45% of the patients with advanced fluorosis had gastrointestinal disorders,[50] a manifestation rarely observed in India. In Morocco[46] where dust from phosphate mines contaminates edibles, the disease differs materially from fluorosis in the Sahara where maritime fossils constitute the source of water and air contamination.

Chizzola maculae

A new approach to the diagnosis of fluorosis has recently opened up with the recognition of bluish-brown lesions, simulating

Table 13-6. Differentiation of Chizzola maculae from bruises

	CHIZZOLA MACULAE	SUFFUSIONS (BRUISES)
History	Exposure to fluoride	Trauma
Shape	Round or oval	Any shape
Size	1 to 2 cm diameter	Any size
Color		
At first appearance	Pinkish-red	Dark blue
When fading	Brownish-red	Brown to yellow
Microscopic appearance	Inflammatory changes around capillaries	Extravasation of blood through broken veins

bruises on the skin (Table 13-6), in children and women residing in the vicinity of two Italian aluminum factories (Fig. 13-5).[61,62]

Recent observations[63] on children (Fig. 13-6) and women drinking fluoridated water leave no doubt that the lesions are related to fluoride. They promptly disappear upon eliminating fluoridated water and can be reproduced, at will, upon its resumption. In most of the affected cases, muscular pains and frequent gastrointestinal upsets are associated with the lesions. Unlike bruises, they are always round or oval in shape ranging from a dime to a quarter in size; they change color only slightly when they are fading. The significance of these harmless appearing lesions lies in the fact that they show accumulation of lymphocytes and basophilic cells around capillaries, which are indicative of a local toxic reaction.

In 1958, the Food and Nutrition Board of the National Research Council listed fluoride as a mineral nutrient because the members felt that fluoride is needed to build caries resistance into tooth enamel. On the other hand, several departments of Health Education and Welfare[64,65] do not include fluoride among minerals whose need in human nutrition has been established.

From the above data it appears that exposure to environmental fluoride is much more far reaching than is generally recognized. Contrary to widespread belief, den-

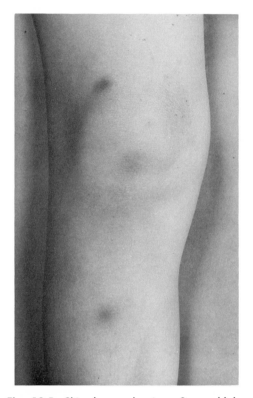

Fig. 13-5. Chizzola maculae in a 3-year-old boy living close to a fluoride-emitting area in Detroit. The reddish-brown lesions mimic bruises but can be readily distinguished from them by their size, shape, color, and by their fleeting character. They are always round or oval and are rarely larger than a twenty-five cent piece.

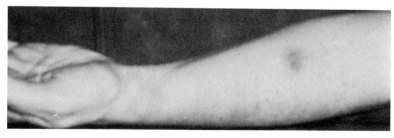

Fig. 13-6. Recurrent "maculae" in a 58-year-old physician residing for 15 years within 300 feet of an iron foundry.

tal and skeletal changes are not the only manifestations of fluoride poisoning. A large variety of preskeletal symptoms gives rise to diagnostic difficulties and accounts for the fact that little attention has been given to the early stage of chronic poisoning. Our data indicate that the early manifestations of chronic poisoning are not uncommon. The question whether or not fluoride in organic form in food and drugs enters into the causation of symptoms requires foremost attention.

When and why fluoride accumulates in soft tissue and whether or not excess storage damages the respective organs, constitutes a major field for further exploration.

CADMIUM

In the October 1970 issue of the *Annals of Internal Medicine,* Dr. B. T. Emmerson[66] reported an unusual disease described by Dr. K. Tsuchiya[67] in the city of Toyama on Japan's Inland Sea. A group of residents had been complaining for several years of lumbago that had gradually turned into extreme bone pain. As the disease progressed, osteomalacia (softening of bones) developed with multiple bone fractures and a wadling gait. The pains became so severe that the inhabitants called the disease "itai-itai byo," which, in its literal translation, means "ouch-ouch disease."

A consistent finding in these patients was the presence of protein in the urine, a sign of kidney involvement. The urine also contained sugar, amino acids, and considerable calcium, the usual concomitant of bone softening. The calcium concentration of the blood serum, however, was normal. The activity of alkaline phosphatase in the blood, an enzyme associated with bone growth, was elevated. The whole skeleton was subject to abnormal softening. Death was usually attributed to kidney failure.

When autopsies revealed unusually high cadmium (Cd) concentrations in body tissues, a search was initiated for the source of cadmium in the environment. It was established that high levels of the metal in rice and soybeans grown in the endemic area had been derived from the soil. A lead and zinc mining operation, situated upstream from the Fuchu-machi farming community, emitted cadmium fumes and particulate matter. From this plant, cadmium had been carried downstream over the years and had been deposited in the rice paddies. The most seriously afflicted persons were residing where the highest levels of cadmium were found in the soil. Even after additional contamination by cadmium had been reduced sharply, sufficient waste residues from the mine remained in the soil to account for the high cadmium content of rice grown in the area and for the accumulation of cadmium in the bodies of the residents. Most vulnerable to the disease were malnourished persons who were deficient in calcium and women who had been under stress because of frequent pregnancies or because of their menopause.

Near another Japanese zinc smelter at Ishinosawa village near Bandai, where another focus of "itai-itai" disease was reported recently, rice contained 1.6 ppm cadmium.[68] Cadmium levels as high as 11,472 ppm in the ash of ribs of victims have been reported.[71]

Properties of cadmium

Cadmium, a silver-white metal, is soft, ductile, and highly resistant to corrosion. It is mined in conjunction with other metals, mainly zinc sulfide, and recovered from flue dusts in copper and lead smelting plants and in the electrolytic purification of zinc. When metal is heated with a welding torch, cadmium forms a yellow-golden film in contrast to the smoky gray film of melting zinc.

Uses of cadmium

In the mid-1920s cadmium was used pharmaceutically in the treatment of syphilis and malaria.[69] Once its toxic properties became recognized, cadmium therapy was abandoned. Nowadays, of the 12.6 million pounds of cadmium consumed in the United States[70] approximately 50% is used for electroplating, another 20% as a constituent of stabilizers for polyvinyl chloride. Most other uses are in conjunction with alloys, particularly with gold in making jewelry. In soldering, cadmium is combined with copper, lead, tin, zinc, and silver.

Cadmium-nickel batteries are employed in military aircraft, in guided missiles, and in refrigerated railway cars; cadmium-copper is used in the overhead wires of street cars and railroads. The automobile and aircraft industries use cadmium in engine parts. It is also employed in radio and television manufacturing. Much of the metal is emitted into the atmosphere during the manufacture of fertilizers and pesticides. Furthermore, cadmium metal and cadmium nitrate are used in reactors to control the rate of nuclear fission. Incineration and melting down of cadmium-containing products, especially scrap steel, automobile radiators, plastic bottles, auto seats, furniture, floor coverings, and rubber tires, constitute 52% of 4.6 million pounds of cadmium emitted into the United States air per year.[70]

Sources

Man's principal sources of cadmium intake are food, water, and polluted air.

In food. In food, cadmium levels vary considerably. Mollusks, crustaceans, and grains, especially rice, the germ-free portion of wheat and certain varieties of tea and coffee, show a high cadmium (above 1 ppm) content.[71] Very high cadmium levels have been found in beef kidneys. Vegetables and grains produced with heavy applications of commercial fertilizers contain between 9 and 36 ppm cadmium.[72] Natural phosphate rock, the source of fertilizers, is partly composed of the hard parts of marine animals that have accumu-

lated cadmium from sea water.* Among 846 food samples purchased in Vancouver, Toronto, and Montreal and analyzed by the Canadian health authorities, 76 contained more than 0.5 ppm cadmium.[73] In this survey, egg, fish, and milk products were named as important sources of cadmium in the diet. More than 70% of the contaminated food came from the vicinity of a British Columbia zinc refinery.

In water. Cadmium is found in drinking water in traces of less than 1 ppb.[71] Many rivers and lakes in the United States are contaminated by cadmium, which is derived mainly from the manufacture of nickel-cadmium batteries. Mud from a stream near such a factory in the Hudson River contained 16.2% cadmium and 22.6% nickel by dry weight. Mud from sediment dredged from lake Erie contained 130 ppm cadmium.[70] In water standing in galvanized and black polyethylene pipes, from 0.15 to 6 ppb is found.[71] Flushing out the water system will lower the cadmium content of water to undetectable amounts. A survey of 950 United States water supply systems in 1970[74] revealed three that exceeded 10 ppb, the Public Health Service's mandatory top allowable limit of cadmium.

In air. The yearly cadmium emission into the air is estimated to be more than 4.6 million pounds.[70] In urban ambient air, cadmium levels range from 0.0 to 0.062 μg/meter^3.[75] Smoking of cigarettes is a source of cadmium inhalation, one pack of which contains approximately 30μg of cadmium; 70% of this amount escapes into the air with the smoke.[76]

Body burden of cadmium

Cadmium has no known biologic function. It is toxic to practically all systems and functions of the human and animal organism.[77] It is absorbed into the human organism without regard to the amount al-

---

*Superphosphate fertilizer contains up to 8.9 ppm cadmium.[70]

ready stored, nor does there appear to be a mechanism to maintain a constant level in blood and body fluids.[78] Of 50 to 60 μg taken into the system daily, about 2 μg is retained mainly in kidney and liver, the rest is eliminated with the feces.[79] At autopsy, the "average" American shows approximately 30 mg cadmium in his body, 33% of which is stored in the kidneys, 14% in the liver, 2% in the lungs, and 0.3% in the pancreas.* In the kidneys of Japanese, on the other hand, about twice as much cadmium has been found.[70] Cadmium inhibits the functions of enzymes containing the sulphydrile (SH) groups, which are dependent on the presence of zinc, cobalt, and other metals. There is evidence that cadmium acts upon the smooth muscle of the blood vessels, either directly or indirectly[78] through the agency of the kidneys.

Hypertension and cadmium

During the past two decades Schroeder[81] studied the biologic action of cadmium in experiments on literally thousands of rats and mice. Newborn animals, kept in an environment free of cadmium were administered traces of cadmium in drinking water (5 μg/1000 ml, or 5 ppb) from the time of weaning. After about a year hypertension (high blood pressure) developed, the severity of which increased with age. Softness of drinking waters appeared to contribute to the disease. When cadmium was removed from the rat's system by means of zinc chelate, the blood pressure decreased. Although the incidence of hypertension was higher in female than in male animals, the mortality in male rats with hypertension exceeded that of females. Death was the result of heart involvement. The kidneys showed microscopic evidence of a vascular disease and concentrations of

---

*Swedish investigators[80] noted higher storage in the pancreas of mice. They also found a close correlation to cadmium in air with storage in the whole body.

cadmium of 600 ppm (ash), whereas the kidneys of the control animals were cadmium free.

Schroeder extended his work to humans and found that accumulation of cadmium in the human kidney rises up to the fifth decade.[82] Humans with arterial hypertension excrete some 40 times more cadmium in their urine than individuals with normal blood pressure.[87] Like in the animals, Schroeder found an increased ratio of cadmium and zinc in the kidneys of humans with arterial hypertension compared to normal individuals[83] both in the United States and abroad. Confirmatory data on the role of cadmium in human and experimental hypertension were presented recently by Thind.[84]

Acute cadmium intoxication

The first case of acute cadmium poisoning was reported by Sovet[85] in 1858 in three servants who were polishing silverware with cadmium carbonate. One of them had been exposed to the cadmium dust throughout the day. After 3 to 4 hours he developed vomiting, diarrhea, spastic colitis, a bladder infection, and abdominal pains that persisted for 3 days, followed by diarrhea. Subsequently numerous other reports, mostly occupational in nature, have been recorded as the result of smelting impure zinc and cadmium. In most cases, respiratory tract disturbances, namely bronchitis and pneumonia, were associated with the gastrointestinal disorders.

Four men, for instance, were exposed to cadmium fumes while they were cutting cadmium-coated bolts with an oxygen-propane torch in an underground vault.[86] One of them contracted pneumonia from which he gradually recovered; but loss of appetite, shortness of breath on exertion, and excessive thirst persisted for about 3 months. A second patient died of arteriosclerotic coronary artery disease. He had thrombi (blood clots) in the coronary artery. In addition, the autopsy showed extensive changes in the lungs such as emphysema, fibrosis, and evidence of an acute bronchopneumonia. The cadmium concentration in the air was believed to be well above the threshold limit value of 0.1 mg/meter[3].

More significant as an environmental problem is the fact that persons not directly exposed to cadmium by reason of their occupation inhale or ingest it in sufficient amounts to cause chronic poisoning.[87] Periodically, epidemics of poisoning have occurred from accidental contamination of acid foods and drinks with soluble cadmium. Lemonade, homemade punch, and raspberry gelatin dessert, stored in cadmium-plated ice trays, were found to contain from 67 to 530 ppm of the metal.[87]

Twenty-nine school children suffered nausea and vomiting after consuming popsicles containing as little as 13 to 15 ppm cadmium; they recovered completely after 6 hours.[87] Larger amounts induce choking attacks, vomiting, diarrhea, dizziness, salivation (excessive secretion of saliva) and loss of consciousness.

In some patients the disease develops gradually with nausea, chest pain, cough, and sore throat followed by a pulmonary infection. In others, blood clots appear in the heart. They originate in blood vessels that had been attacked by the metal and lead to cardiac infarct (destruction of heart muscle tissue). Cadmium poisoning of occupational origin with massive doses can result in pulmonary edema and destructive changes of the kidney cortex.[88] If patients recover from an acute episode, physicians rarely attribute the long-term and occasionally permanent aftereffects of cadmium poisoning to its cause.

Chronic poisoning

Kidneys. A characteristic feature of chronic cadmium poisoning is the presence in the blood and elimination in the urine of two or more cadmium-binding proteins with a very high sulfur containing amino

acid cystein.[79] They are described as "mini-proteins," because of their low molecular weight (10,000 to 30,000).[89] They are not encountered in other kidney diseases. Damage to kidney substance itself is relatively minute, although kidneys constitute the principal target organ in which a steady build-up of the metal takes place. Only during the early months of cadmium intake does the liver accumulate more cadmium than the kidneys accumulate.

Recent studies on cadmium pigment workers show excretion of sugar, amino acids, and cadmium in the urine, impairment of the concentrating ability of the kidneys, and an excess acidity of the urine, features indicative of damage to the renal tubules.[90]

Respiratory organs. Following repeated inhalation of cadmium fumes, chronic nasal catarrhs and pulmonary emphysema are likely to ensue. Paralysis of the olfactory nerve (responsible for the sense of smell) is common after long-term exposure.[91] Cadmium emphysema differs from emphysema from other causes. Cough and expectoration are minimal in the face of severe breathlessness and, at autopsy, the peripheral portions of the lungs are free of emphysema. Changes in the heart have been reported[75] at atmospheric concentrations of 0.002 μg/meter[3]. (The MAC value is 100 μg/meter[3].)

Hard tissue organs. Persistent cadmium intake leads to a disturbance of the calcium mechanism. As long ago as 1942, Nicaud and co-workers[92] described osteoporosis (bone softening) and spontaneous fractures caused by cadmium, a condition probably identical with Itai-Itai disease. In 1950, Pindborg[93] demonstrated experimentally that cadmium interferes with the development of tooth enamel.

Mutagenic and carcinogenic effects. Cadmium passes the placental barrier. It has induced malformation of the upper jaw and face in newborn rats.[94] It interferes with reproduction and has been identified with induction of toxemia in pregnancy.[95] Long-term uptake of cadmium salts likewise gives rise to damage to the vasculature of the testicles.[96] It destroys the seminiferous tubules (the tubes through which the sperms are ejected from the testicles) and leads to sarcoma of the testicle (a fast growing malignant tumor).[96]

Application of zinc or selenium,[97-99] metals of the same group of the periodic table as cadmium, can inhibit or prevent these disturbances.

Because of the expansion of the cadmium industry and our increasing knowledge of illness caused by cadmium, this metal will probably be playing a much greater role in the study of air pollution in the future than it has in the past.

REFERENCES

1. Waldbott, G. L., and Cecilioni, V. A.: "Neighborhood" fluorosis, Fluoride **2**:206-213, 1969.
2. Hall, G. E., Winegard, W. C., and McKinney, A.: Report of the committee appointed to inquire into and report upon the pollution of air, soil and water, Toronto, September 1968, Frank Fogg, Queen's Printer.
3. Yunghans, R. S., and McMullen, T. B.: Fluoride concentrations found in NASN samples of suspended particles, Fluoride, **3**:143-152, 1970.
4. Cholak, J.: Current information on the quantities of fluoride found in air, food and water, Arch. Industr. Health, **21**:312, 1960.
5. Agate, J. N., Bell, G. H., Broddie, G. F., and others: Industrial fluorosis, Medical research council memorandum, London, 1949, His Majesty's Stationary Office.
6. Hodge, H. C.: The concentration of fluorides in drinking water to give the point of minimum caries with maximum safety. J. Amer. Dent. Ass. **40**:436-439, 1950.
7. Garber, K.: Fluoride in rainwater and vegetation, Fluoride **3**:22-26, 1970.
8. Waldbott, G. L.: Fluoride in clinical medicine, Int. Arch. Allerg. **20**(Suppl.):1-60, 1962.
9. Cross, F. L., and Ross, R. W.: Fluoride uptake from gypsum ponds, Fluoride **3**:97-101, 1970.
10. Natural fluoride content of communal water supplies in the United States, Washington, D. C., 1959, Public Health Service Publication No. 655, Division of Dental Public Health.
11. Oelschlager, W.: Fluoride in food, Fluoride **3**:6-11, 1970.
12. Martin, D. J.: The Evanston dental caries study VIII: fluorine content of vegetables cooked in fluorine containing water, J. Dent. Res. **30**:676, 1951.
13. Oelschlager, W.: Fluoride uptake in soil and its depletion, Fluoride **4**:80, 1971.
14. Cheng, J. Y., Yu, M. H., and Miller, G. W.: Fluoorganic acids in soybean leaves exposed to fluoride, Environ. Sci. Technol. **2**:368-370, 1968.
15. Lovelace, J., Miller, G. W., and Welkie, G. W.: The accumulation of fluoroacetate and fluorocitrate in forage crops collected near a phosphate plant, Atmospher. Environ. **2**:187-190, 1968.
16. McClure, F. J.: Fluoride in foods: survey of recent data, Pub. Health Rep. **64**:1061, 1949.
17. Elliott, C. F., and Smith, M. D.: Dietary fluoride related to fluoride in teeth, J. Dent. Res. **39**:93, 1960.
18. Marier, J. R., and Rose, D.: The fluoride content of some foods and beverages: a brief survey using a modified Zr-Spadns method, J. Food Sci. **31**:941-946, 1966.
19. Spencer, H., Osis, D., Wiatrowski, E., and others: Availability of fluoride from fish protein concentrate and from sodium fluoride in man, J. Nutr. **100**:1415-1424, 1970.
20. Krepkogorskii, L. N.: Fluoride in the traditional diet of the population of the Democratic Republic of Vietnam and endemic fluorosis, Gig. Sanit. **28**:30-35, 1963.
21. Collings, G. H., Jr., Fleming, R. B. L., May, R., and others: Absorption and excretion of inhaled fluorides, further observations, Arch. Industr. Hyg. **6**:368-373, 1952.
22. Wallace-Durbin, P.: The metabolism of fluorine in the rat using F_{18} as a tracer, J. Dent. Res. **33**:789-800, 1954.
23. Lawrenz, M., and Mitchell, H. H.: The effect of dietary calcium and phosphorus on assimilation of dietary fluorine, J. Nutr. **22**:91-101, 1941.
24. Singer, L., and Armstrong, W. D.: Determination of fluoride in blood serum, Anal. Chem., **31**:105-109, 1959.
25. Taves, D. R.: Normal human serum fluoride concentrations, Nature **211**:192-193, 1966.
26. McClure, F. J., Mitchell, H. H., Hamilton, T. S., and others: Balance of fluorine ingested from various sources of food and water by five young men, J. Industr. Hyg. Toxicol. **27**:159-170, 1945.

27. Spencer, H., Lewin, I., Fowler, J., and others: Effect of sodium fluoride on calcium absorption and balances in man, Amer. J. Clin. Nutr. **22**:381, 1969.

28. Largent, E. J.: Fluorosis, Columbus, 1961, Ohio State University Press, p. 54 and Table 17.

29. Gedalia, I.: Urinary fluorine levels of children and adults, J. Dent. Res. **37**:601-604, 1958.

30. Gedalia, I., Brzezinski, A., and Bercovici, B.: Urinary fluorine levels in women during pregnancy and after delivery, J. Dent. Res. **38**: 548-557, 1959.

31. Likens, R. C., McClure, F. J., and Steere, A. C.: Urinary excretion of fluoride following defluoridation of a water supply, Public Health Rep. **71**:217-220, 1956.

32. Roholm, K.: Fluorine intoxication: a clinical hygienic study, London, 1937, H. K. Lewis and Co., Ltd.

33. Weidmann, S. M., Weatherell, J. A., and Jackson, D.: The effect of fluoride on bone, Proc. Nutr. Soc. **22**:105-110, 1963.

34. Singh, A., Jolly, S. S., and Bansal, B. C.: Skeletal fluorosis and its neurological complications, Lancet **1**:197-200, 1961.

35. Posen, G. A., Marier, J. R., and Jaworski, Z. F.: Renal osteodystrophy in patients on long-term hemodialysis with fluoridated water, Fluoride **4**:114-128, 1971.

36. Trace elements in enamel and dentin, Nutr. Rev. **17**:259-261, 1959.

37. Herman, J. F., Mason, B., and Light, F.: Fluorine in urinary tract calculi, J. Urol. **80**: 263-267, 1958.

38. Waldbott, G. L.: Fluoride and calcium levels in the aorta, Experientia **22**:835, 1966.

39. Faccini, J. M.: Review, fluoride and bone calcium, Tiss. Res. **3**:1-16, 1969.

40. McLaren, J. R.: Fluoride and the thyroid gland, Fluoride **2**:192-194, 1969.

41. Bowie, J. Y., Darlow, G., and Murray, M. M.: The effect of sodium fluoride on gastric acid secretion, J. Physiol. **122**:203, 1953.

42. Waldbott, G. L.: Acute fluoride intoxication, Acta Med. Scand. **174**(Suppl. 400):1-42, 1963.

43. Waldbott, G. L.: "Neighborhood" fluorosis, Clin. Toxicol. **2**:387-396, 1969.

44. Russell, A. L.: Dental fluorosis in Grand Rapids during the seventeenth year of fluoridation, J. Amer. Dent. Ass. **65**:608-612, 1962.

45. Jolly, S. S., Prasad, S., Sharma, R., and others: Human fluoride intoxication in Punjab, Fluoride **4**:64-79, 1971.

45a. Jolly, S. S.: An epidemiological, clinical and biochemical study of endemic, dental and skeletal fluorosis in Punjab, Fluoride **1**:65-75, 1968.

46. Pinet, A., and Pinet, F.: Endemic fluorosis in the Sahara, Fluoride **1**:86-93, 1968.

47. Soriano, M.: Periostitis deformans due to fluorine in wine, Radiology **87**:1089-1094, 1966.

48. Jowsey, J., Schenk, R. K., and Reutter, F. W.: Some results of the effect of fluoride on bone tissue in osteoporosis, J. Clin. Endocr. **28**:869, 1968.

49. Webb-Peploe, M. M., and Bradley, W. G.: Endemic fluorosis with neurological complications in a Hampshire man, J. of Neurol. Neurosurg. Psychiat. **29**:577-585, 1966.

50. Fradà, G., Mentesana, G., and Nalbone, G.: Richerche sull 'idrofluorosi, Minerva Med. **54**:451-59, 1963.

51. Linsman, J. F., and McMurray, C. A.: Fluoride osteosclerosis from drinking water, Radiology **40**:474-84, **41**:497, 1943.

52. Sauerbrunn, B. J., Ryan, C. M., and Shaw, J. F.: Chronic fluoride intoxication with fluorotic radiculomyelopathy, Ann. Intern. Med. **63**:1074-78, 1965.

53. Bacon, J. F.: Arterial calcification in infancy, J.A.M.A. **181**:933-935, 1964.

54. Report of the committee appointed to inquire and report upon the pollution of air, soil and water, Toronto, Ontario, September 1968, Queen's Printer.

55. Moser, E.: The treatment of fumes from primary aluminum reduction plants: International Conference on Air Pollution and Water Conservation in the Copper and Aluminum Industries,, London, 1969. Paper No. 12 British Non-Ferrous Metals Research Association.

56. Murray, M. M., and Wilson, D. C.: Fluorine hazards with special reference to some social consequences of industry processes, Lancet **2**:821-824, 1946.

57. Transcript of record in the case of Reynolds Metal Co. vs the Paul Martin family, Nos. 14990-14991-14992 in the U. S. Court of Appeals for the Ninth District, 1968.

58. Balazova, G., Macuch, P. and Rippel, A.: Effects of fluorine emissions on the living organism, Fluoride **2**:36, 1969.

59. Midttun, O.: Bronchial asthma in the aluminum industry, Acta Allerg. **15**:208-221, 1960.

60. Siddiqui, A. H.: Fluorosis in Nalgonda district Hyderabad Deccan, Brit. Med. J. **2**:1408, 1955.

61. Colombini, C., Mauri, C., Olivo, R., and

others: Observations on fluorine pollution due to emissions from an aluminum plant in Trentino, Fluoride 2:40, 1969.

62. Steinegger, S.: Endemic skin lesions near an aluminum factory, Fluoride 2:37, 1969.

63. Wallbott, G. L., and Cecilioni, V. A.: Chizzola maculae, Cutis 6:331-335, 1970.

64. Mangels, J. M., Consumer inquiries staff, Office of Education and Information, March 17, 1967, U. S. Food and Drug Administration.

65. Bonds, R. W.: Community fluoridation section: disease control branch, Division of Dental Health, May 10, 1966, Public Health Service.

66. Emmerson, B. T.: "Ouch-Ouch" disease: the osteomalacia of cadmium nephropathy, Ann. Intern. Med. 73:854, 1970.

67. Tsuchiya, K.: Causation of Ouch-Ouch disease (Itai-Itai Byo): Part I, nature of the disease. Part II, epidemiology and evaluation, Keio J. Med. 18:181-194, 195-211, 1969.

68. Gayn, M.: Smoke from a smelter adds a Japanese town to a long horror list, Toronto Daily Star, August 15, 1970.

69. Prodan, L.: Cadmium poisoning: Part I, the history of cadmium poisoning and uses of cadmium, J. Industr. Hyg 14:132-155, 1932.

70. McCaull, J.: Building a shorter life, Environment 13:2-15, 1971.

71. Schroeder, H. A., and Balassa, J. J.: Abnormal trace metals in man: cadmium, J. Chron. Dis. 14:236, 1961.

72. Schroeder, H. A., and Balassa, J. J.: Cadmium: uptake by vegetables from superphosphate in soil, Science 140:819-820, 1963.

73. Vancouver Sun, February 13, 1961.

74. McCabe, L. J., Symons, J. M., Lee, R. D., and others: Survey of community water supply systems, J. Amer. Water Works Ass. 6:670-687, 1970.

75. Carroll, R. E.: The relationship of cadmium in the air: cardiovascular disease death rate, J.A.M.A. 198:267-269, 1966.

76. Nandi, M., Gick, H., Slone, D., and others: Cadmium content of cigarettes, Lancet 2:1329-1330, 1969.

77. Tipton, I. H.: The distribution of trace metals in the human body, in metal binding. In Seren, M. J., editor: Medication, Philalelphia, 1960, J. B. Lippincott Co., p. 27.

78. Cotzias, G. C., Borg, D. C., and Seleck, B.: Virtual absence of turnover in cadmium metabolism, Cd^{109} studies in the mouse, Amer. J. Physiol. 201:139, 1957.

79. Friberg, L., Piscator, M., and Nordberg, G.: Symposium on cadmium in the environment: a toxicologic and epidemiologic appraisal, New York, June, 1971, University of Rochester.

80. Nordberg, G. F., and Nishiyama, K.: Whole body and hair retention of cadmium in mice, Arch. Environ. Health 24:209-214, 1972.

81. Schroeder, H. A.: Cadmium hypertension in rats, Amer. J. Physiol. 207:62-66, 1964.

82. Perry, H. M., Jr., and Schroeder, H. A.: Concentration of trace metals in urine of treated and untreated hypertensive patients compared with normal subjects, J. Lab. Clin. Med. 46:936, 1955.

83. Schroeder, H. A.: Cadmium as a factor in hypertension, J. Chron. Dis. 18:647-656, 1965.

84. Thind, G. S.: Role of cadmium in human and experimental hypertension, J.A.P.C.A. 22:267-270, 1972.

85. Sovet, A.: Empoisonnement par une poudre à écurer l'argenterie, Presse Med. Belge 10:69, 1858.

86. Zavon, M. R., and Meadows, C. D.: Vascular sequelae to cadmium fume exposure, Amer. Industr. Hyg. Ass. J. 31:180-182, 1970.

87. Frant, S., and Kleeman, S.: Cadmium "food poisoning," J.A.M.A. 117:86-89, 1941.

88. Kendrey, G., and Roe, F. J. C.: Cadmium toxicology, Lancet 1:1206-1207, 1969.

89. Lucis, O. J., Shaikk, Z. A., and Embril, J. A. Jr.: Cadmium as a trace element and cadmium binding compounds in human cells, Experimentia 26:1109-1110, 1970.

90. Kazantzis, G., Flynn, F. V., Spowage, J. S., and others: Renal tubular malfunction and pulmonary emphysema in cadmium pigment workers, Quart. J. Med. 32:165-192, 1963.

91. Louria, D. B., Joselow, M. M., and Browder, A. A.: The human toxicity of certain trace elements, Amer. Int. Med. 76:307-319, 1972.

92. Nicaud, P., Lafitte, A., and Gros, A.: Les troubles de l'intoxication chronique par les cadmium, Arch. Mal. Prof. 4:192-202, 1942.

93. Pindborg, J. J.: Den kroniske fluorog cadmiumforgiftnings, Copenhagen, 1950, Ejnar Munksgaard.

94. Carpenter, S. J.: Teratogenic effect of cadmium and its inhibition by zinc, Nature 216:1123, 1967.

95. Parizek, J.: The peculiar toxicity of cadmium during pregnancy in an experimental toxemia pregnancy induced by cadmium salts, J. Reprod. Fertil. 9:111-112, 1965.

96. Parizek, J.: The destructive effect of cadmium on testicular tissue and its prevention by zinc, J. Endocr. 15:56-63, 1957.

97. Parizek, J., and Zahor, A.: Effect of cadmium salts on testicular tissue, Nature 177:1036, 1956.

98. Gunn, S. A., Gould, T. C., and Anderson, W. A. D.: Effect of zinc on cancerogenesis by cadmium, Proc. Soc. Exp. Biol. Med. **115**:653-657, 1964.

99. Gunn, S. A., Gould, T. C., and Anderson, W. A. D.: Mechanism of zinc, cysteine and selenium protection against cadmium induced vascular injury to mouse testis, J. Reprod. Fertil. **15**:65-70, 1968.

14

SYSTEMIC POISONS: selenium, vanadium, phosphorus, boron, titanium, and tellurium

SELENIUM

Occurrence in nature

Selenium (Se) a nonmetallic element of the sulfur group, is distributed widely in nature. It occurs mainly in sulfide minerals and in soil but only in minute concentrations (average, 0.09 ppm).[1] Levels of selenium above 120 ppm have been found in volcanic sulfur deposits in some of the western states of the United States,[3] in carbonaceous siltstone in western Wyoming (680 ppm), and in phosphate rock (212 ppm).[4]

Certain plants, such as milk vetch (Astragalus) and woody aster (Xylorhiza), which emit an offensive garliclike odor, contain sizeable amounts of selenium (1000 to 10,000 ppm).[5] Known as "primary" indicator plants for selenium, they require the metal for growth[5] and accumulate it from the soil regardless of the form in which it occurs. However, selenium content of soil does not parallel that of vegetation.[2] Grains, vegetables, grasses, and other vegetation that accumulate water-soluble selenium compounds from the soil can cause acute and chronic poisoning in livestock at concentrations of less than 30 ppm.

Superphosphate, which contains selenium at levels of 20 ppm and above, and ammonium phosphate fertilizers enrich the soil with selenium.[6] In rainwater, its concentration is of the order of 0.21 μg/liter.[7]

Table 14-1. Selenium content of various earth materials*

MATERIAL	SELENIUM CONTENT (PPM)
Earth's crust	0.09
Igneous rocks	.05
Shales	.60
Sandstones	.05
Carbonates	.08
Deep-sea sediments	.17
Soils	.10 to .20

*Adapted from Lakin, H. W.: Selenium accumulation in soils and its absorption by plants and animals, 1971. Geol. Soc. Amer. Bull. 83:181-189, 1972.

Selenium in industry

Selenium is a by-product in the refining of such ores as copper, lead, gold, nickel, and silver and in the manufacturing of sulfuric acid. It is used in the manufacture of pigments, insecticides, stainless steel, photoelectric cells, in rubber compounding, and in the glass industry.[8]

Burning of coal releases into the atmosphere between 0.7 and 7.38 ppm of selenium, combustion of newsprint, cardboard, and tissue paper from 1.6 to 19.5 ppm.[9,10] In tobacco, up to 0.88 ppm of selenium was found.[11] Rubber in automobile tires in the Tokyo area contained 0.7 to 2.0 ppm selenium.[12] Soils in that region showed a content of 1.0 to 1.8 ppm selenium, a level that is considered toxic. In dust from

Table 14-2. Selenium content of various samples of paper, coal, and petroleum*

MATERIAL	SELENIUM AVERAGE	(PPM) MAXIMUM
Newspaper	8.60	18.30
Cardboard	2.80	5.10
Laboratory tissue	7.10	19.50
Cigarette paper	.17	—
Raw petroleum	.92	.95
Heavy petroleum fractions	.99	1.65
Coal (Tokyo market)	1.18	1.30
U. S. crude petroleum	.17	.35
U. S. coal	3.20	10.65

*Adapted from Lakin, H. W.: Selenium accumulation in soils and its absorption by plants and animals, 1971. Geol. Soc. Amer. Bull. **83:**181-189, 1972.

Table 14-3. Selenium content of fish meal*

	AVERAGE (PPM)	RANGE (PPM)
East Canadian herring	1.95	1.30–2.6
Chilean anchovetta	1.35	.84–2.6
Tuna	4.63	3.40–6.2
Smelt	.95	.49–1.23
Menhaden	2.09	.75–4.2

*Adapted from Kifer, R. R., Payne, W. L., and Ambrose, M. E.: Selenium content of fish meals, Part II, Feedstuffs **41:**24-25, 1969.

air-conditioning filters collected at residences, stores, and office buildings in United States cities, selenium levels ranged from 0.05 to 10 ppm.[8]

Additional data on selenium content of materials are given in Table 14-2. The maximum allowable concentration (MAC) of selenium compounds for occupational exposures (40-hour week) was set in 1962 at 0.1 mg/meter^3.[13]

Selenium in food

The selenium content of edible foods depends on the kind of soil in which they are grown, on whether or not they are grown near industrial establishments, and on the manner in which the particular edible plants take up and retain selenium. Food derived from plant life contains between 0.07 and 1.01 ppm selenium.[6]

Sunflowers and wheat tend to accumulate selenium from soil. In hothouse experiments, sunflowers showed levels as high as 500 ppm selenium.[14] Wheat usually contains between 0.1 to 1.5 ppm selenium[6] but near industrial establishments, as much as 18.8 ppm has been found in wheat, 1.0 to 14.9 in corn, 1.6 to 15.7 in barley, and 0.9 to 3.8 ppm in rye.[15]

Selenium levels in meat from cattle raised in exposed areas range between 1.17 and 8.0 mg/kg.[6] Kidneys from cows contain twice as much selenium as those from calves.

In fish, selenium levels vary widely both within and between species. In waters that are very low in selenium, Kifer and associates[16] found unusually high accumulations in tuna fish (Table 14-3), a fact that suggests an ecologic role in the food chain similar to that of mercury.

Highly fertilized agricultural products, such as rice, beans, and grain, may contain more than ten times the usual selenium content. In drinking water, selenium levels range from 1.6 to 5.3 μg/liter (0.0016 to 0.0053 ppm).[6] High levels, such as 9 ppm, have caused chronic selenosis in humans and livestock.[5] Five-tenths ppm in drinking water or 5 mg/kg in food can cause adverse effects.[5]

Selenium metabolism

The action of selenium in humans depends largely on the solubility of the respective selenium compound and the manner in which it is taken up by the system. Elemental selenium is relatively nontoxic.[10] It is converted in the body into a volatile compound, dimethylselenide, which is eliminated through the breath and sweat.[17] Inhaled metallic selenium compounds are less toxic than the more soluble aerosols such as SeO_2, SeO_3, and halogen compounds. Hydrogen selenide (H_2Se), a gas with a strong offensive odor,* and certain organic selenium compounds, such as methyl and ethyl selenide, rank among the most toxic and irritating selenium compounds. They are retained in tissue longer and at greater magnitudes than inorganic compounds.[18]

In the human organism, 50% to 80% of ingested selenium is excreted through the kidneys.[18] On the other hand Schultz and associates[17] indicate that between 17% and 52% of sodium selenate given subcutaneously to cats in doses of 2.5 to 3.5 mg/kg body weight is exhaled within 8 hours. Such variations in results are probably related to dose, compounds, individual susceptibility, and many other factors. The highest amounts of selenium are found in kidneys and liver. Storage takes place also in the spleen, pancreas, muscles, and lungs. Selenium levels in hair serve as a criterion of the length of exposure and the degree of selenium storage in the system.

Persons not exposed to selenium hazard except through normal ingestion of cereals excrete from 0.01 to 0.95 ppm in the urine a day.[20] However, minor symptoms of poisoning have been reported when urinary excretion was 0.069 ppm.[21]

Selenium deficiency

Selenium is considered a micronutrient at levels of 0.02 to 1 ppm, but at slightly higher magnitudes it affects the mammalian hosts adversely. In poultry, a lack of selenium leads to exudative diatheses (a tendency to skin, nasal, and eye irritation) and to dermatitis. In lambs and calves a deficiency causes "white muscle disease,"[22] a condition characterized by progressive muscular dystrophy (muscle wasting and shrinkage), retardation of growth, and decrease in fertility. In New Zealand, approximately 20% to 30% of all sheep are deficient in selenium, which constitutes a threat to wool production.

Selenium is also essential for the functioning of light receptors in the retina. Animals with excellent vision, such as the deer and the sea swallow, contain in their system about 100 times more selenium than animals with lesser visual capacity.[23] Furthermore, selenium is involved in decarboxylation* processes. It increases the capacity of vitamin E to reduce lipids (fat) in the system.[24] Selenium is an antagonist to arsenic,[25] a significant feature that must be taken into account in interpreting environmental behavior of either agent.

Selenium intoxication

Acute selenium poisoning. Acute selenium poisoning in humans is rare in spite of its widespread use in industry. Its toxic action resembles that of arsenic and tellurium. Because it causes immediate and intense irritation of the eyes, nose and throat and because of a peculiar unpleasant, sour, garliclike odor, the presence of selenium in fumes is easily detected and further exposure can be avoided.

At first the victims develop nasal congestion, nosebleed, cough, dizziness, and redness of the eyes. Two to four hours later severe headaches occur, mainly in the frontal (sinus) area, associated with difficult breathing and edema of the throat.[26] In extreme cases, difficult breathing is followed by convulsions, with falling blood pressure and respiratory failure. In such cases selenium may not show up in the urine and the white blood count and hemoglobin may be normal.[25]

Chronic selenosis. In persons with *chronic selenosis,* mental depression, marked pallor, weakness, nervousness, dizziness, gastrointestinal disorders, and excessive perspiration are noted. The skin shows yel-

---

*At 0.001 mg hydrogen selenide per meter³ of air the odor quickly disappears because of paralysis of the olfactory nerve.[19]

*Elimination of carboxyl radicals from an organic acid, with the release of carbon dioxide.

low (jaundice) discoloration. Ascites (fluid in abdomen), liver and splenic damage, followed by progressive anemia, are also encountered.[27] The garliclike odor is the most characteristic symptom of the disease. Kidney and liver disease constitute the long-term effects of selenium poisoning. Protracted exposure to selenium in dust and gases causes fibrosis of the lungs. Long-term intake of selenium through food and water produces dental caries.[28] Dermatitis has been described as a result of contact of selenium with the skin.

Rats fed 10 to 50 ppm selenium for 18 months developed a cancerous tumor of low malignancy in the liver.[29] Whether or not selenium is carcinogenic to humans has not been resolved.

High protein diets, particularly casein, are protective against selenium poisoning and are administered as an antidote. Sodium arsenate is a preventive for liver damage and destruction of hemoglobin, which are caused by toxic amounts.[30]

It appears that the toxicity of selenium varies depending on with what other elements it is combined. Whereas elemental selenium is practically nontoxic, hydrogen selenide and certain organic selenium compounds are powerful poisons. No harm has been reported at the levels of selenium ordinarily encountered in ambient air, but accidental occupational exposure and chronic intake of selenium through food can affect the liver, kidneys, and spleen adversely. Recent work on the relationship of vitamin E to selenium has contributed materially to the understanding of selenium's biologic action.

VANADIUM

In 1911 workers in Peruvian ore mines developed a disease characterized by irritation in the throat, eyes, and nose, and by severe cough with pulmonary hemorrhages. In some, the kidneys were involved,[31] with blood loss through the urine and generalized anemia. Exposure to vanadium (V) dust and fumes was found to be respon-

sible for the disease. During the 1940s and 1950s, the same disease was recorded by several authors from different parts of the world as a result of airborne vanadium pentoxide (V_2O_5) and vanadium trioxide (V_2O_3) present in by-products of residual or crude oil combustion.[32,33] The intensity of the observed effects was directly related to the concentration of the vanadium compound in the air and their particle size. Exposure ranged from 1 to 50 mg of vanadium per meter^3; particle sizes were less than 5 μ, sometimes even less than 1 μ in diameter.

Sources of vanadium

Vanadium has been identified in more than 65 vanadium-bearing minerals. It is usually found combined with iron, nickel, molybdenum, phosphorus, and carbon. In Colorado and Utah mines, vanadium is associated with uranium-containing ores. In Idaho and Montana, from 0.11% to 0.45% vanadium pentoxide is found in phosphate rocks. Burning of coal liberates between 16 and 176 ppm vanadium.[34] After combustion of residual oil and petroleum, from 0.4 to 38.5% vanadium remains in the ash.

Vanadium is emitted into the atmosphere by industries producing the metal and its compounds, by power plants and utilities that consume vanadium-containing crude oils and coal, by industries engaged in refining crude oil, and by the iron, steel, and aluminum industries, which produce vanadium-bearing alloys. The chemical industry utilizes vanadium in the production of numerous chemicals.

In ambient air, the average vanadium concentrations range from a level below detection to 0.9 μg/meter^3 [35] depending largely on burning of heavy fuel oil at power plants. Recent readings in Boston showed up to 2.5 μg/meter^3.[36] The MAC values adopted in 1967 by the American Conference of Governmental Industrial Hygienists are 500 μg/meter^3 for vanadium pentoxide dust and 100 μg for fumes of vanadium pentoxide.

Health effects

In rats vanadium is stored in the body in fat and blood serum. Schroeder and associates[37] detected vanadium in lungs and intestines in minute amounts of 0.01 μg or less per gram of tissue.

In the human organism vanadium has a threefold action:

1. It inhibits the synthesis of cholesterol, of phospholipids, and of other lipids (fat). Cholesterol, a precursor of the all important adrenocortical hormones, affects a great number of metabolic processes, especially the metabolism of salt, water, mineral, and carbohydrate.

2. It inhibits formation of cystine, cysteine, and methionine, the three basic sulfur-containing amino acids. Cystine is the sulfur-containing constituent of skin, hair, and nails. Methionine has a sulfur-bound methyl group that enters into the production of adrenalin, choline, and creatine.

3. It interferes with the utilization of iron in the synthesis of hemoglobin. Vanadium also leads to accumulation of serotonin, a crystalline protein and powerful constrictor of blood vessels found in many body tissues, chiefly in the brain and in the blood.

Experimental data. Rabbits and rats exposed for 2 hours daily to inhalation of vanadium trioxide in concentrations of 40 to 70 mg/meter^3 over a period of 9 to 12 months developed anemia and a reduction in the number of white blood cells. After 2 to 3 months, the albumin content of the blood had decreased and the blood globulin had increased. After 11 months, the amino acids had increased in the blood serum, the vitamin C level of the blood had declined, the tissue respiration in the liver and brain was drastically reduced. At the end of the experimental period, the animal had contracted chronic bronchitis, pulmonary emphysema, and fibrosis.[38]

Clinical data. At the relatively low concentrations recorded for urban atmospheres, to date no clinically observable physiologic changes have been identified. The lethal dose of vanadium through inhalation is believed to range between 60 to 120 mg.[39] Chronic exposure to environmental air concentrations have been associated statistically with a high incidence of chronic bronchitis, cardiovascular disease, and certain kinds of cancers,[40] especially when vanadium occurs in conjunction with other metals such as nickel and cadmium.

Two volunteers who were exposed to vanadium pentoxide dust at a concentration of 1 mg/meter^3 for an 8-hour period developed cough that persisted for 8 days. All of five other volunteers exposed to an average concentration of 0.2 mg/meter^3 for about 8 hours had a loose cough the following day. A maximum urinary vanadium excretion of 0.13 mg/liter and of 3 mg/kg with the bowel content was recorded 3 days following exposure.[41]

In 24 workers exposed to vanadium pentoxide at concentrations ranging from 18 to 925 μg/meter^3, serum cholesterol levels were approximately 10% below normal.[42] Concentrations above 1 mg/meter^3 led to a wide variety of clinically observable adverse effects, mainly gastrointestinal and respiratory symptoms, nausea, cough, pulmonary hemorrhages, damage to the lungs and kidneys, bronchitis, and bronchopneumonia.

A review of the action of vanadium reveals that this element, especially its pentavalent compounds, inhibits the synthesis of cholesterol and other lipids, and of cysteine and other amino acids. Exposure to environmental concentrations leads to cardiovascular disease and to a variety of symptoms involving mainly the gastrointestinal and respiratory systems.

PHOSPHORUS AND PHOSPHATES

In 1832 the first white phosphorus (P) matches were made in Austria and Germany. Almost immediately they became popular throughout the world. This discovery set the stage for one of the greatest tragedies in the history of occupational diseases. Workers in the match factories developed a disease characterized by necrosis (destruction) of the jaw bone and by pus formation around the roots of the teeth. The disease usually began with a toothache often accompanied by a dull red spot on the mucous lining of the mouth. Abscesses formed on the jaw bones and pieces of bones sequestered from the affected areas. Fever and chills followed. Eventually septicemia (blood poisoning) led to the patient's death.[43] Later, when phosphorus was used for fireworks, acute poisoning occurred, occasionally among children when they put such fireworks into their mouths.[44]

White phosphorus, a waxy transparent solid, is soft enough to be cut with a knife. It is highly inflammable and ignites in the air at 30° C. Because of this property, it is especially useful for incendiary warfare. When it comes in contact with air, it is readily oxidized and undergoes yellow discoloration. During this process, it gives off fumes of the very poisonous phosphorus trioxide, (P_2O_3), characterized by a garlic-like odor. In contrast to white and yellow phosphorus, red phosphorus and certain organic (for example, the pesticide malathion) and inorganic phosphorus compounds are comparatively nontoxic even at gram levels.

In recent years phosphorus and its compounds have gained increasing importance as an air pollutant. Elemental phosphorus is an intermediate product in the manufacturing of phosphoric fertilizers and it is widely used in the chemical industry. Phosphorus compounds are used as additives to gasoline and aviation fuels.

Elemental phosphorus occurs in the atmosphere, but most of it reacts to form phosphorus oxides and suboxides. Boilers and furnaces burning crude oils and coals emit phosphorus compounds.

In flue dusts the gases generated by heating contain phosphine fumes (PH_3), a very toxic agent that ignites spontaneously in air. This gas acts on the central nervous system and the blood. At concentrations of 2000 ppm (2800 mg/meter³), phosphine is lethal to man in a few minutes. At lower concentrations, phosphine produces shortness of breath, dizziness, bronchitis, and convulsions. The maximum dose tolerated for 2 hours without appearance of symptoms is 7 ppm.[45]

Unfortunately, only few known phosphorus compounds have been investigated with respect to their effect on humans, animals, and plants.[46] The action of organophosphorus compounds as agricultural chemicals and their significance as toxic air pollutants are discussed in Chapter 18.

BORON AND ITS COMPOUNDS

Compared with other atmospheric pollutants the medical literature on boron (B) and its compounds and data on their role as air pollutants is sparse. It seems that damage to human health by boron compounds is insignificant in spite of the large number of persons who are exposed to them.

Boron is widely distributed in nature but constitutes only an estimated 0.001% of the earth's crust.[47] Deposits of commercially valuable boron minerals are found in regions where volcanic activity has been intense in the past as, for instance, in California and near Trona in the Mohave Desert. It is also a constituent of coal ash, which contains on an average more than 0.1%.[48]

Borax* is used in the manufacture of glass and ceramics and in leather tanning. In gasoline, diesel, and aircraft turbine fuels, it serves as an additive to prevent growth of microorganisms. It is also a constituent of many artificial fertilizers. Borax is particularly useful as a detergent in combination with soaps.

---

*Borax is a white crystalline compound from which boron is derived.

The most common health hazards occur from accidental ingestion of certain compounds such as boric acid and borax used in households. Surgeons have encountered boric acid poisoning following absorption of boric acid from wounds or burns.

Boron dusts in the atmosphere are derived mainly from manufacture of boron compounds, each of which varies in its action. Air contamination is liable to occur from the use of boron hydrides, or so-called boranes. They are highly toxic gases employed in fuels for rocket motors and jet engines. Inhalation of these compounds can cause severe disturbances of the central nervous system and lead to permanent injury and death. A syndrome resembling metal fever has been described after exposure to diborane in a limited number of workers.[49] Pentaborane affects mainly the central nervous system inducing dizziness and headaches. Inhalation of boric acid and boron oxide in the form of dust can cause respiratory distress but is not likely to induce permanent damage.[50]

Threshold limit values for boranes in industry for a 40-hour week for healthy workers are 100 μg/meter^3 of air for diborane, 10 μg/meter^3 for pentaborane, and 300 μg/meter^3 for decaborane.[47]

TITANIUM

Titanium (Ti) is a trace metal the biologic action of which has been little explored to date. It ranks third in abundance on the earth's crust after aluminum and iron[51] and is found in beach sands and rock deposits, usually associated with iron.

Industrially it is employed mainly in making pigments, welding-rod coatings, and alloys, particularly carbides, ceramics, and fiber glass. Titanium-containing paints are currently in wide use; titanium oxides are employed in paper sizing and in the metallurgical industry.

Exposure to titanium dust and fumes occurs in the operation of electric furnaces, in various kinds of machining, and in metal fabrication. Tabor and Warren[52] recorded values of less than 0.01 μg/meter^3 up to 0.3 μg/meter^3 in the atmosphere.

Titanium is a constituent of most human foods, especially of vegetation growing in forests where it is derived from soil. The green portions of a plant contain more of the metal than do the roots and stems.[53] Schroeder and associates[54] found little titanium in milk, cheese, lamb, beef, and whole grains; they found large amounts (up to 2.49 μg/gm wet weight) in butter and corn oil. About 300 μg is ingested with an average daily diet, approximately 3% of which is absorbed into the bloodstream and excreted in the urine.[54] By inhalation through the lungs, the normal intake of titanium varies from almost zero to 4.5 μg.

According to Vinogradov[55] algae, plankton, spongeous corals, and starfish, absorb titanium from the environment. Fish, however, do not store much of the metal. The integument of seafood and chicken contains titanium. Values in water range from nondetectable amounts to 0.14 ppm.

A normal human body contains less than 15 mg titanium, most of which has accumulated in the lungs and in the skin. Newborn babies have little if any titanium in their bodies. Urinary values were found to be 10.2 μg/liter (0.010 ppm) in pooled normal urine.[56] Blood levels are about 3 μg/100 cc of blood plasma.

In rats, titanium salts suppress conversions of cysteine to cysteic acid by rat liver, kidneys, and brain.[57] At concentrations as low as 0.46 mM, titanium interferes with the activity of serum alkaline phosphatase, the enzyme involved in bone growth. Titanium also inhibits invertase and amylase, two enzymes concerned with carbohydrate metabolism. Formation of the yellow pigmentation of the skin has been attributed to titanium.[58] Schroeder and associates[54] found much of the metal in human hair.

Thus far, no toxicity has been recorded in the literature at levels present in the air.

TELLURIUM

Tellurium (Te) is a brownish-black powder that occurs in sulfide ores in conjunction with selenium, gold, silver, lead, and bismuth. During the electrolytical refining of copper, it is present in the sediment at the anode. Industrially, it serves to improve rubber, to harden the surface of car wheels and to enhance ductility of steel. It is present in tellurium vapor "daylight" lamps and is employed in the electronic industry. Fumes of tellurium and tellurium oxides contaminate the air in industrial establishments, mainly through handling the chemical.

The body takes up tellurium largely through inhalation but also through the skin. Most of it accumulates in the kidneys. Although very little is excreted from the body, whatever excretion occurs takes place through the lungs, urine, and sweat. Excretion through the lungs accounts for a characteristic garliclike smell similar to that of selenium.[59]

When tellurium salts are given by mouth, they are reduced by the action of bacteria to elemental tellurium in the intestinal tract. DeMeio[60] found 63% to 84% of a given dose of elemental tellurium in the feces. The garlic smell is caused by a volatile tellurium compound, dimethyl telluride.[61]

Toxicity. Little is known about the action of tellurium as an air pollutant. After long-time exposure of iron foundry workers to concentrations of tellurium between 0.1 and 1.0 mg/10 meter^3 of air over a period of 22 months, Steinberg and co-workers[62] noted the typical garliclike odor of the breath and sweat and found tellurium in the urine in concentrations between 0.01 to 0.06 ppm in workers and their families. In addition dryness and metallic taste of the mouth, sleepiness, and loss of appetite were recorded.

A toxic tellurium compound is hydrogen telluride gas, the odor of which is similar to that of hydrogen sulfide. Inhalation of large doses of this gas causes acute pneumonia.[63]

It has been found that administration of vitamin C eliminates the garliclike breath in persons exposed to tellurium. This however may not be desirable, since toxicity of tellurium dioxide is enhanced by vitamin C.[64] The workers' maximum allowable concentration for tellurium in air is 0.01 to 0.1 mg/meter^3.[65]

REFERENCES

1. Goldschmidt, V. M.: Geochemistry, Oxford, 1954, Clarendon Press, p. 730.
2. Lakin, H. W.: Selenium accumulation in soils and its absorption by plants and animals, Geol. Soc. Amer. Bull. 83:181-189, 1972.
3. Byers, H. G.: Selenium occurrence in certain soils in the United States, with a discussion of related topics, U. S. Dept. Agr. Tech. Bull. 482:48, 1935.
4. Beath, O. A., Hagner, A. L., and Gilbert, C. S.: Some rocks and soils of high selenium content, Geol. Survey Wyoming Bull. 36:23, 1946.
5. Rosenfeld, I., and Beath, O. A.: Selenium, New York, 1964, Academic Press, Inc.
6. Oelschlager, W., and Menke, K. H.: Über Selengehalte Pflanzlicher, Tierischer und Anderer Stoffe. Z. Ernährungswiss. 9:216-222, 1969.
7. Hashimoto, Y., and Winchester, J. W.: Selenium in the atmosphere, Environ. Sci. Technol. 1:338, 1967.
8. Lakin, H. W., and Davidson, D. R.: The relation of geochemistry of selenium to its occurrence in soils. In Muth, O. H., editor: Symposium: selenium in biomedicine, Westport, Conn., 1967, AVI Publishing Co.
9. Johnson, H.: Determination of selenium in solid waste, Environ. Sci. Technol. 4:850-853, 1970.
10. Stahl, Q. R., and others: Air pollution aspects of selenium and its compounds, PB 188 077, Bethesda, Maryland, 1969, Litton Industries, Inc.
11. Olson, O. E.: Selenium in papers and tobaccos, Environ. Sci. Technol. 4:686-687, 1970.
12. Hashimoto, Y., Hvang, J. Y., and Yanagisana, S.: Possible source of atmospheric pollution of selenium, Environ. Sci. Technol. 4:157-158, 1970.
13. Documentation of threshold limit values, Cincinnati, Ohio, 1962, American Conference of Governmental Industrial Hygienists Committee on Threshold Limit Values.
14. Oelschlager, W., and Menke, K. H.: Über Selengehalte Pflanzlicher, Tierischer und

Anderer Stoffe I: Selengehalte der Futtermittel, Z. Ernährungswiss. **9:**208-215, 1969.

15. Underwood, E. J.: The mineral nutrition of livestock, Aberdeen, Scotland, 1966, pp. 202-222.

16. Kifer, R. R., Payne, W. L., and Ambrose, M. E.: Selenium content of fish meals, II, Feedstuffs **41:**24-25, 1969.

17. Schultz, J., and Lewis, H. B.: The excretion of volatile selenium compounds after the administration of sodium selenite to white rats, J. Biol. Chem. **133:**199, 1940.

18. Smith, M. I., Westfall, B. B., and Stohlman, E. E.: Studies of the fate of selenium in the organism, Public Health Rep. **53:**1199, 1938.

19. Cerwenka, E. A., Jr., and Cooper, W. C.: Toxicology of selenium and tellurium and their compounds, Arch. Environ. Health **3:**189-200, 1961.

20. Sterner, J. H., and Lidfelt, V.: Selenium content of normal urine, J. Pharmacol. Exp. Ther. **73:**205, 1941.

21. Dudley, H. C.: Toxicology of selenium: Part II, the urinary excretion of selenium, Amer. J. Hyg. **23:**181, 1936.

22. Glover, J. R.: Selenium in urine, Ann. Occup. Hyg. **10:**3, 1967.

23. Siren, M. J.: Science tools, The LKB Instrument J. **11:**37, 1964.

24. Stokinger, H. E.: The spectre of today's environmental pollution—U. S. A. brand: new perspectives from an old scout, Amer. Indust. Hyg. Ass. J. **30:**195-217, 1969.

25. Rhian, M., and Moxon, A. L.: Chronic selenium poisoning in dogs and its prevention by arsenic, J. Pharmacol. Exp. Ther. **78:**249, 1943.

26. Clinton, M., Jr.: Selenium fume exposure, J. Industr. Hyg. Toxicol. **29:**225, 1947.

27. Moxon, A. L., and Rhian, M.: Selenium poisoning, Physiol. Rev. **23:**305, 1943.

28. Hadjimarkos, D. M.: Effect of selenium on dental caries, Arch. Environ. Health **10:**893, 1965.

29. Nelson, A. A., Fitshugh, O. G., and Calvery, H. O.: Liver tumors following cirrhosis caused by selenium in rats, Cancer Res. **3:**220, 1943.

30. Moxon, A. L., Paynko, C. R., and Halverson, A. W.: Effect of route of administration on detoxication of selenium by arsenic, J. Pharmacol. Exp. Ther. **84:**115-119, 1945.

31. Athanassiadis, Y. C.: Air pollution aspects of vanadium and its compound, PB 188 093, Bethesda, Maryland, 1969, Litton Systems, Inc.

32. McTurk, L. C., Hirs, C. H. W., and Eckardt, R. E.: Health hazards of vanadium-containing residual oil ash, Ind. Med. Surg. **25:**29, 1956.

33. Thomas, D. L. G., and Stiebris, K.: Vanadium poisoning in industry, Med. J. Aust. **1:**607, 1956.

34. Abernathy, R. F., and Gibson, F. H.: Rare elements in coal. U. S. Bureau of Mines Information Circular 8163, 1963.

35. NASN, hi-vol samples of urban and non-urban sites, Cincinnati, Ohio, 1966-1967, Air Quality and Emissions Data Division, N.A.P.C.A.

36. Sillerly, R. H.: Trace elements in air and water, Sci. News **97:**538, 1970.

37. Schroeder, H. A., Balassa, J. J., and Tipton, I. H.: Abnormal trace metals in man—vanadium, J. Chron. Dis. **16:**1047, 1963.

38. Roshchin, I. V.: Toxicology of vanadium compounds used in modern industry, Gig. Sanit. **32:**4-6, 1967.

39. Stokinger, H. E.: Vanadium. In Patty, F. A., editor: Industrial hygiene and toxicology, New York, 1963, Interscience Publishers.

40. Stocks, P.: On the relation between atmospheric pollution in urban and rural localities and mortality from cancer, bronchitis and pneumonia, with particular reference to 3, 4 benzo[a]pyrene, beryllium, molybdenum, vanadium and arsenic, Brit. J. Cancer **14:**397, 1960.

41. Zenz, C., and Berg, B. A.: Human responses to controlled vanadium pentoxide exposure, Arch. Environ. Health **14:**709, 1967.

42. Lewis, C. E.: The biological actions of vanadium. Part III, the effect of vanadium on the excretion of 5-hydroxy-indolacetic acid and amino acids and the electrocardiogram of the dog, Arch. Industr. Health **20:**455, 1959.

43. Hunter, D.: The diseases of occupations, London, 1969, The English Universities Press Limited.

44. Heimann, H.: Chronic phosphorus poisoning, J. Industr. Hyg. Toxicol. **28:**142-150, 1946.

45. Jacobs, M. B.: The analytical toxicology of industrial inoganic poisons, New York, 1967, Interscience Publishers.

46. Athanassiadis, Y. C.: Air pollution aspects of phosphorus and its compounds, PB 188 073, Litton Industries, Inc., Bethesda, Maryland, 1969, U. S. Dept. of Commerce, National Bureau of Standards.

47. Durocher, N. L.: Air pollution aspects of boron and its compounds, PB 188 085, Litton Industries, Inc., Bethesda, Maryland, 1969, U. S. Dept. of Commerce, National Bureau of Standards.

48. Abernathy, R. F., and Gibson, F. H.: Rare elements in coals, Bureau of Mines Informa-

tion Circular IC 8163, 1963, U. S. Dept. of Interior.

49. Rozendaal, H. M.: Clinical observations on the toxicology of boron hydrides, Arch. Industr. Health Occup. Med. 4:247-260, 1951.
50. Saks, H. I.: Dangerous properties of industrial materials, ed. 3, New York, 1968, Van Nostrand Reinhold Co.
51. Mason, B.: Principles of geochemistry, ed. 2, New York, 1958, John Wiley & Sons.
52. Tabor, E. C., and Warren, W. V.: Distribution of certain metals in the atmosphere of some American cities, Arch. Industr. Health 17:145, 1958.
53. Bibliography of the Literature on the Minor Elements and their Relation to Plant and Animal Nutrition. Vol. II, New York, 1958, Chilean Nitrate Educational Bureau.
54. Schroeder, H. A., Balassa, J. J., and Tipton, I. H.: Abnormal trace metals in man: titanium, J. Chron. Dis. 16:55-69, 1963.
55. Vinogradov, A. P.: The elementary composition of marine organisms memorandum No. 2, New Haven, 1953, Sears Foundation for Marine Research, Yale University.
56. Perry, H. M., Jr., and Perry, E. F.: Normal concentrations of some trace metals in human urine: changes produced by ethylenediaminetetraacetate, J. Clin. Invest. 38:1452, 1959.
57. Bernheim, F., and Bernheim, M. L. C.: The effect of titanium on the oxidation of sulfhy-

dryl groups by various tissues, J. Biol. Chem. 127:695, 1939.
58. Kikkawa, H., Ogita, Z., and Fujito, S.: Nature of pigments derived from tyrosine and tryptophan in animals, Science 121:43, 1955.
59. DeMeio, R. H., and Henriques, F. C., Jr.: Tellurium IV: excretion and distribution in tissues studied with radio-active isotope, J. Biol. Chem. 169:609-623, 1947.
60. DeMeio, R. H.: Tellurium: effect of ascorbic acid on tellurium, J. Industr. Hyg. Toxicol. 29:293-295, 1947.
61. Cerwenka, E. A., Jr., and Cooper, W.: Toxicology of selenium and tellurium and their compounds, Arch. Environ. Health 3:189-200, 1961.
62. Steinberg, H. H., Massari, S. C., Miner, A. C., and others: Industrial exposure to tellurium: atmospheric studies and clinical evaluation, J. Industr. Hyg. Toxicol. 24:183-192, 1942.
63. Dennis, L. M., and Anderson, R. P.: Hydrogen telluride and the atomic weight of tellurium, J. Amer. Chem. Soc. 36:882-909, 1914, p. 890.
64. Amdur, M. L.: Tellurium oxide: an animal study in acute toxicity, Arch. Industr. Health 17:665-667, 1958.
65. Sax, N. I., Schultz, W. W., and O'Herin, M. J.: Handbook of dangerous materials, New York, 1951, Reinhold Publishing Corp.

15
ALLERGENIC AGENTS

In 1928 Figley and Elrod[1] reported an epidemic of asthma in East Toledo, Ohio, involving 85 patients. Most of them were residing within ½ to 1½ miles of a linseed and castor oil factory. Because its characteristic odor permeated the area, linseed oil was first thought to be the noxious agent. However it was soon determined that clouds of fine dust residue of the odorless castor bean had been issuing from the chimneys of the plant. Dust derived from processing flaxseed contains about 9% oil, which renders the flaxseed particles too heavy to be windborne.

None of the 85 persons had had asthma before they moved into the district. They had resided in the neighborhood between 1 and 17 years before the attacks developed. All patients gave strongly positive skin tests to castor oil bean dust. In seven, the reactions produced wheals of 8 cm in diameter.

In the factory itself numerous workers, who had had contact with the dust for years, had not contracted the diseases. The 85 victims, therefore, were believed to have had a special disposition to the development of an allergic disease from the castor oil dust, a strongly sensitizing agent.

Similar episodes of asthma caused by so-called allergenic agents were reported from Minneapolis where grain dust is stored. Students at the University of Minnesota developed intermittent asthmatic attacks from grain and from the fungous spores that are abundantly present in grain elevators.[2]

Other epidemics, presumably caused by grain dust, occurred in New Orleans in 1958 and 1962.[3]

A somewhat different kind of "asthma" made its appearance in 1946, during the American occupation of Japan, when servicemen stationed in Yokohama began to suffer attacks of cough and wheezing. In distinction to true allergic asthma, very few of these sufferers had had allergic manifestations previously nor, according to the history, was allergy prevalent in their families, which is usually the case in *allergic* asthma. The afflicted soldiers improved temporarily when they left the vicinity of Yokohama. Flying personnel reported relief as soon as they reached an altitude of 5000 feet. The disease also occurred in two other cities among the Japanese inhabitants, namely in Tokyo and Zama, where American military installations were located. All three cities situated in the Kanot plain, a large bowl surrounded by high mountains, are ideally suited for thermal inversions as a result of weak winds and stagnation of pollutants. About 64% of the "Tokyo-Yokohama disease" sufferers continued to have respiratory symptoms after they returned to the United States although they had shown improvement temporarily.

The asthma of the East Toledo castor oil bean epidemic and that in Tokyo-Yokohama differ profoundly. The Toledo asthma was a true allergic disease. The description of the Yokohama episode suggests that the asthmatic wheezing represented a chronic irritation of the air passages of chemical origin, which led to constriction of bronchi, simulating the condition that prevails in allergic asthma.

MECHANISM OF ALLERGIC DISEASES

In a person who is allergic to a specific substance, the precipitating source is called the antigen. It may be a single item or, more frequently, a combination of many antigens such as pollen, animal hair, and fungi, which induce allergic manifestations. The capillary blood vessels in the mucous lining of the respiratory tract become distended; fluid permeates into the surrounding tissues and attracts certain cells, mainly eosinophiles (white blood cells that stain with the dye eosin), lymphocytes, and mast cells. This response in the capillary blood vessels is brought about by the presence of histamine or histaminelike substances, which originate as the result of a reaction of the antigen with its respective antibody, another specific agent formed in the system.

Histamine and similar substances especially an agent called SRSA (Slow Reacting Substance of Anaphylaxis) also produce spasm of the bronchial musculature, which account for the wheezing and shortness of breath of the asthmatic. The same mechanism leads to waterlogging and swelling of the lining of the sinuses and nasal passages. This so-called edema interferes with the normal flow of secretions; the retained mucus and the waterlogged tissue form a fertile soil for bacterial invasion precipitating chronic sinusitis, bronchitis, and pneumonitis, a condition similar to pneumonia.

The tendency to form an allergic hive (wheal) is utilized by physicians to ferret out the cause or causes of allergic reactions, that is, the antigens responsible for the disease. In skin testing, a number of suspected antigens (pollen, food, and others) are either injected or scratched into the skin. If the test material induces a hive, an allergy to the respective agent is indicated. The degree of sensitivity can be estimated according to the size of a wheal and the concentration of the injected antigen.

MANIFESTATIONS OF ALLERGY

The major manifestations of airborne allergens are bronchial asthma and upper respiratory allergy, which involve the nose, sinuses, and pharyngeal structures. Airborne allergenic agents also induce certain skin diseases, mainly hives and so-called atopic and contact dermatitis. The latter two are often called eczema. Atopic dermatitis is caused by inhalation or ingestion of an antigen, contact dermatitis by direct contact. Many other organs of the body can be the seat of allergic reactions that manifest themselves as allergic colitis and enteritis (bowel inflammation), allergic urinary tract disease, or certain kinds of migraine headaches. If the allergic wheals are formed in the appendix or gallbladder they can elicit conditions simulating appendicitis or gallstones. The degree of sensitivity varies widely from person to person and is often dependent on an inherited factor.

Bronchial asthma

Asthmatic wheezing in the lungs is brought about by air passing through narrowed bronchial tubes similar to the manner in which musical sounds originate in the narrowed tubes of a woodwind or a brass instrument. Spasm of the bronchi and the presence of mucus in the bronchial tree account for the narrowing of the tubes and the wheezy sounds. Asthmatics usually obtain much relief if they can cough up mucus.

Three different situations may confront us:

1. Allergic asthma can be caused by allergenic pollutants, that is, agents with a tendency to sensitize a person.

2. In persons afflicted with allergic asthma, asthmatic attacks may be precipitated by a nonallergenic gaseous or particulate pollutant. A local irritant has a caustic effect on the mucous lining of the bronchial tree, which has been rendered irritable by the underlying allergy. No allergic mechanism may be involved. The Tokyo-Yokohama cases may have originated in this manner.

3. Air pollutants can produce bronchospasm, cough, wheezing, and shortness of breath, which simulate allergic asthma.

Allergic asthma can be precipitated or aggravated by any irritant. Formerly, during a few days late in October I was aware that practically all my allergy patients experienced an aggravation of their disease although atmospheric pollen and fungous spore counts were not excessive. They identified their attacks with the burning of leaves near their homes. This condition ceased after the city of Detroit banned leaf burning. Skin tests with extracts of the respective leaves were negative in several patients. The many gases and particulates present in the smoke were believed to have irritated the sensitive mucous membranes rather than to have induced an allergic reaction.

On a particular day in 1967, three of my patients from the Dearborn, Michigan, area developed asthmatic attacks exactly at the same time, within a short time after the area where they resided had been sprayed from an airplane with Aldrin to eradicate the corn borer. This chemical is not known to exhibit allergenic properties and was, therefore, likely to have acted upon allergic mucous membranes of the respiratory tract by irritating them.

Formerly *nonallergic* chronic respiratory diseases for which no tangible source was identified, have been termed "intrinsic" or "idiopathic asthma" or asthma without a known cause. Some authors have attributed this condition to bacterial infection, to an endocrine gland disturbance, or to other causes.

During the past decades a large segment of the cases of so-called "intrinsic" asthma has been recognized to be caused by smoking.[4] I have recently observed patients in whom this heretofore progressive disease cleared up by the simple expedient of discontinuing smoking. If atmospheric pollution could be eliminated as promptly as smoking, the cause of many more cases of so-called intrinsic asthma would undoubtedly be identified.

Allergic shock

A patient may be so sensitive that the "wheal" or hive reaction is not confined to a single organ; it may involve practically every part of his body. This condition,

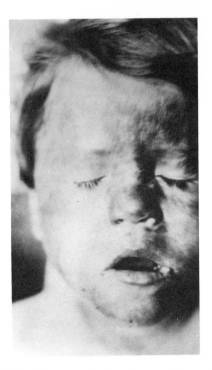

Fig. 15-1. Allergic shock in a 6-year-old boy. He was so sensitive to egg that the kiss of his mother who had eaten egg immediately prior to the incident caused severe shock. Edema appeared to involve every part of his body. The condition was promptly relieved with an injection of epinephrine.

called "allergic shock," usually starts suddenly with generalized hives and severe shortness of breath. In rare instances it can become fatal, when spasm and swelling of the larynx (voice box) and bronchi lead to asphyxiation. Extremely small amounts of vapors or particulates that emanate from boiling such items as fish, peanuts, and other harmless food substances or inhalation of animal dander and airborne chemicals can induce allergic shock (Fig. 15-1).[5] Certain drugs, especially penicillin, aspirin, and local anesthetics can cause allergic shock in predisposed individuals.[6]

Allergic nasal and sinus disease

These diseases are estimated to involve between 5% and 10% of the population in the United States. They are much less common in Europe where ragweed, the major source of respiratory allergy in the United States, is not known.

Allergic nasal and sinus disease, either the perennial form or hayfever or rose fever,* which is limited to specific seasons is characterized by sneezing, watery nasal discharge, itching of the eyes, nose, and mouth. Especially at the height of the hayfever season, this condition is often associated with recurrent periodic paroxysms of asthmatic wheezing, shortness of breath, choking sensation, cough, and obstruction of the expiratory air flow.

Urticaria (hives)

Hives occur as a part of a reaction known as serum sickness 3 to 9 days after an injection of an animal serum of the kind used in prophylaxis for tetanus and for other infectious diseases. Certain drugs and probably some airborne chemical agents can induce this kind of hive.[7] The other, more common type of hives, occurs within minutes to a few hours after exposure to, or ingestion of, an allergenic agent. In the

*Rose fever is not caused by roses but by grasses. The simultaneous pollination of the grass with that of roses has led to the misnomer.

latter type of hives, skin tests are usually positive. They can, therefore, be traced much more readily to their source than the serum sickness type of reaction. Hives may occur seasonally as the result of allergy to hayfever pollen.

Atopic dermatitis

Atopic dermatitis, often called eczema, occurs mainly in infancy and early childhood up to 2 years of age but can, in rare instances, persist throughout a person's early life or even his entire lifetime. It can be readily differentiated from the contact type of dermatitis by its characteristic appearance on the inner surface of elbows and knees and occasionally by lesions below the ear lobes.

Contact dermatitis

So-called contact dermatitis[8] is a skin disease caused by contact of the causative

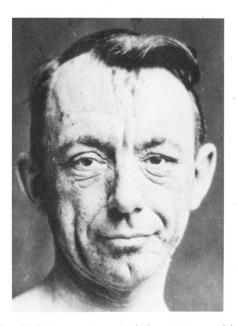

Fig. 15-2. Recurrent seasonal dermatitis caused by ragweed pollen involving only the exposed areas of the body. Each individual pointlike lesion in the face is produced by a single pollen grain. The substance in ragweed responsible for this skin disease is a lipid (oily ingredient of the pollen).

agent with the skin. It is caused by a large variety of agents. Among airborne pollutants chromium, nickel, formaldehyde, epoxy (a resin), lead, arsenic spray, and certain pollen must be considered as possible sources (Fig. 15-2). Small, extremely itchy and oozing blisters arise at the site of contact. They gradually dry up within 1 to 2 weeks if no further contact with the irritant takes place. When such lesions are confined to parts of the body not covered by clothes such as arms, legs, and face, contact with an air pollutant should always be considered. Burning of poison ivy plants can produce dermatitis through spreading the resinous particles of the plants into the atmosphere, which are responsible for the skin eruption.

MODE OF ONSET OF RESPIRATORY ALLERGY

There are several distinct patterns in the onset of respiratory allergy. Most allergic persons have an inherited tendency to allergy. Their condition starts in early childhood with a tendency to frequent "colds." Especially on days of high pollen or fungus counts, a dry nonproductive cough develops, which gradually turns into wheezing. Frequently this condition is complicated by low-grade fever associated with secondary bronchial and pulmonary infection. Repeated and prolonged episodes of this kind may be followed by deformities of nasal structures such as deviation of the nasal septum, the cartilage that separates the two nasal passages, and of enlargement of the nasal turbinates (bones shaped like an inverted cone in each nasal passage).

In patients who acquire sensitivity without an allergic family background, asthma may occur at any time in life. Intensive exposure to an animal, to pollen, or to certain allergenic chemicals are often precipitating factors.

In infants and young children, the onset of the disease differs materially from that in adults. Sometimes even within the first

week of life an infant starts sniffling and coughing and manifests an eczematous skin rash, usually caused by food, which may persist until 1½ to 2 years of age. Throat, nasal, and chest "colds" recur; tonsils, adenoids, and lymph glands at the neck become enlarged. Instead of the typical asthmatic attacks, these children develop a dry hacking cough, which simulates whooping cough,[9] or a condition somewhat resembling pneumonia called bronchiolitis. After a number of such episodes, which usually occur at the height of the hayfever season, wheezing or full-fledged asthmatic attacks develop.

AIRBORNE ALLERGENS

The most common airborne allergens are pollen, spores of molds or fungi, particles of plants and insects, emanations from animals, and, particularly, house dust. Allergic respiratory and skin diseases also occur from a number of chemicals.

Pollen. By far the most important source of allergic respiratory diseases is ragweed, a plant that grows in nearly all 50 of the United States whenever soil has been disturbed (Fig. 15-3).

The ragweed plant produces a great abundance of pollen, which is readily windborne because of its small size (20μ) and its light weight. Tiny spicules on its surface render the respiratory mucous membranes particularly vulnerable to its action (Fig. 3-6).

In most of the United States[*] the peak of the pollinating season of certain hayfever plants (Table 15-1) coincides with specific holidays: at Easter time most trees pollinate; Decoration Day is the beginning of the grass season; and Labor Day marks the height of the ragweed season (Fig. 15-4).

Flowering plants and blossoms of trees do not produce hayfever unless a person is

---

[*]Variations caused by climate and local flora occur in different sections of the country.

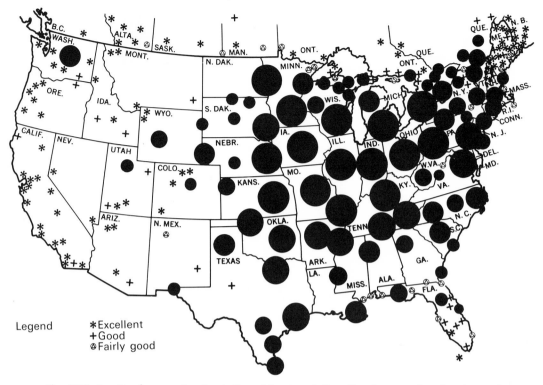

Fig. 15-3. Density of ragweed pollen indicated by size of discs. Heaviest growth is found in midwestern and prairie states. The asterisks indicate low ragweed pollen areas. (Courtesy Abbott Laboratories, North Chicago, Illinois.)

Legend

* Excellent
\+ Good
⊕ Fairly good

close to the plant. Their pollen is heavier than that of hayfever plants and is therefore not windborne. Because of its resinous surface it adheres to insects, particularly bees.

Pollen enters buildings through windows and doors. It is carried to high altitudes over hundreds of miles. Air-conditioning, especially electrostatic filters, reduce its concentration in buildings. Keeping weeds cut close to the ground to reduce the amount of pollen in a particular area has not been found effective in alleviating the symptoms of hayfever patients.

Fungi. Spores of fungi are the other major allergenic pollutant (Fig. 2-2). They grow in a moist atmosphere, preferably in the presence of carbohydrates, on damp food, damp hay, damp wood, and on many other organic substances. They also arise

from soil, particularly during the summer months.

Unlike pollen, their presence in the atmosphere shows no seasonal pattern. In the first annual fungus survey made in the United States by Waldbott and others[10] in 1938 to 1939 (Fig. 15-5), alternaria was the only fungus, with a strong sensitizing property, which exhibited a distinct trend to seasonal occurrence. Starting with the harvesting season in June-July, it continued until fall. Yeast and yeastlike spores were more prevalent early in the spring when the snow melts. Spores of smut, the black fungus seen on the ears of corn and other grains, occur in the atmosphere mostly in late fall at the end of the harvesting season (Fig. 15-6). Rust spores, which grow on the stem of grains and grasses, are found in the air for only a short period in Febru-

Table 15-1. Hayfever plants

COMMON NAME	BOTANICAL NAME	DIAMETER* (MICRONS)	SPECIFIC GRAVITY
Giant ragweed	*Ambrosia trifida*	19.25	0.52
Burweed marsh elder	*Iva xanthifolia*	19.30	0.79
Short ragweed	*Ambrosia elatior*	20.00	0.55
False ragweed	*Franseria acanthicarpa*	22.00	0.75
Marsh elder	*Iva ciliata*	23.00	0.58
Southern ragweed	*Ambrosia bidentata*	23.00	0.50
Western ragweed	*Ambrosia psilostachya*	26.40	0.57
Cocklebur	*Xanthium commune*	27.00	0.45
Russian thistle	*Salsola pestifer*	23.60	0.90
Palmer's amaranth	*Amaranthus palmeri*	25.80	1.02
Western water hemp	*Acnida tamariscina*	27.50	1.01
Mexican fireweed	*Kochia scoparia*	32.70	0.97
Annual sage	*Artemisia annua*	20.40	1.02
Tall wormwood	*Artermisia caudata*	21.00	1.04
Sagebrush	*Artemisia tridentata*	25.85	1.03
Nettle	*Urtica gracilis*	14.00	0.77
Red sorrel	*Rumex acetosella*	21.45	0.78
Hemp	*Cannabis sativa*	25.00	0.82
English plantain	*Plantago lanceolata*	27.50	0.97
Bluegrass	*Poa pratensis*	30.00	0.90
Bermuda grass	*Capriola dactylon*	28.50	1.01
Orchard grass	*Dactylis glomerata*	34.00	0.91
Timothy	*Phleum pratense*	34.00	0.90
Rye	*Secale cereale*	49.50	0.98
Corn	*Zea mays*	90.00	1.00
Sycamore	*Platanus occidentalis*	22.22	0.92
Mountain cedar	*Juniperus sabinoides*	22.80	1.08
Hazelnut	*Corylus americana*	23.60	1.09
Birch	*Betula nigra*	24.60	0.94
Alder	*Alnus glutinosa*	26.00	0.97
Ash	*Fraxinus americana*	27.10	0.90
Cottonwood	*Populus virginiana*	30.00	0.79
Elm	*Ulmust americana*	31.20	1.00
Bur oak	*Quercus macrocarpa*	32.30	1.04
Shingle oak	*Quercus imbricaria*	33.10	1.04
Walnut	*Juglans nigra*	35.75	0.93
Beech	*Fagus grandifolia*	44.00	0.94
Hickory	*Carya ovata*	45.00	0.79
Scotch pine	*Pine sylvestris*	52.00	0.45
Bull pine	*Pinus ponderosa*	60.00	0.45

*The relatively large size of pollens prevents them from reaching beyond the large bronchi. The products of their reaction, however, can reach the bloodstream within minutes.

ary.[10] In the above-mentioned survey, penicillium was identified as the most common of all fungi, with wide fluctuations from day to day.

Fungi produce two kinds of respiratory diseases: as antigens similar to pollen, they precipitate allergic reactions mainly in the respiratory tract and on the skin. On rare occasions they can also induce pulmonary infections, similar to those caused by bacteria and viruses, characterized by fever and gradually increasing shortness of

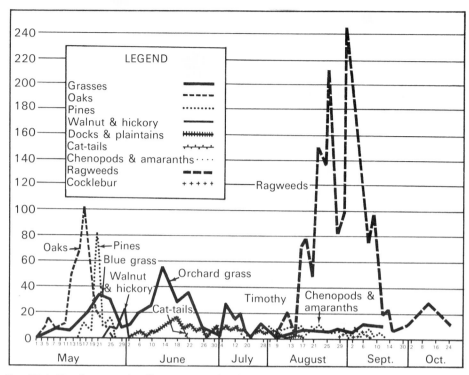

Fig. 15-4. The first annual pollen survey undertaken in Michigan in 1929 revealed three major pollen seasons: trees up to and through May, grasses in June and July, and ragweed in August and September. In contrast to the distribution of fungus spores, the levels of atmospheric pollens are remarkably consistent year after year.

breath. *Aspergillus* and *Monilia* are the two most common species causing this kind of illness (Fig. 15-7, *A* and *B*).

Insects. Among other airborne allergens, scales of moths and butterflies, particles of insects and of vegetation are frequently encountered on exposed slides. A few species, such as caddis flies (Trichoptera) and fish flies (Ephemerida),[11] appear in large numbers in the Great Lakes region on certain days in June and July, respectively. Extracts of these insects can produce marked skin reactions. Aggravation of respiratory allergy, at the time of their prevalence in the atmosphere, is common. Strongly positive skin reactions are also obtained from extracts of moths.

House dust. Among airborne allergenic agents, house dust plays an important role, particularly when the indoor heating systems are started in fall because they promote circulation of dust throughout the homes. House dust embraces a wide variety of substances mainly cotton, wool, and other fabrics, dyes from materials such as carpets, food particles and other substances. In spite of a vast amount of research, the chemical nature of the sensitizing power of house dust has not been clearly established. Recently, its sensitizing properties have been attributed to the presence of a mite,[12] extracts of which appear to be highly antigenic and productive of strong skin reactions (Fig. 15-8).

Chemicals. It was formerly believed that only protein substances could precipitate allergic reactions. Now it is recognized that many chemical compounds can be aller-

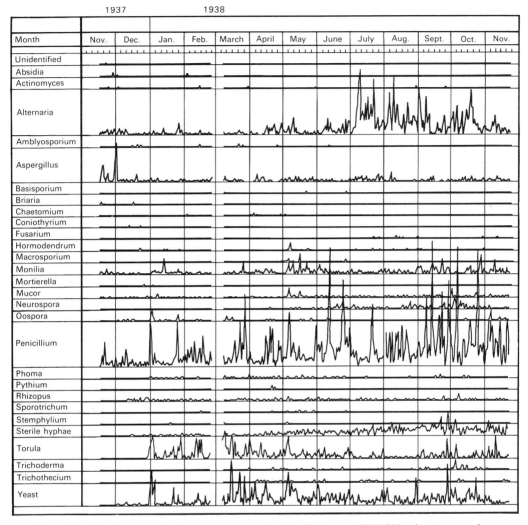

Fig. 15-5. The first annual fungus survey in the United States, 1937-1938, showing no clear seasonal trend of fungus growth except for *Alternaria* and *Monilia,* which prevail from May through November. *Penicillium* was found to be the most abundant fungus throughout the year. The graph represents the mean values of three exposures on every third day: one at the top of the highest building in Detroit (640 ft.), the second at the roof of a three-story building in the center of Detroit, and the third at a field 60 miles northwest of Detroit. Each curve represents the count of an individual mold during one year.

genic as well. They combine with the body's protein and thus induce an antigen-antibody reaction similar to that of other allergens. Most chemical substances, however, do not give positive skin reactions, and, for detection of allergy to chemical agents, more sophisticated tests must be used.

An example of allergic asthma caused by a chemical atmospheric pollutant is the case of J. M. a six-year-old girl who consulted me on July 27, 1966, because of severe wheezing. In May 1966, shortly after an Ontario chemical plant began its operations within 1½ miles of her residence, she developed episodes of cough, itchy

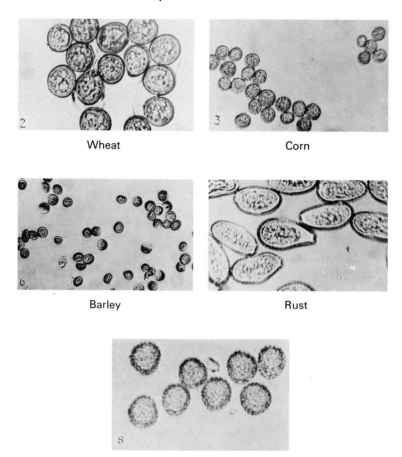

Wheat

Corn

Barley

Rust

Ragweed for comparison

Fig. 15-6. Smut and rust spores, common causes of respiratory allergy. These smut spores are prevalent in the air throughout the year, especially during harvesting season and near grain elevators. ($\times$430.)

eyes, a watery nose, and asthmatic wheezing. This usually happened on days when other residents in the area complained of the "rotten fish" odor caused by methylamines that emanated from the plant. Several other children experienced allergic symptoms but only while they were attending a school located $\frac{6}{10}$ mile from the plant. A skin test with a solution of methylamine produced a strong reaction. Measures intended to relieve this condition were to no avail. The family was eventually forced to move to western Canada where the asthma promptly subsided.

ISOCYANATES

One of the most characteristic groups of chemical air pollutants with strong allergenic properties[13] is the isocyanates.

During the past two decades a vast new industry has originated here and abroad with the creation of plastic polyurethane. This substance is developed from the reaction between isocyanates and a wide variety of compounds that contain active hydrogen atoms. The degree of the "foamy" character of polyurethane is determined by the amount of carbon dioxide and the kinds of isocyanates and resins of which it

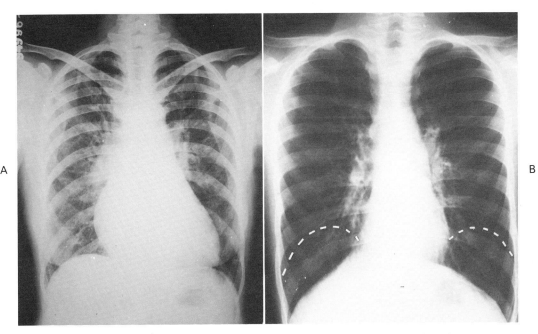

Fig. 15-7. A, Roentgenogram of a 52-year-old white female with a chronic *Monilia* infection. Repeated cultures for the fungus showed pure *Monilia* growth without the presence of any other microorganisms. **B,** In contrast is a roentgenogram of a 15-year-old asthmatic boy with severe emphysema who is very allergic to numerous pollens, food, and fungi, including *Monilia*. The position of his diaphragm is compared with the normal position (dotted outline).

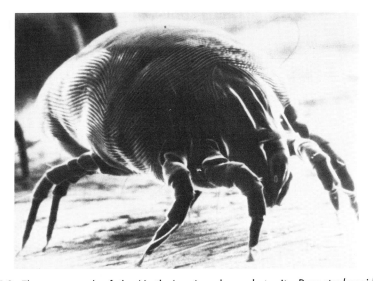

Fig. 15-8. The protonymph of the North American house-dust mite *Dermatophagoides farinae*, which is one of the major allergic constituents of house dust and produces strong allergic reactions. (×300.) (Courtesy G. W. Wharton: Mites and commercial extracts of house dust, Science **167**:1382, 1970.)

Table 15-2. U. S. consumption of polyurethanes in 1970*

FLEXIBLE FOAM		RIGID URETHANES	
Bedding	74	Appliances	57
Furniture	220	Building and construction	71
Rug and underlay	22	Furniture	12
Textile laminates	66	Marine flotation	12
Transportation	190	Transportation	43
Miscellaneous	26	Miscellaneous	28
Total	598	Total	223

*Compiled from Booming growth seen for polyurethanes, Chemical and Engineering News, Feb. 21, 1972.

consists. In addition to plastics, surface-coating fibers and adhesives are made from polyurethanes.

Uses of polyurethane

Flexible polyurethane foam is now displacing traditional upholstery materials both in furniture and in automobile seats (Table 15-2). The use of polyurethane foam as a packaging material in chemical plants and coal mines, and in aircraft, automobile, and boat construction, is rapidly increasing. The *rigid* foams are finding wide application for insulation and refrigeration of portable containers, deepfreezes, and refrigerators. Soft toys, surface-coating varnishes, and paints contain polyurethane.

All isocyanates are made by reaction of primary organic amines with phosgene. Toluene diisocyanate (TDI), the most important building stone of isocyanates, is most significant toxicologically. In the process of manufacturing toluene diisocyanate its vapor can appear in the atmosphere in concentrations substantially above the current occupational threshold limit value, which has been set at 0.02 ppm. Furthermore, unreacted isocyanates often appear in finished polyurethane products thus giving rise to low-grade toxic manifestations.[14]

A danger of toluene diisocyanate as an environmental pollutant is its fire hazard during manufacturing and storage. When burned in refuse dumps with other trash it releases toxic gases. There is also danger of spontaneous combustion when the foam is incorrectly formulated or processed.

Furthermore "instant polyurethane foam" kits, which are available for household use, may be responsible for exposure to TDI fumes at levels exceeding those permitted in factories.[15] Residual amounts of phosgene have been found in barrels containing toluene diisocyanate.[16]

Acute intoxication

The acute effect of toluene diisocyanate on human health is described by McKerrow and associates,[17] in thirty-six firemen who were confronted with extinguishing a fire at a polyurethane foam factory. They were exposed to high concentrations of TDI when approximately 1000 gallons of the liquid leaked to the floor of the burning building during a period of about 2 hours. Eighteen developed immediate illness; in the others, the symptoms occurred after an 8-hour delay. Cough and tightness in the chest, breathlessness, nausea, vomiting, euphoria, and ataxia (unstable gait) were immediate effects. Two of the men lost consciousness. The delayed symptoms were shortness of breath and features indicative of brain damage, such as inability to concentrate, poor memory, odd behavior, and headaches. In two of the men, the residual chest symptoms persisted for several months.

Chronic intoxication

The effects of long-term inhalation of minute amounts of TDI are those of typical allergic asthma, often associated with allergic eye and nasal symptoms. Pulmonary function studies in workers exposed to levels of toluene diisocyanate below the current threshold limit of 0.02 ppm indicate that frequent exposures have a cumulative action. Significant impairment of the pulmonary function may have already occurred in spite of only minor, or lack of, symptoms.

That asthma encountered following exposure to TDI represents a true allergic sensitization was demonstrated by Taylor[13] who identified antibodies specific for TDI in four individuals following exposure to the chemical. Clinical observations also point to this fact. Re-exposure to even minimal concentrations of toluene diisocyanate by patients who have completely recovered following their first exposure produces a recurrence of symptoms so severe that they are obliged to discontinue their work.[18] Such aggravation has occurred at exposures below 0.1 ppm. Other allergic manifestations such as hives[19] and dermatitis caused by toluene diisocyanate[20] have been observed.

Nearly all patients reported by Brugsch and Elkins[21] had no past history of allergy. Thus it is likely that their asthma originated as the result of exposure to toluene diisocyanate. The following history of a patient who gave an excellent account of the development of his disease bears out this point.

A 52-year-old professor of chemistry had never manifested pulmonary symptoms nor was there a history of any allergic disease in the family, as is usually the case in allergic asthma. The first asthmatic attacks occurred in 1956 after repeated exposures in his poorly ventilated laboratory to levels of 50 to 100 ppm toluene diisocyanate. The patient was unable to avoid intermittent exposure to the chemical. Gradually the asthma assumed a more persistent course with marked restriction of pulmonary ventilation. When the condition first developed, skin tests for the usual allergenic agents were negative, and the attacks occurred only upon exposure to toluene diisocyanate. When I examined him in 1971, unusually strong skin test reactions were obtained to a wide variety of antigens. At first, the attacks occurred only on exposures for 2 or more hours' duration. Fresh air provided prompt relief, alcoholic beverages aggravated the symptoms. Now, even very small concentrations of toluene diisocyanate for less than 1 minute elicit severe asthmatic attacks. In addition numerous other antigenic agents (food, pollen, and others) are now contributing to the asthmatic condition. This case suggests that toluene diisocyanate may have been instrumental in inducing this patient's general allergic state.

REFERENCES

1. Figley, K. D., and Elrod, R. H.: Endemic asthma due to castor oil bean dust, J.A.M.A. **90**:79, 1928.
2. Goppers, V., and Paulus, H. G.: Allergenic compounds in nature, Intern. Arch. Allerg. **31**:546, 1967.
3. Lewis, R., Gilkeson, M., and McCaldin, R. O.: Air pollution and New Orleans asthma, Public Health Rep. **77**:947, 1962.
4. Waldbott, G. L.: Smoker's respiratory syndrome, J.A.M.A. **151**:1398-1400, 1953.
5. Waldbott, G. L.: The prevention of anaphylactic shock, J.A.M.A. **98**:446-449, 1932.
6. Waldbott, G. L.: Allergic shock from local and general anesthetics, J. Anesth. Anal. **14**:199-204, 1935.
7. Waldbott, G. L., and Ascher, M. S.: Urticaria of the serum sickness type, J. Allerg. **9**:584-592, 1938.
8. Waldbott, G. L.: Contact dermatitis, Springfield, Ill. 1953, Charles C Thomas, Publisher.
9. Waldbott, G. L.: Allergic bronchitis, J. Lab. Clin. Med. **13**:943, 1928.
10. Waldbott, G. L., Blair, K. E., and Ackley, A. B.: An evaluation of the importance of fungi in respiratory allergy, J. Lab. Clin. Med. **26**:1593-1599, 1941.
11. Urbach, E., and Gottlieb, P. M.: Allergy, New York, 1943, Grune & Stratton, Inc., p. 293.
12. Voohorst, R., Spieksma, F. T. M., Varekamp, H., and others: The house-dust mite (*Dematophagoides pteronyssinus*) and the allergens

it produces: identity with house-dust allergen, J. Allerg. 39:325, 1967.

13. Taylor, G.: Immune responses to toluene diisocyanates (TDI) exposure in man, Proc. Roy. Soc. Med. 63:379-380, 1970.

14. Frish, K.: Personal communication, 1971.

15. Peters, J. M., and Murphy, R. L. H.: Pulmonary toxicity of isocyanates, Ann. Intern. Med. 73:654, 1970.

16. Peters, J. M.: Acute respiratory effects in workers exposed to low levels of toluene diisocyanate, T.D.I., Arch. Environ. Health 16:642-647, 1968.

17. McKerrow, C. B., Davies, H. J., and Jones, A. P.: Symptoms and lung function following acute and chronic exposure to toluene diisocyanate, Proc. Roy. Soc. Med. 63:376, 1970.

18. Munn, A.: Hazards of isocyanates, Ann. Occup. Hyg. 8:163-169, 1965.

19. Shur, E.: Schädigung durch Desmodur-Lacke, Reizgas oder Allergie? Med. Klin. 54:168, 1959.

20. Woodbury, J. W.: Asthmatic syndrome following exposure to toluene diisocyanate, Industr. Med. Surg. 25:540-543, 1956.

21. Brugsch, H. G., and Elkins, H. B.: Toluene diisocyanate (TDI) toxicity, New Eng. J. Med. 268:353-357, 1963.

16
CARCINOGENS

The development of a malignant tumor can be classified as a host-specific process, since there seems to be a conditioning of organ tissue by chronic irritation in those who contract the disease. In contrast to the allergic reaction, however, not all tumors are alike, although they manifest essentially the same kind of response regardless of the precipitating source: the tendency to unlimited cell growth, higher than normal metabolic rates, and abnormal chromosomes.

In 1775 the British surgeon Percivall Pott, in a treatise entitled *The Cancer of the Scrotum,* related the occurrence of cancer in chimney sweeps caused by soot lodged in the crevices of the skin of male genitalia.[1]

Not until 1918 was it possible to reproduce cancer experimentally when Japanese investigators induced skin cancer in rabbits by repeated painting of the inner surface of the earlobes with tar.[2] Subsequently, certain polynuclear aromatic hydrocarbons (PAH), particularly the ubiquitous benzo[a]pyrene (BaP), were isolated as the carcinogenic substance in tar.[3]

Identification of a cancer-producing environmental agent is difficult: many years elapse between exposure to a pollutant and the occurrence of visible signs of cancer. Interactions between numerous pollutants in the atmosphere either interfere with, or enhance, the action of a particular substance. Thus the problem of establishing that the disease has been caused by a particular pollutant is very complex. Furthermore, the tendency for families to move from one locality to another results in a change of exposure of the individuals to carcinogens.[4] Because smoking of cigarettes by a large segment of a given population in itself favors cancer growth, this factor often precludes an accurate statistical assessment of a suspected pollutant.

MORTALITY STATISTICS

Although no specific single agent has been definitely proved to cause lung cancer in humans,[5] an association between air pollution and mortality rates has been shown repeatedly.

In large industrial metropolitan areas, the rate of lung cancer is higher than in rural regions[6] regardless of whether or not an individual smokes.[7] Teleki[8] recorded the results of a statistical study in the German industrial Rhein area in the late 1920s, which revealed a death rate from cancer of the bladder (Anilinkrebs) six times higher in the town of Leverkusen with large chemical plants than in München-Gladbach without such industry, namely 38.0 deaths per 100,000 male inhabitants versus 6.2 deaths. A similar relationship among females (4.8 and 0.8, respectively) not employed at the factories suggested that the carcinogenic agents are airborne. Likewise a higher trend to lung cancer in persons who move from a rural to an urban community implies that the greater air pollution in cities aids in the development of the disease.[9]

According to statistics, Los Angeles smog does not appear to precipitate cancer. A 10-year study on 70,000 persons revealed a lower lung cancer ratio for Los Angeles County (96.6 per 100,000) where smog concentrations were higher than in San Francisco and San Diego (106.3 per 100,000). Lung cancer death rates in all three cities, however, were higher than for the state at large (79.9 per 100,000).[10]

Since most air pollutants enter the body through inhalation primarily, the lungs are the major target of malignant tumors caused by air pollutants. However, other parts of the body can be affected likewise as, for instance, the male genitalia by cadmium, the pleura and peritoneum (lining of the chest and abdominal cavities) by asbestos, and the bone marrow by radioactive pollutants. Mortality rates from cancer of the stomach have been reported to be twice as high in an industrial area as in an area with little pollution.[11]

INTERACTION OF CAUSATIVE AGENTS

Lung cancer is not believed to be caused by a single irritating agent but by an interplay of multiple environmental factors.

In experimental animals a combination of sulfur dioxide with benzo[a]pyrene inhalation, for instance, results in production of squamous-cell carcinomas (cancer consisting of platelike cells)[12] whereas no such effect occurs when each agent is administered separately. Chronic exposure to ozonized gasoline vapor increases[13] the tumor incidence. Infection with an influenza virus strain induced malignant tumors in the lungs.[14] Soot, an otherwise harmless substance, has been identified as a powerful carcinogenic agent because of its tendency to adsorb many known cancer-producing substances, especially polynuclear aromatic hydrocarbons.[15] The particle size determines the ability of these agents to penetrate the tracheobronchial tree.[16] Pylev[16] noted rapid disappearance of benzo[a]pyrene from lungs of rats when he administered coarsely dispersed soot particles, 0.3 μ in diameter, into the upper air passages; on the other hand, the finely dispersed soot particles (0.01 μ) impeded elimination of benzo[a]pyrene from the lungs and aided in its decomposition. Similarly, iron oxide and other so-called inert particles act as vehicles to transport benzo[a]pyrene through the lining of the bronchial tree into the lung tissue where it is eluded by cell plasma.[17] Extracts of certain airborne dusts, that is, combinations of many agents, have given rise to cancer experimentally. Campbell,[18] for instance, produced benign lung tumors by exposing mice in dust chambers to asphalt road sweepings.

Horton and associates[19] have shown that certain petroleum products in water and air, aliphatic and aromatic hydrocarbons, act as accelerators for agents that cause skin cancer. A similar mechanism is believed to operate with respect to other kinds of cancer. Conversely, a number of agents present in the atmosphere inhibit the development of tumors.[20]

CARCINOGENIC SUBSTANCES

Many respiratory irritants contribute to the development of cancer. By interfering with ciliary activity and retarding the flow of mucus in the bronchi, they enhance retention of carcinogenic particles in the lungs and, in this way, encourage tumor formation.[21] Substances that thus trigger the production of cancer without being themselves carcinogenic are presented in the list below. The carcinogenic property of some has been questioned. Others have not been identified as carcinogens mainly because the quantities in which they are present in the air are insufficient for bioassays. The tools currently available to us for definitely pinpointing a pollutant as the cause of cancer are inadequate.

Carcinogenic air pollutants fall into 3 groups: organic, inorganic, and radionuclides. The last-mentioned group is discussed in Chapter 20.

Organic carcinogens

The principal organic air pollutant carcinogens are shown in the following list. Among some forty aromatic hydrocarbons known to occur in polluted atmospheres, those with less than 3 or more than 6 condensed benzene rings, as a rule, do not exhibit carcinogenic activity.[22]

Principal organic air pollutant carcinogens

I. Polynuclear aromatic hydrocarbons (PAH)
   A. Benzo[a]pyrene (BaP)
   B. Benz [a] anthracene
   C. Benz [e] acephenanthrylene
   D. Benzo [b] fluoranthene
   E. Benzo [j] fluoranthene
   F. Dibenzo [e,l] pyrene
   G. Dibenzo [a,h] pyrene
   H. Ideno [1,2,3-cd] pyrene
II. Polynuclear aza-heterocyclic compounds
   A. Dibenz [a,h] acridine
   B. Dibenz [a,j] acridine
III. Polynuclear imino-heterocyclic compounds

Some airborne polynuclear aromatic hydrocarbons, mainly products of imperfect combustion, originate primarily from burning of coal and refuse, from heat generation in industrial processes such as steel and coke production, and from motor vehicle exhaust. Tars and asphalts used in surfacing roads release aromatic hydrocarbons. However, because of relatively limited dust production, their concentration in ambient air is believed to be too low to cause harm.

A group of cancer-inducing organic

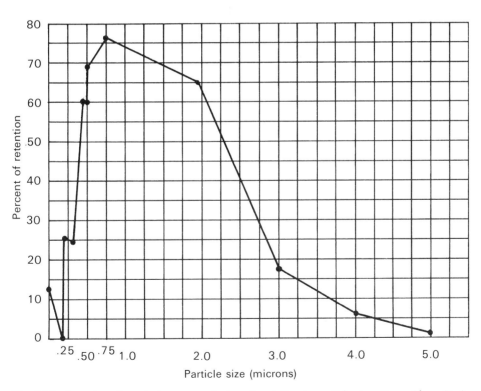

Fig. 16-1. Retention of particulate matter in lung in relation to particle size. (From Olson, D. A.: Air pollution aspects of organic carcinogens, Litton Industries, Inc., Bethesda, Maryland, 1969, U. S. Department of Commerce, PB 188-090.)

agents, namely epoxides, hydroperoxides, peroxides, and lactones, is derived from olefins. According to the United States Public Health Service, the concentration of aromatic hydrocarbons per 1000 meter³ of atmosphere in over fourteen American cities ranged from 5 to 146 μg compared with benzo[a]pyrene, which was found in concentrations from 0.25 to 31 μg/meter³.[23] Certain airborne nitrogen-containing agents have been identified with production of cancer in mice.[24]

West[25] suspected a large number of organic pesticides as carcinogens including DDT, aldrin, dieldrin, endrin, and heptachlor. Although they induce cancer in animals at relatively high concentrations, they have not been established as carcinogens in humans at the concentrations found in ambient air, a difficult task in view of our present day lack of adequate diagnostic tools.[25]

A large number of nitrosamines are formed by the reaction of nitrites with so-called secondary amines, under conditions of acidity in the stomach.[26]

Their concentrations in grains and alcoholic beverages where they are found mainly, are 5 ppm or less.[27] Experimentally, they exhibit systemic effects involving specific organs. For instance, one compound, nitrosopiperidine, produces cancer in the esophagus (an organ connecting the oral cavity with the stomach) in rats regardless of whether it is administered by mouth or intravenously. Some cause malignant tumors in lungs and others in the stomach of hamsters.[27]

The so-called secondary amines such as dimethylamine and diethylamine occur in fish products, cereals, tea, tobacco, and tobacco smoke.[28] Cooking of food is believed to be a source of secondary amines. They also originate in the preparation of various flavoring agents, including those present in bread and meat; some toothpastes contain carcinogenic substances of the same category.[29]

Mancuso and Brennan[30] named certain nitrosamines, namely diethyl-nitrosamine, p-nitroso-N,N-dimethylaniline, and N,4-dinitrosomethylaniline (Elastopar) as possible causes of a higher than normal mortality rate from cancer of the gallbladder, bile ducts, and salivary glands in rubber factory workers. At this time it is impossible to establish whether or not these substances are emitted into the atmosphere in sufficient magnitude to damage populations residing near rubber factories.

Although the methods for detection of nitrosamines are not very sensitive, their widespread environmental distribution has been demonstrated as well as that of their precursors, nitrites and secondary amines.

Further data on organic carcinogens are given in the discussions on hydrocarbons and on smoking in Chapters 19 and 21.

Inorganic carcinogens

Among inorganic airborne pollutants, industrial chromates, nickel, asbestos, beryllium, arsenic, selenium, and cobalt have been linked with the production of malignant tumors in animal experiments.

The action of only four organic carcinogens—asbestos, nickel, chromium compounds, and arsenic—is presented here, because they are generally considered sources of cancer in humans.

ASBESTOS

In 1906 the German scientist Marchand[31] noted "peculiar pigment crystals" within the alveoli of the lungs. They were rod-shaped structures with clubbed ends, light yellow to reddish brown, 30 to 200 μ long and 1 to 6 μ thick. Their bodies were segmented into discs interconnected by colorless threads (Fig. 16-2, A and B).[32] Because they turned black near the areas where they disintegrated, Marchand suspected and subsequently confirmed that the yellow pigment contained iron. Twenty years later Cooke[33] rediscovered what he called "curious bodies" throughout the lungs of an asbestos worker. He felt that they might be fungi, which they resemble.

In 1965 Gough[34] termed them mineral fiber bodies because they were not solely identified with asbestos. Their iron-containing coating led Gross and associates[35]

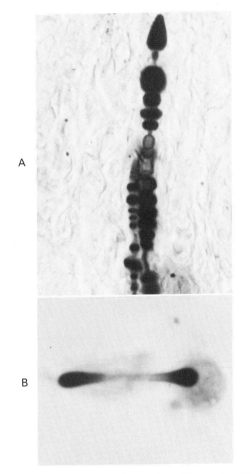

A

B

Fig. 16-2. A, Specimen from a lung biopsy of a 42-year-old rubber shredder, with diffuse widespread pulmonary fibrosis. This "asbestos body" was associated with talc crystals throughout the specimen. Commercial talcum powder contains approximately 20% asbestos. B, A "ferruginous" body with macrophages attached at each end. Smear was taken after washing a hamster lung with saline solution 9 months afer injection with ceramic aluminum silicate. (×1300.) (From Gaensler, E. A., and Addington, W. W.: Asbestos or ferruginous bodies, New Eng. J. Med. 280:488-491, 1969.)

to designate them "ferruginous bodies." Actually, they consist of a combination of protein and iron, which is found in their coating; usually less than 5% of their content is asbestos. The iron is believed to originate from hemosiderin, a constituent of red blood cells, the protein from the phagocytes of the alveoli-scavanger cells that are mobilized in response to the inhalation and lodging in the alveoli of asbestos fibers.

Graphite, carborundum, and other materials that are not related to asbestos can produce structures resembling asbestos bodies. In Capetown, South Africa, during routine lung smears Thomson[36] found ferruginous bodies in 26.4% of 500 consecutive autopsies of persons above 15 years of age. More recently, the bodies were encountered by Gold[37] in 336 of 629 lung specimens and by Langer and associates[38] in two thirds of 3000 consecutive autopsies in New York City. Their presence, therefore, is widespread in the population.

Gross and co-workers[39] found a variety of asbestos bodies in the lungs of people not occupationally exposed to asbestos. These bodies are generally round or oval, 4 to 30 μ in diameter, and vary in color from translucent light yellow to semitranslucent red-gold. Their central core is either composed of a single large or multiple small particles. They are believed to originate from inhalation of particles of smoke derived from burning leaves, paper, wood, or coal.

Properties and uses of asbestos

Asbestos is not a single material. It is the generic name for several varieties of fibrous mineral silicates that occur in nature. The main varieties are chrysotile asbestos (white), crocidolite (blue), and amosite (brown). Properties of the asbestos fiber that make it valuable in industry are its resistance to heat, friction, and acid, its flexibility and great tensile strength.

Two thousand years ago, asbestos was used for making lamp wicks. Now, with more than a thousand different applications, the world's consumption is over three million tons each year.[40] The principal asbestos mines are in Canada, U.S.S.R., South Africa, and Cyprus.

Asbestos is relatively inexpensive. Its tensile strength can be compared with that of steel. About two thirds of all asbestos production is used in cement work. Asbestos cement will withstand weathering much better than cement alone. Asbestos also protects the steel framework of modern buildings against fire. It has been common practice to spray fireproofing material containing 10% to 30% asbestos onto girders, spandrels, and decking of high-rise buildings. Asbestos is also employed in the formation of pipes and ducts for water, air, and chemicals, in brake pads and brake linings, in corrugated roofing, and in making garden ornaments and furniture.

It insulates ceilings against noise. In roofs and pipes, it prevents condensation. In homes and offices, air-conditioning ducts are lined with soft asbestos. The use of unsealed ceiling tile is a minor but continuous source of air pollution. Asbestos is also spun and woven into fire protection clothes, oven cloths, wicks for oil stoves, and other items. Filters of certain types of gas masks are made of asbestos. Customarily, waste asbestos rock has been used in South African mining areas for surfacing roads.[41] Tremolite asbestos is an ingredient of some talcum powders. Asbestos is even being added to the fabric of women's coats. Rubbing or brushing such material increases the atmospheric level of asbestos considerably. Some air contamination occurs naturally from abrasion and weathering of serpentine rock, which contains fibrous material believed to be chrysotile.[42]

Chronic asbestosis

Elmes[43] described a woman, age 53, whose pulmonary fibrosis (scarring of lungs) of several years duration was associated with increasing breathlessness and was complicated by a spontaneous pneumo-thorax. He suspected asbestosis, but the patient denied occupational exposure. Subsequently, she recalled that her husband had built two asbestos bungalows, one in 1947 and the other in 1948. She had held the asbestos sheets while her husband sawed them. They had resided in one of the bungalows for about 2 years before painting the sheets that lined the walls and ceilings. Subsequently, the diagnosis of asbestosis was confirmed in her case as well as in that of her husband, who had never been occupationally exposed to asbestos. Once asbestos particles reach the lungs, they are neither expelled nor dissolved.

Like other cases of "dust lung" diseases, asbestosis develops slowly. It becomes manifest usually 20 to 30 years after the first exposure, often long after exposure to asbestos has completely ceased.

Unexplained breathlessness on exertion and productive cough often precede the disease by many years. The tightness in the chest is frequently associated with pain. In the advanced stage, the patients show cyanosis (a bluish discoloration of the skin), restricted chest expansion, and the barrel type of chest seen in emphysema. The tips of the fingers become enlarged and assume a bluish dark color, a condition called club fingers.

The roentgenogram shows typical scarring of lungs and, occasionally, a honeycomb appearance at their bases.[44,45] A characteristic feature of the disease is the unusually extensive thickening of the pleura (the lining surrounding the lungs). The thickened tissue is often replaced by calcium deposits, which are visible on x-ray examination. Their localization in the lower third of the lungs makes it possible for physicians to detect industrial or environmental exposures in a given area.[46]

Warts develop on fingers of asbestos workers whose hands have cuts or abrasions. Elmes[43] reports that as many as 42% of a group of 100 insulators are liable to have cuts and abrasions on their hands.

Lung cancer caused by asbestos

More significant is the development of lung cancer caused by exposure to asbestos. In 1947 it was discovered in England that over 50% of patients diagnosed as having asbestosis eventually die of lung cancer. More recently, exposure to asbestos without development of asbestosis has been shown to increase the risk of lung cancer.[47] Other kinds of dusts in addition to asbestos most likely contribute to this development. In asbestos workers who smoke, a 90-fold increase in the incidence of lung cancer over that in nonsmokers has been recorded.[47] Cancer caused by asbestos localizes most often in the lower lobes of the lungs in contrast to the more common site of lung cancer in the upper lobes.

Another type of cancer that affects the gastrointestinal tract was reported by Selikoff and associates[48] in a survey on 1117 insulation workers in New York City. The source of the tumor could be consumption of food contaminated by asbestos and the swallowing of sputum containing asbestos particles. However more data are needed in order to establish uneqivocally relationship of such tumors to asbestos.

Mesothelioma

An otherwise rare tumor, called *mesothelioma*,[49] has been identified with asbestos. It has been reported in patients who had never worked in asbestos mines but who had resided in mining areas 1 to 2 years as children.[50] In the town of Bergedorf near Hamburg, Germany, where an asbestos works was located, 119 such cases were detected.[51] Sixty-four of these persons had never worked in the factory itself. In the remaining ones, the average interval between the first exposure and the development of the tumor was 35.2 years. Specifically, the blue asbestos mineral fiber called crocidolite has been identified with mesothelioma. Near the Quebec asbestos mines, which produce chrysolite, no excess incidence of the tumor has been reported.

Mesotheliomas usually involve the pleura but also originate in the peritoneum (lining of the abdominal wall and of the abdominal organs). This malignant tumor spreads rapidly over the whole abdominal cavity and into the lymph glands of the body.

As in other kinds of lung cancer, the condition starts slowly with chest pain and breathlessness: the patients seldom survive more than a year from the time the diagnosis is established.

With the expanding role of asbestos in industry, it is likely that both mesothelioma and asbestosis will continue to take their toll of lives.

NICKEL

Nickel (Ni), a grayish-white metallic element, has been found to produce cancer of the lungs and nose in humans[52] and in animal experiments.[53] Resistant to corrosion and oxidation, it is present in a wide variety of alloys among which are the so-called white gold of a wedding ring, stainless steel, the zipper in a woman's dress, the lustrous grill of an automobile. Nickel creates a glossy finish on metals.

Airborne nickel

Sources of airborne nickel compounds are mining and smelting. Nickel is also present in chrysolite, the common asbestos mineral, in a range of approximately 1.5 to 1.8 mg/gm (1500 ppm).[54] In coal ash, its concentration varies from 3 to 10 mg/gm[55]; in fly ash from residual fuel oil, from 1.8 to 13.2 mg/gm. Cigarettes contain traces of nickel.[56]

Nickel oxide (NiO) is released from the operation of municipal incinerators. Nickel sulfide (NiS) and nickel carbonyl ($Ni[CO_4]$) are important carcinogens. The latter is formed when nickel reacts with carbon monoxide under certain temperature and pressure conditions. In Milwaukee, incinerator ash contained 1% to 10% nickel.[57] According to McMullen of the

National Air Sampling Network, nickel concentrations in urban air (1957 to 1964) averaged from 0.035 to 10.045 μg/meter^3.[58] In rural areas, the level is believed to be much lower.[59]

Nickel in food

According to Schroeder and associates,[60] buckwheat (6.45 ppm) and other cereals contain the largest amounts of nickel; legumes, tea, and cocoa show lesser amounts; fish and food of mammalian origin contain very little nickel. Some foods, namely baking powder, cider, and breakfast cereals can become contaminated, during processing, with nickel and nickel alloys. A few milligrams of nickel are consumed daily from nickel and nickel alloy-containing cookware.[61] The average daily exposure to nickel on a normal diet is estimated at about 0.5 mg or less.[60] Whether or not such minute compounds of nickel in food constitute a risk in humans has not been established.

Toxicity

The oral tolerance of metallic nickel, that is, the dose that produces no ill-effect in dogs when given by mouth, ranges between 1 and 3 gm/kg body weight. Although the metal nickel is relatively nonpoisonous, most of its salts, particularly gaseous nickel carbonyl, are extremely toxic. This slightly yellow volatile liquid with a musty odor is believed to be lethal to man at a concentration of 30 ppm for 30 minutes. Exposure to 3 ppm for 30 minutes is believed to be the short-term safe limit.[62]

Acute exposure. Acute exposures to nickel carbonyl fumes induce dizziness, shortness of breath, frontal headaches, nausea, and vomiting, which usually disappear when the individual is exposed to fresh air. However, after 12 to 36 hours the white blood count becomes elevated, and the temperature may rise. Chest pains, dry cough, shortness of breath, and extreme weakness set in. Fatalities have occurred

4 to 11 days after accidental exposures.[63] They are usually preceded by convulsions and mental confusion.

Chronic exposure. Nickel and its compounds in high doses have produced cancer of the sinuses and of the lungs in nickel workers in Wales[52] and in Ontario.[64] In an Ontario nickel refinery covering the period 1930 to 1957, 245 workers were exposed to the nickel fumes for more than 5 years. Furnace workers with more than 3 years of exposure had a death rate 200 times higher than expected. The disease may not develop for 22 years after exposure.[62] Cancer of the lungs has been induced in rats by exposure to nickel carbonyl.[53] However, nickel cannot be considered the exclusive cause of cancer in these cases because of the simultaneous presence in the atmosphere of other airborne poisons, particularly arsenic and fluoride. Nor has it been determined to what extent the population near such establishments has been affected by the metal.

Contact dermatitis. A common manifestation caused by direct contact of the skin with nickel is contact dermatitis. Next to poison ivy, nickel compounds are probably the most common causes of contact dermatitis.[65] This skin disease has also been designated wristwatch, garter clasp, earring, and zipper dermatitis.[65] Tiny, highly itchy nodes or blebs appear at the areas of contact. They fill up with a yellow-brown fluid and eventually turn into a confluent area. In persons severely allergic to the metal, airborne nickel compounds emitted from factories might conceivably cause a dermatitis limited to the exposed parts of bodies, mainly the face, arms, and hands.

According to the National Air Pollution Survey, emission of nickel and nickel compounds into the United States air has been reduced considerably in recent years, undoubtedly as the result of precautionary measures instituted by industry and government.

CHROMIUM

For several decades, chromium compounds, the decorative finish of chrome plating, have been known to be carcinogenic[66] in chromate-producing industries and in animal experiments.[67]

Chromium (Cr) is never found in pure form in nature. It is usually associated with silica, iron oxide, and magnesium oxide. Ambient air shows only minute amounts of chromium which range from 0.15 μg/meter^3 to as high as 0.35 μg/meter^3.[66]

Food contains very little chromium, ranging on an average between 0.02 to 0.11 ppm.[68] Only certain condiments (black pepper and thyme) show higher ranges (up to 10 ppm). Refined sugar contains little or no chromium, whereas commercial syrups provide as much or more chromium as the raw or brown sugar. In soils, the chromium content varies from a trace to as high as 2.4%. In vegetables, chromium is found in concentrations from 10 to 1000 μg/kg (0.01 to 1 ppm) of dry matter.

The chromium metal itself and the trivalent chromium are stable and relatively nontoxic.[69] However, the water-soluble hexavalent compounds are extremely irritating, corrosive, and toxic to human body tissue.[70] They penetrate surface tissue before they react.[71] Insoluble chromium compounds, on the other hand, are retained in the lungs[72] over extended periods of time and play a role in the production of lung cancer.

Chromium, which is present in all human tissue, is at its highest level at the time of birth.[68] Although in most organs, chromium levels decrease during a person's lifetime, the respiratory tract and fat tissue accumulate the metal. According to Schroeder[73] the skin, muscle, fat, and pancreas contain high levels throughout life. Less chromium is found in Americans than in people living in Africa and eastern countries (Table 16-1).

Health effects

Chromium, a trace element essential for sugar and fat metabolism,[75] is necessary for the action of insulin. Chromium deficiency in the diet of animals causes a syndrome simulating diabetes.[74] A lack of chromium has also been associated with atherosclerotic heart disease, elevated cholesterol levels in the blood, and high fat content of the aorta (main artery of the heart).[74] In areas where atherosclerosis is mild or absent, more chromium is found in body tissue than where the disease is endemic.[74]

A Russian scientist[76] exposed 250 volunteers to 12 different chromium aerosols in concentrations of 1.5 to 40 μg/meter^3. Levels from 10 to 24 μg/meter^3, even for brief periods, caused shock (failure of circulation) and irritation of the upper respiratory tract. For the most sensitive individuals, a level below 2.5 μg/meter^3 constituted the threshold of perception. At this concentration eye adaptation to dark was inhibited.

A classical finding of chrome-plating workers exposed to chromium dust or chromic acid mist is perforation of the nasal septum,[77] a hole in the cartilage that divides the two nasal passages. This condition, which occurs without pain, is occasionally associated with ulcers, sometimes with atrophy (wasting) of the lining of the nose as well as the nasal skeleton. It is often accompanied by chronic catarrhs, congestion in the larynx, polyps in the respiratory tract, chronic inflammation in the bronchi, and, sometimes, bronchopneumonia. The above manifestations constitute

Table 16-1. Body burden of chromium (mg)*

United States	1.72 to 1.86
Africa	2.73
Middle East	9.63
Far East	7.70

*Compiled from Schroeder, H. A., Mason, A. P., and Tipton, I. H.: Chromium deficiency as a factor in atherosclerosis J. Chron. Dis. **23:**123-142, 1970.

the precursor of cancer of the respiratory tract. Czechoslovakian physicians described wartlike swellings in the mouth and larynx in workers exposed for an average of 6.6 years to a mist containing 4 mg/meter³ of chromium.[78]

Chromium and nickel, ingredients of snuff tobacco in common use in certain African countries, have given rise to cancer of the antrum (the sinus in the upper jaw bone).[79]

Contact dermatitis is the other major health effect of chromium and chromium compounds (chromates). Sensitivity to the metal develops following an exposure of several weeks to 6 months. Even the minute amounts of chromates that are present in the atmosphere can cause dermatitis on exposed portions of the skin in individuals who have been previously sensitized through occupational contact, such as workers in woolen mills, automobile plants, garages, aircraft plants, locomotive maintenance, and air-conditioning equipment shops, manufacture of chromate compounds, tanning, photographic, and lithographic plants.[80] Residual scars in individuals afflicted with ulcers on the hands, arms and feet serve as a criterion to physicians in the diagnosis of chromium sensitivity. Cement contains sufficient chromium (0.03 to 7.8 µg/gm) to cause dermatitis in hypersensitive people.

ARSENIC

About 5 months following the opening of a gold mine and smelter in a western state, 32 of 40 children contracted a dermatitis associated with irritation of the eyes and the nasal passages. Older children in the same community, who were being bussed into a high school in a distant town, were not afflicted. Workers at the mine had similar dermatologic manifestations. In some, the nasal septum (the cartilage that separates the two nasal passages) became perforated, a characteristic feature of arsenic poisoning. A yellow-gray dust on the ground gave evidence of fallout from the plant. Air samples taken at the plant showed 0.06 to 13 mg/meter³ of arsenic (As); flue dust from the base of the plant's stack showed a concentration of 44% arsenic; dust near the mill between 1.2 to 4.4% arsenic; and tap water, 30 µg arsenic per liter.[8]

In the late 1940s a more serious environmental contamination, which involved soil and air,[82] occurred near a copper mine in northern Chile. Of 124 workers exposed to the arsenic hazard at the roasting plant and the smelter, 7.2% had arsenical melanosis, a black discoloration of the skin; 5.6% had other skin lesions, and 1.6% had a perforated nasal septum. In 21 persons, residing from 1 km to 50 meters below the plant, the skin was unaffected. Arsenic levels in the urine of the two groups were 0.3 and 0.26 mg/liter, respectively, as compared to 0.04 mg/liter in the control groups of residents of the city of Santiago.

The entire population residing near the plant reacted positively to patch tests (applied to the surface of the skin) composed of a 10% aqueous solution of sodium arsenite, whereas the tests in the control group were negative. Dogs and chickens developed ulcers of the feet. The mineral copper arsenic sulfide contained arsenic in a concentration of 1.64%. The dust from the stack of the plant showed an arsenic content of 16.64%. The problem was resolved when the mine was exhausted.

Sources of environmental pollution

Arsenic is a common industrial nuisance in the vicinity of factories where ore, particularly gold and copper, are being smelted. Burning of coal releases from 0.08 to 16 µg arsenic per gram of coal. Since lead arsenate sprays are being abandoned and organic pesticides substituted for them, there has been little economic incentive to salvage arsenic from the fumes produced by a smelter. Sodium arsenate sprays are still in limited use to sterilize vegetation around fence posts, bridges, radar sites, tennis courts, roadways, and other non-agricultural areas.[83] Smoke from burning the pesticide containers contributes to the presence of arsenic in the atmosphere. Several common phosphate presoaks and household detergents containing arsenic in concentrations as high as 10 to 70 ppm drain into river waters.[84] Ordinarily arsenic occurs in surface waters at concentrations of less than 10 ppb (μg/liter).[85]

The range of atmospheric arsenic is between 0.02 μg/meter^3 to 1.4 μg/meter^3 with the highest urban value in 1964 in El Paso, Texas.[83]

The most common commercial form is arsenic trioxide (As_2O_3), which is readily suspended in small particles in the air. Metallic arsenic, in its original form, is nontoxic.

Effect on humans

Arsenic enters the human body by means of inhalation, ingestion, and absorption through the skin. Excretion takes place mainly through the urine, some through the feces, hair, nails, and skin. Arsenic content of hair serves as an indicator of exposure to the metal.

Up to four decades ago, arsenic was a popular medication for certain skin diseases. Prolonged intake of the drug led to keratosis (scaling) of hands and feet and to dermatitis, especially in the moist areas of the skin (groins, arm pits). Following inhalation of arsenic, a mild bronchitis and nasal irritation ensued.

More concentrated exposures, particularly among workers with arsenic, lead to perforation of the nasal septum. Nausea, pain in the stomach, diarrhea, or constipation are the symptoms caused by eating food contaminated by arsenic. The intestinal symptoms are associated with a loss of protein from the system and a tendency to fluid accumulation (edema) in the body.[86] The fatal dose is in the range of 70 to 180 mg. Arsine (AsH_3), one of the most toxic arsenical compounds is formed wherever hydrogen is produced in the presence of arsenic, as for instance in pickling of arsenic-containing metals. It causes hemolytic anemia, a condition characterized by jaundice and destruction of red blood cells at occupational exposures of less than 1.5 ppm.[87]

Hueper[88] recognized arsenic as a cause of cancer of the skin, lungs, and liver. This association with cancer was supported by the frequent occurrence of lung cancer in German vineyard workers[89] who had been exposed to lead arsenate dust. Other sporadic case reports from long-term ingestion of arsenic trioxide[90] and recent reports on mutagenic effects on human lymphocytes qualify arsenic for inclusion among carcinogenic agents. (See Chapter 17.)

There is evidence[91] that arsenic causes abnormalities in offspring (teratogenic effects). (See Chapter 17.) The antagonistic effect of selenium to arsenic is well established.[92]

REFERENCES

1. Pybus, F. C.: Cancer and atmospheric pollution, Med. Proc. **10**:242, 268, 1964.
2. Yamagira, K., and Ichikawa, K.: Experimental study of the pathogenesis of cancer, J. Cancer Res. **3**:1, 1918.
3. Cook, J. W., Hieger, I., Kennaway, L. E., and Mayneord, W. V.: Production of cancer by pure hydrocarbons, Proc. Roy. Soc. London (Series B) **111**:455-484, 1932.
4. Air conservation, Publication No. 80, Washington, D. C., 1965, American Association for the Advancement of Science.
5. Olson, D. A.: Air pollution aspects of organic carcinogens. Litton Industries, PB 188-090 Bethesda, Maryland, September, 1969, U. S. Department of Commerce.
6. Hueper, W. C., Kotin, P., Tabor, E. C., and others: Carcinogenic bioassays on air pollutants, Arch. Pathol. **74**:89, 1962.
7. Hammond, E. C., and Horn, D.: Smoking and death rates: report on 44 months of follow-up of 187,783 Men, J.A.M.A. **166**:1159-1294, 1958.
8. Teleki, L.: Nebel und Nebel Katastrophen, Arch. Gewerbepathol. Gewerbehyg. **13**:6-28, 1954.
9. Haenzel, W., and Shimkin, M.: Lung cancer

among women, Acta Unio Internat. Contra Cancrum **15**:493, 1959.

10. Stokinger, H. E.: The spectre of today's environmental pollution, U.S.A. brand, Amer. Industr. Hyg. Ass. J. **30**:195-217, 1969.

11. Winkelstein, W., Jr., and Kantor, S.: Stomach cancer, Arch. Environ. Health **18**:544, 1969.

12. Nelson, N.: Inhalation carcinogenesis in man; environmental and occupational hazards, symposium. Relation of inhalation exposure to carcinogenesis. Gatlinburg, Tenn., October 8-11, 1969, Oak Ridge National Conference Laboratory.

13. Kotin, P., Falk, H. L., and Thomas, M.: Production of skin tumors in mice with oxidation products of aliphatic hydrocarbons, Cancer **9**:910, 1956.

14. Kotin, P., and Wiseley, D. V.: Production of lung cancer in mice by inhalation exposure to influenza virus and aerosols of hydrocarbons. In Homburger, F., editor: Progress in experimental tumor research, vol. 3, Basel, 1962, Karger.

15. Kotin, P., and Falk, H. L.: The role and action of environmental agents. In the pathogenesis of lung cancer: Part I, air pollutants, Cancer **12**:147, 1959.

16. Pylev, L. N.: Effect of the dispersion of soot in deposition of 3,4-benzpyrene in lung tissue of rats, Hyg. Sanit. **32**:174, 1967.

17. Saffioti, U., Cefis, F., and Kolb, L. H.: A method for the experimental induction of bronchogenic carcinomas, Cancer Res. **28**:104, 1969.

18. Campbell, J. A.: Cancer of skin and increase in incidence of primary tumors of lung in mice exposed to dust obtained from tarred roads, Brit. J. Exp. Pathol. **15**:287, 1934.

19. Horton, A. W., Denman, T., and Trosset, R. P.: Carcinogenics of the skin: Part II, the accelerating properties of aliphatics and related hydrocarbons, Cancer Res. **17**:758, 1957.

20. Falk, H. L., Kotin, P., and Thompson, S.: Inhibition of carcinogenesis, Arch. Environ. Health **9**:169, 1964.

21. Dautrebande, L., Beckman, H., and Walkenhorst, W.: Lung deposition of fine dust particles, Arch. Industr. Health **16**:179, 1957.

22. Air conservation, Washington, D. C., 1968. American Association for Advancement of Science.

23. Sawicki, E., Fox, F. T., Elbert, W. C., and others: Polynuclear aromatic hydrocarbon composition of air polluted by coal-tar pitch fumes, Amer. Industr. Hyg. Ass. J. **23**:137, 1962.

24. Wada, S., Nishimoto, Y., Miyanishi, M., and others: Mustard gas as cause of respiratory neoplasia in man, Lancet **1**:1161-1163, 1968.

25. West, I.: Biological effect of pesticides in the environment. In Organic pesticides in the environment, (Advances in Chemistry No. 60) Washington, D. C., 1966, American Chemical Society.

26. Lijinsky, W., and Epstein, S. S.: Nitrosamines as environmental carcinogens, Nature **225**:21-23, 1970.

27. Neurath, G.: Zur Frage des Vorkommens von N-Nitroso-Verbindungen in Tabakrauch, Experimentia **23**:400-404, 1967.

28. Neurath, G., Dünger, M., Gewe, J., and others: Untersuchung der Flüchtigen Basen des Tabakrauches, Beitr. Tabakforsch **3**:563-569, 1966.

29. Druckrey, H., Preussmann, R., Ivankovic, S. and others: Organotrope Carcinogene Wirkungen bei 65 Verschiedenen N-Nitroso-Verbindungen an BD-Ratten, Z. Krebsforsch **69**:103-201, 1967.

30. Mancuso, T. F., and Brennan, M. J.: Epidemiological considerations of cancer of the gallbladder, bile ducts and salivary glands in the rubber industry, J. Occupat. Med. **12**:333-341, 1970.

31. Marchand, F.: Ueber Eigentümliche pigmentkristalle in den Lungen, Verh. Deutsch. Path. Ges. **10**:223-228, 1906.

32. Gaensler, E. A., and Addington, W. W.: Asbestos or ferruginous bodies, New Eng. J. Med. **280**:488-92, 1969.

33. Cooke, W. E.: Fibrosis of lungs due to inhalation of asbestos dust, Brit. Med. J. **2**:147, 1924.

34. Gough, J.: Differential diagnosis in pathology of asbestosis, Ann. N. Y. Acad. Sci. **132**:368-372, 1965.

35. Gross, P., deTreville, R. T., Cralley, L. J., and others: Pulmonary ferruginous bodies: development in response to filamentous dusts and a method of isolation and concentration, Arch. Pathol. **85**:539-546, 1968.

36. Thomson, J. G.: Asbestos and urban dweller, Ann. N. Y. Acad. Sci. **132**:196-214, 1965.

37. Gold, C.: Asbestos levels in human lungs, J. Clin. Path. **22**:507, 1969.

38. Langer, A. M., Selikoff, I. J., and Sastre, A.: Chrysotile asbestos in the lungs of persons in New York City. Arch. Environ. Health **22**:348-361, 1971.

39. Gross, P., Tuma, J., and deTreville, R. T.: Unusual ferruginous bodies, their formation from non-fibrous particulates and from carbonaceous fibrous particles, Arch. Environ. Health **22**:534-537, 1971.

40. Hendrey, N. W.: The geology, occurrences and major uses of asbestos, Ann. N. Y. Acad. Sci. **132:**12, 1965.

41. Wagner, J. C., Sleggs, C. A., and Marchand, P.: Diffuse pleural mesothelioma and asbestos exposure in the northwestern Cape Province, Brit. J. Industr. Med. **17:**260-271, 1960.

42. Selikoff, I. J., Nicholson, W. J., and Langer, A. M.: Asbestos air pollution, Arch. Environ. Health **25:**1-13, 1972.

43. Elmes, P. C.: The epidemiology and clinical features of asbestos and related diseases, J. Postgrad. Med. **42:**623-635, 1966.

44. Newhouse, M. L.: The medical risk of exposure to asbestos, Practitioner **199:**285-293, 1967.

45. Hourihane, D., Lessof, L., and Richardson, P. C.: Hyaline and calcified plural plaques as an index of exposure to asbestos, Brit. Med. J. **1:**1069-1074, 1966.

46. Sluis-Cremer, G. K.: Asbestosis in South Africa in certain geographical and environmental considerations, Ann. N. Y. Acad. Sci. **132:**215, 1965.

47. Selikoff, I. J., Churg, J., and Hammond, E. C.: Asbestos exposure and neoplasia, J.A.M.A. **188:**22-32, 1964.

48. Selikoff, I. J., Bader, R. A., Bader, M. E., and others: Asbestosis and neoplasia, Amer. J. Med. **42:**487-496, 1967.

49. Wagner, J. C., Slagg, C. A., and Marchand, P.: Diffuse pleural mesothelioma and asbestos exposure in North Western Cape Province, Brit. J. Industr. Med. **17:**260-71, 1960.

50. Hourihane, D. O'B., and McCaughey, W. T. E.: Pathological aspects of asbestosis, Portland Med. J. **42:**613-622, 1966.

51. Dalquen, P., Dabbert, A. F., and Heinz, Y.: On the epidemiology of the pleura mesothelioma, preliminary report, 119 cases from the Hamburg area, Prax. Pneumol. **23:**548-558, 1969.

52. Sullivan, R. J.: Air pollution aspects of nickel and its compounds, PB 188 070, Bethesda, Maryland, September 1969, Litton Systems, Inc.

53. Sunderman, F. W., and Donnelly, A. J.: Studies on nickel carcinogenesis, metastasizing pulmonary tumors induced by inhalation of nickel carbonyl, Amer. J. Path. **6:**1027-1041, 1965.

54. Bridge, J. C.: Annual report of the chief inspector of factories and workshops for the year 1932, London, 1939, Her Majesty's Stationery.

55. Abernethy, R. F., and Gibson, F. H.: Rare elements in coal, Bureau of Mines Information Circular IC-8163, Wash., D. C., 1963.

56. Schroeder, H. E.: Metals in the air, Environment **13:**18-32, 1971.

57. Chass, R. L., and Rose, A. H.: Discharge from municipal incinerators. Preprint, presented at the 46th Annual Meeting, Air Pollution Control Association, 1953.

58. McMullen, T. B.: Concentrations of nickel in urban atmosphere (1957-1964). Preprint 1966, E.P.A., Triangle Park, N. C.

59. Lee, R. E., Jr., Patterson, R. K., and Wagman, J.: Concentration and particle size distribution of metals in urban and rural air, Cincinnati, 1969, Preprint, U. S. Department of Health, Education and Welfare, National Air Pollution Control Administration.

60. Schroeder, H. A., Balassa, J. J., and Tipton, I. H.: Abnormal trace metals in man—nickel, J. Chron. Dis. **15:**51, 1962.

61. Stokinger, H. E.: Nickel, Ni. In Patty, F. A., editor: Industrial hygiene and toxicology, vol. II, ed 2, New York, 1963, Interscience.

62. Brief, R. S., Blanchard, J. W., Scala, R. A., and others: Metal carbonyls in the petroleum industry, Arch. Environ. Health **23:**373-384, 1971.

63. Sunderman, F. W., and Kincaid, J. F.: Nickel poisoning. Part II, studies of patients suffering from acute exposures to vapors of nickel carbonyl, J.A.M.A. **155:**889, 1954.

64. Sutherland, R. B.: Respiratory cancer mortality in workers employed in an Ontario nickel refinery covering the period 1930 to 1957, Division of Industrial Hygiene, Ontario Department of Health. Unpublished report, November 1959, with additions.

65. Waldbott, G. L.: Contact dermatitis, Springfield, Ill., 1953, Charles C Thomas, Publisher.

66. Sullivan, R. J.: Air pollution aspects of chromium and its compounds, PB 188 075, Bethesda, Md., September 1969, Litton Systems, Inc.

67. Laskins, S., Kuschner, M., and Drew, R. T.: Studies on pulmonary carcinogenesis in inhalation carcinogenesis, Proceedings of the Oak Ridge National Laboratory Conference, Gatlinburg, Tenn. Oct. 8-11, 1969.

68. Schroeder, H. A., Balassa, J. J., and Tipton, I. H.: Abnormal trace metals in man—Chromium, J. Chron. Dis. **15:**941, 1962.

69. Baetjer, A. M.: Relation of Chromium to Health. In Udy, M. J., editor: Chromium, vol. 1, American Chemical Society Monograph 132, New York, 1956, Reinhold.

70. Gafafer, W. M., editor: Health of workers in chromate-producing industry, Division of Oc-

cupational Health, U. S. Public Health Service Publication 192, 1953.

71. Samitz, M. H., Katz, S., and Schrager, J. D.: Studies of the diffusion of chromium compounds through skin, J. Invest. Derm. **48**:514, 1967.

72. Mancuso, T. F., and Hueper, W. C.: Occupational cancer and other health hazards in a chromate plant. A medical appraisal: Part I, lung cancer in chromate workers, Ind. Med. Surg. **20**:359, 1951.

73. Schroeder, H. A.: The role of chromium in mammalian nutrition, Amer. J. Clin. Nutr. **21**:230-244, 1966.

74. Schroeder, H. A., Mason, A. P., and Tipton, I. H.: Chromium deficiency as a factor in atherosclerosis, J. Chron. Dis. **23**:123-142, 1970.

75. Mertz, W.: Chromium occurrence and function in biological systems, Physiol. Rev. **49**: 165-239, 1969.

76. Cooperman, E. F.: Maximal permissable concentration of hexavalent Chromium in Atmospheric Air. Translated by Levine, B. S., U.S.S.R. Literature on Air Pollution and Related Occupational Diseases, **12**:249, 1963.

77. Kleinfeld, M., and Rosso, A.: Ulcerations of the nasal septum due to inhalation of Chromic acid mist, Ind. Med. Surg. **34**:242, 1965.

78. Hanslian, L., Nadratil, J., Jurak, J., and others: Upper respiratory tract lesions from chromic acid aerosol, Czech. Pracovni Lekar. **19**:294, 1967.

79. Baumslag, N., and Keen, P.: Trace elements in soil and plants, and antral cancer, Arch. Environ. Health **25**:23-25, 1972.

80. Winson, J. R., and Walsh, E. N.: Chromate dermatitis in railroad employees working with diesel locomotives, J. Amer. Med. Ass. **147**: 1133, 1951.

81. Birmingham, D. U., Key, M. M., Holaday, D. A., and others: An outbreak of arsenical dermatosis in a mining community, Arch. Derm. **91**:457, 1965.

82. Ovanguren, H., and Perez, E.: Poisoning of industrial origin in a community, Arch Environ. Health **13**:185-189, 1966.

83. Sullivan, R. J.: Air pollution aspects of arsenic and its compound, PB 188 071, Bethesda, Maryland, 1969, Litton Systems, Inc.

84. Angino, E. E., Magnuson, L. M., Waugh, T. C., and others: Arsenic in detergents—possible danger and pollution hazard, Science **168**:389, 1970.

85. Durum, W. H., Hem, J. I., and Heidel, S. G.: Reconnaissance of selected minor elements in surface waters of the United States, October 1970, Geological Survey Circular 643, Washington, D. C., 1971, U. S. Bureau of Sport Fisheries and Wildlife, Department of Interior.

86. Akio, K., and Ohbe, Y.: Protein-losing enteropathy associated with arsenic poisoning, Amer. J. Dis. Child. **121**:515-517, 1971.

87. Arsine, hygienic guide series, Amer. Ind. Hyg. Ass. J. **26**:438-441, 1965.

88. Hueper, W. C.: Environmental carcinogenesis in man and animals, Ann. N. Y. Acad. Sci. **108**:963, 1963.

89. Braun, W.: Carcinoma of skin and internal organs caused by arsenic, German Med. Monthly **3**:321, 1958.

90. Novey, H., and Martell, S. H.: Asthma arsenic and cancer, J. Allerg. **44**:315-9, 1969.

91. Holmberg, R. E., and Ferm, V. H.: Interrelationships of selenium, cadmium and arsenic in mammalian teratogenesis, Arch. Environ. Health **18**:873, 1969.

92. Ferm, V. H., and Carpenter, S. J.: Malformation induced by sodium arsenate, J. Reprod. Fertil. **17**:199, 1968.

17
MUTAGENIC POLLUTANTS

Carcinogenic and mutagenic (producing genetic aberrations)* air pollutants have certain features in common, namely their insidious nature, the relatively long time lag between exposure and overt manifestations, the irreversible course of the disease, the greater susceptibility of immature tissue, and the production of pathologic changes. These features are characteristic of each of the two groups regardless of the kind of pollutant involved. All these factors contribute to the complexity of relating genetic effects to their cause.

KINDS OF GENETIC EFFECTS

Mutagenic effects may manifest themselves immediately at birth as defects of the offspring,[1] or they may not make their appearance for many decades.[2] Examples of such diseases are achondroplasia (a disease that interferes with skeletal growth), deafness associated with albinism, Marfan's syndrome (a disease characterized by displacement of the lens of the eye and changes in the development of fingers). The current state of our knowledge renders it very difficult to assess to what extent air pollution will affect future generations.

Prolonged exposure to pollutants as well as a single acute episode during pregnancy are involved in spontaneous abortions, stillbirths, and reduction of birth weight, which has been documented repeatedly in

*Carcinogenics can be mutagenic, since they may induce mutations in the growing cell.

domestic animals (Chapter 4). It can also lead to high death rates at birth and during childhood and to retardation of growth and development of children.

Since every cell of the body and every single metabolic process is susceptible to genetic changes, a pollutant does not necessarily elicit a single effect in a particular organ or organ system (Table 17-1). Hundreds of inherited defects can be attributed to mutagenic poisons as, for instance, disturbances in bone growth, crippling of limbs, and abnormalities of the spine, the central nervous system, and the kidneys.

MODE OF ACTION

The physical determinants of hereditary characteristics are called the genes. They are identified with the chromosomes (Fig. 17-1, A) of the cell nuclei. Mutagenic agents can affect both the sex chromosomes[2] and autosomes. They affect the development of the fertilized egg[2] and of the embryo. They can either produce an abnormal number of chromosomes, or they can alter the structural arrangement of the chromosome itself.[3]

Changes in number of chromosomes (aneuploidy). When a cell divides (division of cells takes place continuously in gametes, in the developing embryo, and throughout life) delicate structures called spindles aid in the movement of the sister chromatids (the longitudinal half of the chromosome) to the opposite poles of the dividing cell (Fig. 17-1, B). Under normal conditions

Table 17-1. Major congenital malformations reported among 1,135,156 live births in Missouri, 1953-1964*

BIRTH DEFECT	INCIDENCE
Cleft lip and/or cleft palate	2,242
Clubfoot	1,482
Polydactyly (more than 5 fingers)	817
Congenital heart disease	734
Spina bifida (defective spine)	712
Epispadias or hypospadias (deformity of external genitalia)	572
Syndactyly (abnormal union of fingers)	451
Mongolism	423
Bones and joint deformities	386
Hydrocephalus (excess fluid about brain)	314
Anencephaly (absence of brain tissue)	254
Omphalocele and eventration (naval hernia and protrusion of bowels)	229
Head and trunk deformities	225
Imperforate anus	188
Ear deformities	185
Tracheo-esophageal deformities	144
Atresia of intestines (bowel obstruction)	115
Skin	104

*Adapted from Silberg, S. L., Marienfeld, C. J., Wright, H., and others: Surveillance of congenital anomalies in Missouri, 1953-1964: a preliminary report, Arch. Environ. Health **13:**641-644, 1966.

each daughter cell will have a complete set of 23 pairs of chromosomes (Fig. 17-2). When spindles are damaged (Fig. 17-1, *C*) the two cells receive an unequal number of chromosomes either in excess of, or less than, 46. The mechanism most commonly causing aneuploidy, however, is nondisjunction of the chromosomes. Proliferation of cells, which show changes in the number of chromosomes, induce birth defects in humans. One typical airborne poison that inhibits the formation of the spindle fibers is mercury.[4] In Table 17-1 the incidence of some of the common birth defects is presented. Any toxic agent, for example, drugs, contaminants of food, water, or air, might be responsible for such lesions. How much air pollutants contribute to the development of these conditions has not been determined.

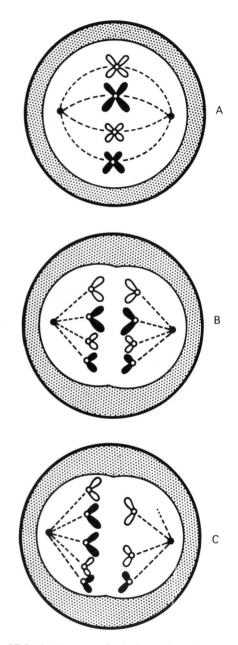

Fig. 17-1. A, Diagram of spindles pulling the two sets of chromosomes to opposite ends of a cell about to divide. Chromosomes are lined up in pairs along the center. **B,** Normal cell division. **C,** Damaged spindles in "nondisjunction." The two cells receive an unequal number of chromosomes. This can produce personality defects in mammalians.

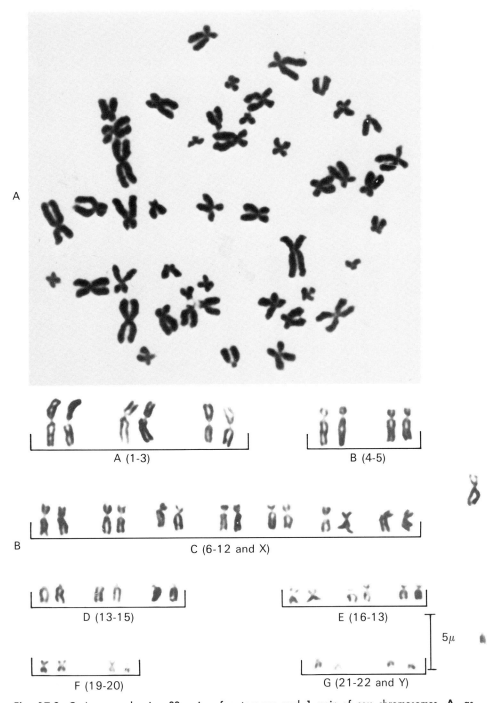

Fig. 17-2. Cariograms showing 22 pairs of autosomes and 1 pair of sex chromosomes, **A,** as they appear in the cell, and, **B,** in the order of their classification according to size and shape.

Structural aberration. Damage to chromosomes consists in so-called chromosome breakage (Fig. 17-3). One or both of the two chromatids can be involved in chromosome breaks. If both chromatids are damaged, the defect is called "chromosome breaks" or "isochromatid breaks"; whereas involvement of only one chromatid is termed a single "chromatid break." Chromosome breaks may also be classified according to the number of chromosomes involved—homosomal breaks, which affect only one chromosome and heterosomal breaks, which affect more than one chromosome. It is estimated that about 1% of live-born infants suffer from effects of chromosomal aberrations that arise spontaneously. How much natural radiation and other air contaminants contribute to this incidence is not known.[6]

Damage can occur at any phase of the embryonic development. The toxic agent can induce changes in the mother or in the father, that is, it may damage the sperm or the egg. It can also affect the embryo directly. Carbon monoxide, for instance, reaches the embryo through the mother's bloodstream, although the saturation of the fetal hemoglobin with carbon monoxide lags behind that of the mother.[7] Mature male germ cells, the spermatozoa, are more sensitive to damage than their precursors,

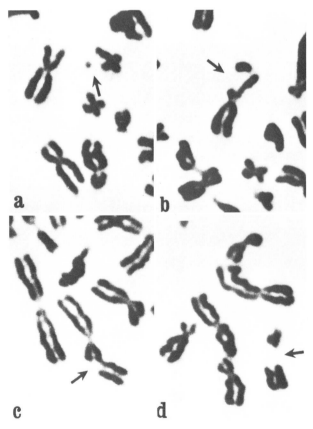

Fig. 17-3. Breakage of chromosomes (arrows) in the blood cells of humans who consumed very large amounts of fish contaminated by mercury. (Preparations made and furnished by the Clinical Genetic Laboratory of the Karolinska Hospital, Stockholm, Sweden; courtesy Schubert, J.: A program to abolish harmful chemicals, Ambio 1:79-89, 1972.)

the spermatogonia.[8] After irradiation of the testis up to several hundred rads* recovery of spermatozoa can be expected, whereas the recovery of irradiated ovarian germ cells is uncertain and erratic.[9] In some instances, damage to the placenta interferes with placental transfer of nutrients to the embryo, which may account for defects in the newborn.[10]

Interval between conception and exposure. The interval between conception and exposure to a pollutant is a prime factor influencing the frequency and degree of mutations. In general, the longer the interval,[11] the less is the hazard. The early weeks of pregnancy, when the major organs of the fetus are being laid down, appear to be the most sensitive period to irradiation with fission products. During the late stages of its development the embryo is much more resistant to damage although some tissues, such as the retina and the brain, remain susceptible to low doses of radiation throughout the entire period of pregnancy. Birth defects caused by thalidomide (the well-known teratogenic drug) occurred relatively late, namely when the medication was taken between the thirty-fourth and fiftieth day of pregnancy at the time of formation of the limbs.[12] The changes produced by thalidomide are similar to those produced by genes but are not inherited.

METHODS OF TESTING

Fruit fly. Much information concerning mutagenic effects is based upon experimental data with the fruit fly *(Drosophila melanogaster),* which produces large numbers of offspring within a few days. In 1927 Muller demonstrated that mutations could be produced in fruit flies by x-radiation.[13] Subsequent experiments, which showed more extensive and more frequent abnormalities in mice[8] than in fruit flies, indi-

cated that the genetic hazard to mammalians, inclding man, was greater than that which had been initially anticipated.

For the study of teratogenic poisons, a suspected substance is administered to pregnant animals. Shortly before the anticipated birth, the fetuses are removed and examined. The incidence of abnormal litters, of abnormal fetuses per litter, of specific congenital abnormalities, and of fetal mortality are assessed. Additional observations are made on the newborn animals.

Human cells. In humans one of the most reliable methods of demonstrating mutagenic effects is the direct observation of the chromosome karyotypes (the chromosomal constitution of the nucleus in a cell) in lymphoid blood cells. Cytologic analyses show a wide range of abnormalities from slight chromosomal damage to the death of the cells.

Another approach in the study of chromosome breaks pertains to whether or not healing or reunion occurs. An open break or a nonhealing defect is called a "simple break," a reuniting one is called a "gap." Such "aberrations" of chromosomes have been reported in human white blood cells from exposures to x-radiation at levels employed for diagnosis.[14] Gaps may produce minute deficiencies and eventually the loss of some genes.

DNA synthesis. In evaluating the mutagenic status of a cell another significant parameter is whether or not the cell retains its ability to synthesize deoxyribonucleic acid (DNA). DNA is a long-chain molecule, the major ingredient of chromosomes, which contains the genetic codes necessary for the development and functioning of the organism. It controls the formation of different proteins and enzymes.

Epidemiologic data. In humans, data on genetic effects have been gleaned from records of women who have undergone radiotherapy during pregnancy, and from newborn children in Japan whose mothers were exposed to atomic bomb radiation during

---

*Rad: standard unit for measuring radiation exposure, namely the dose absorbed by radiation.

pregnancy. Considerable information was obtained from patients given x-ray treatment over the spine[15] for relief of spondylitis (arthritis in spine). Epidemics of poisoning, such as the methyl mercury intoxication in Minamata, Japan (Chapter 12), permit observations on the offspring of mothers who consumed or were exposed to toxic agents during their pregnancy.

In a review of 135,156 birth records in Missouri extending from 1953 to 1964, Silberg and associates[5] reported an overall incidence of abnormalities of 7.4 in 1000 live births. The same incidence namely 7.4 per 1000 live births were found in Ohio in 1953 among 1560 infants born alive[16] and a higher incidence namely of 10.7 per 1000 in New York state, exclusive of New York City, from 1948 through 1955.[17] The Missouri study suggested that the variations from one county to another were the result of an environmental factor. Over one half of the congenital anomalies (52.7%) consisted of cleft lip or cleft palate, clubfoot, craniospinal (skull and spine), and external urethral anomalies.[5] At the present state of our knowledge it is impossible to identify the causes of these defects. Besides air pollutants, other toxic agents such as infections, drugs, natural and artificial irradiation, food additives, and polluted water must be considered.

Airborne mutagens. The following are examples of airborne mutagens:

1. Organic agents. *DDT and other insecticides* derived from phosphates and phosphoramides are mutagenic upon viruses, bacteria, fungi, and wheat.[2] They also alter the cultures of human lymphocytes.

Two popular weed killers *2,4,5-T* (trichlorophenoxyacetic acid) and its closely related *compound 2,4-T* (which contains one chlorine atom less than 2,4,5-T) have caused birth defects in animals.[18] Several esters of these agents are also teratogenic.[19] Potent *dioxin* compounds that are contaminants of 2,4-T and 2,4,5-T have produced deaths and gastrointestinal hemorrhages in

the fetuses when pregnant rats were treated with doses of .125 to 8 μg. The mutagenic effects of these extremely toxic substances is brought about through interaction with DNA.[20]

2. Inorganic agents. Among inorganic chemicals, *nitrous oxide* can cause abnormalities in vertebrae (spine) and ribs and malformation of the intestinal tract; *fluorides* induce a variety of teratogenic defects in rats (Fig. 17-4). In hamsters, 5-hour exposure to 0.02 ppm *ozone* caused chromosome aberrations of circulating lymphocytes.[21] The frequency of the chromosome breaks in these experiments (1.6×0.001 breaks per cell per minute) is in agreement with that obtained from exposures of human cells in the test tube. Indeed, applying these values to a human exposed for 40 hours to the permitted 0.1 ppm ozone, a greater frequency in chromosome breaks will occur than that resulting from permitted radiation exposure.

A single large intravenous dose of *sodium arsenate* (20 mg/kg) injected into hamsters on the eighth day of pregnancy led to various kinds of malformations, mainly exencephaly (protrusion of brains through the skull). Doses of 5 mg/kg produced no malformations, whereas 40 mg/kg killed all embryos.[22]

On the other hand when arsenate was added to drinking water of mice and rats in a concentration of 5 ppm for three generations, little damage was noted except for a slight reduction in the size of the litters and an increase in the ratio of males to females.[23] This is in contrast to the many abnormalities and failure to reproduce, when concentrations of 3 ppm selenium, 10 ppm cadmium, 10 ppm molybdenum, and 25 ppm lead were administered.

Pregnant hamsters that were injected with *cadmium* sulfate in doses of 2.0 mg/kg body weight gave birth to defective offspring and embryos failed to develop.[24] Injections of *lead* salts into hamsters produced many abnormalities in the offspring especially stunted or complete absence of

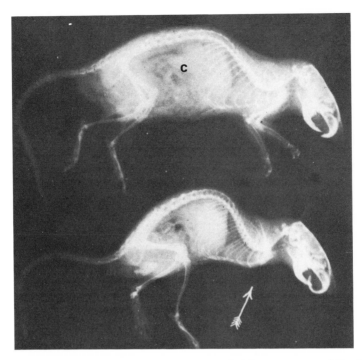

Fig. 17-4. Roentgenogram of rats whose mothers were fed large amounts of fluoride. Note the absence of forelegs in lower animal (arrow) with marked curvature of the spine. C is the normal control rat.

the tailbones.[25] Addition of 1% lead acetate to the diet of young mice for 2 weeks showed an increased number of chromosome gaps and breaks.[26]

OBSERVATIONS IN HUMANS

Although the experimental phase of mutagenicity caused by air pollutants has received increasing attention in recent years, only few clinical data in humans are available.

In a study of 34 patients attending the University of Freiburg, Germany, skin clinic, who had hyperkeratosis (excess scaling) on feet and hands caused by *arsenic* poisoning, chromosomal abnormalities were found in lymphocytes. The patients, who had been working in the vineyards, had been poisoned through exposure to arsenical sprays; others had taken arsenicals as medication for psoriasis (a chronic skin disease of unknown origin)

as long as 20 years previously. Some had cancer of the skin.[27]

A Czechoslovakian physician, Kauzal,[28] reported hemorrhages in the duodenum (upper bowel) of five newborn infants whose mothers had been working in an industry where they were exposed to air contaminated by *fluoride*. The ulcers in the upper gastrointestinal tract, which are otherwise rare in infants, were of the kind experimentally produced in acute fluoride intoxication by large doses.[29] Such observations suggest the possibility of a causal relationship between the hemorrhages and the mothers' exposure to fluoride.

More significant are the studies of Rapaport[30] who reviewed official birth records in four midwestern states in 1956 and a total of 333,350 births in Illinois in 1959.[31] He found only 23.6 mongoloid births per 100,000 from mothers whose drinking water at their permanent residence was nearly fluoride free (0.0 to 0.1 ppm), compared to 71.6 mongoloid births per 100,000* from mothers whose water supplies contained 1.0 to 2.6 ppm. In 1963[32] he presented further supporting evidence for the causal relationship between fluoride and mongolism.† New data showed a significantly elevated fluoride content of teeth in relation to dental fluorosis and a lower caries rate among mongoloid children. Furthermore he showed that fluoride can induce mutations in the fruit fly *Drosophila melanogaster*,[33] which seem to be analogous to the trisomy‡ of chromosome 21, a defect associated with mongolism in humans.

Thirty-two patients who had recovered from a blood disease (bone marrow impairment) caused by *benzene* poisoning had significantly increased rates of "unstable" and "stable" chromosomes. Aberrations of chromosomes were present for several years after cessation of the exposure and after recovery from poisoning.[34] Persistence of an increase of the "stable" changes was particularly remarkable.

It has already been pointed out that *methyl mercury,* which inhibits formation of spindle fibers, caused serious illness in newborn Japanese children of Minamata. *Organic lead* has induced abortions, stillbirths, and premature births (see chapter 12).

Smoking tobacco accounts for a reduction of weight in newborn children[35] but benzo[a]pyrene, a constituent of tobacco smoke and of other combustion products and a proven carcinogen in mice has not been tested for its effect on chromosomes. In the blood of pregnant women, *carbon monoxide* concentrations were higher in

smokers than in nonsmokers.[36] The oxygen carrying capacity of the maternal and umbilical cord blood of these smoking women was significantly reduced.

Many studies indicate harm to the fetus of expectant mothers who had been exposed to *x-radiation* during pregnancy. For instance, an investigation at the Harvard School of Public Health, involving 500,000 infants from 30 United States hospitals, showed a 30% increase in cancer, mainly leukemia, and malignancy of the central nervous system in children whose mothers were irradiated during pregnancy.[37] Another study, involving 216 families with mongoloid children born and residing in the city of Baltimore, showed that mothers of the mongoloid children had been exposed to x-radiation seven times as frequently as a group of "control" mothers.[38]

Probably the most reliable data on genetic effects in humans are those garnered following the *atomic bomb* blasts in Hiroshima and Nagasaki where large populations were involved.

Gamma rays from atomic explosions are potent mutagens. Some of the radioactive isotopes such as Iodine 131, Plutonium 238, Tritium H-3, and Carbon 14 are stored in the spleen, bone marrow, liver, and lymph nodes[39] where they produce chromosome breaks in body tissues, especially in the reproductive organs. *Carbon atoms* make up about 37% of DNA. If a ^{14}C atom becomes incorporated in a DNA molecule, further damage occurs by the transmutation of Carbon 14 to Nitrogen 14.

Abortions, stillbirths, and an increase in the natal and infantile death rate followed the bomb explosion.

In a subsequent survey[40] children, whose mothers while pregnant were within 1200 meters of the center of the explosion, developed microcephaly, an otherwise rare deformity of the skull associated with mental retardation (Table 17-2). Other birth defects involved the skeletal system. Of 30 mothers who were within 2000 meters of

---

*This contrasts with an incidence of 37.2 per 100,000 reported by Silberg and associates.[5]

†These figures showed the highest degree of probability recognized by the Chi square formula.

‡In a normal cell nucleus chromosomes occur in pairs. However in mongolism the number 21 chromosome occurs in triplicate. This abnormality is termed trisomy.

Table 17-2. Twenty-five children with congenital anomalies among 205 exposed to atomic bomb blast prior to birth*

ANOMALY	NUMBER OF CHILDREN	DISTANCE OF MOTHER FROM CENTER OF BLAST (METERS)
Microcephalic mental retardation	6	<1200
Mongoloid mental retardation	2	<1200
Congenital dislocation of hips	5	One between 2500 and 3000 One <1000 One between 1600 and 1800 Two >2500
Congenital heart disease	3	Questionable
Hydrocele	2	>2000
Deformed chest	1	1200 to 1400
Talipes calcaneovalgus (clubfoot)	1	>3000
Deformed iris	1	1600 to 1800
Deformed ear	1	>3000
Congenital strabismus (squinting)	1	>3000
Congenital glaucoma	1	>2000
Partial albinism	1	1600

*Compiled from Plummer, G.: Anomalies occurring in children exposed in utero to the atomic bomb in Hiroshima, Pediatrics 10:687-692, 1952.

the center of the detonation and who had major signs of radiation sickness, 7 miscarried and the offspring of 6 died. Four of 6 surviving children were mentally retarded.[41] Concrete provided an effective shield against irradiation, whereas wood was ineffective. Further details on radionuclides are given in Chapter 20.

The above defects resulted from a single massive exposure. With respect to pollutants present in ambient air, it should be borne in mind that the levels of toxic agents in animal experiments exceed, by far, those with which we are confronted through polluted air. However accidental exposures to high levels during human pregnancy can occur. Furthermore, persistent intake of minute quantities of a toxic agent for extended periods of time are apt to induce, in predisposed individuals, effects similar to or identical with those elicited by a single sudden massive exposure.

On the other hand, numerous natural mutagenic agents, such as natural radiation and products of decomposition, have been present in the air for ages. There are no means of comparing their effects with those inherent to our industrial development.

REFERENCES

1. Neel, J. V.: Mutations in the human population. In Burdette, W. J., editor: Methodology in human genetics, San Francisco, 1962, Holden-Day Inc.
2. Epstein, S. S.: Control of chemical pollutants, Nature **228**:816-819, 1970.
3. Neel, J. V., and Bloom, A. D.: The detection of environmental mutagens, Med. Clin. N. Amer. **53**:1243-1256, 1969.
4. Ramel, C., and Magnusson, J.: Genetic effects of organic mercury compounds: Part II, chromosome segregation on *Drosophila melanogaster,* Hereditas **61**:231-254, 1969.
5. Silberg, S. L., Marienfeld, C. J., Wright, H., and others: Surveillance of congenital anomalies in Missouri, 1953-1964; a preliminary report, Arch. Environ. Health **13**:641-644, 1966.
6. Report of the United Nations Scientific Committee on the Effects of Atomic Radiation, New York, 1966, United Nations.
7. Curtis, G. W., Algeri, E. J., McBay, A. J., and others: The transplacental diffusion of carbon monoxide, Arch. Path. **59**:677-690, 1955.
8. Russel, W. L.: Studies in mammalian radiation genetics, Nucleonics **23**:53, 1965.

9. Carter, T. C.: Radiation-induced gene mutation in adult female and foetal male mice, Brit. J. Radiol. **31**:407-411, 1958.

10. Sullivan, F. M.: Mechanism of action of teratogenic drugs, Proc. Roy. Soc. Med. **63**: 42-43, 1970.

11. Chadwick, D. R., and Abrahams, S. P.: Biological effects of radiation, Arch. Environ. Health **9**:643-8, 1964.

12. Lenz, W.: Thalidomide and congenital abnormalities; Lancet **1**:271-272, 1962.

13. Muller, H. J.: Artificial transmutation of the gene, Science **66**:84, 1927.

14. Schmickel, R.: Chromosome aberrations in leucocytes exposed in vitro to diagnostic levels of x-rays, Amer. J. Hum. Genet. **19**:1-11, 1967.

15. Court-Brown, W. M., and Doll, R.: Leukemia and aplastic anemia in patients irradiated for ankylosing spondylitis, Medical Research Council Special Report Series No. 295, 1957.

16. Hendricks, C. H.: Congenital malformations: analysis of 1953 Ohio records, Obstet. Gynec. **6**:592-598, 1955.

17. Gentry, J. T., Parkhurst, E., and Bulin, G. V.: An epidemiological study of congenital malformations in New York, Amer. J. Public Health **49**:497-513, 1959.

18. Report of the Secretary's Commission on Pesticides and Their Relationship to Environmental Health, Washington, D. C., 1969, U. S. Department of Health, Education and Welfare.

19. Epstein, S. S.: A family likeness, Environment **12**:16-25, 1970.

20. Hussain, S., Ehrenberg, L., Löfroth, G., and others: Mutagenic effects of TCDD on bacterial systems, Ambio **1**:32-33, 1972.

21. Zelac, R. E., Cromroy, H. L., Bolch, W. E., Jr., and others: Inhaled Ozone as a mutagen: Part 1, chromosome aberrations induced in chinese hamsters' lymphocytes, Environ. Res. **4**:262-282, 1971.

22. Ferm, V. H., and Carpenter, S. J.: Malformations induced by sodium arsenate, J. Reprod. Fertil. **17**:199-201, 1968.

23. Schroeder, H. A., and Mitchener, M.: Toxic effects of trace elements on the reproduction of mice and rats, Arch. Environ. Health **23**: 102-106, 1971.

24. Holmberg, R. E., Jr., and Ferm, V. H.: Interrelationships of selenium, cadmium and arsenic in mammalian teratogenesis, Arch. Environ. Health **18**:873-877, 1969.

25. Ferm, V. H., and Carpenter, S. J.: Development malformations resulting from the administration of lead salts, Exp. Molec. Path. **7**:208-213, 1967.

26. Muro, L. A., and Goyer, R. A.: Chromosome damage in experimental lead poisoning, Arch. Path. **87**:660-663, 1969.

27. Petres, J., Schmid-Ulrich, K., and Wolf, U.: Chromosome abnormalities in human lymphocytes due to chronic arsenic exposure, Deutsch. Med. Wschr. **95**:79, 1970.

28. Kauzal, G.: Fluoride as an etiopathogenic factor in the development of duodenal ulcers in the newborn, Rozhl. Chir. **42**:379-382, 1963.

29. Waldbott, G. L.: Acute fluoride intoxication, Acta Med. Scand. **174**(Suppl. 400):1-42, 1963.

30. Rapaport, I.: Mongolism and fluoridated drinking water, Bull. Nat. Acad. Med. (Paris) **140**:529, 1956.

31. Rapaport, I.: Mongolism and fluoridated drinking water, Bull. Nat. Acad. Med. (Paris) **143**:367, 1959.

32. Rapaport, I.: Mongolian oligophrenia and dental caries, Rev. Stomat. (Paris) **64**:207-218, 1963.

33. Rapaport, I.: Apropos of infantile mongolism: a deviation of tryptophan metabolism induced by fluorine, Bull. Nat. Acad. Med. (Paris) **145**:450-453, 1961.

34. Forni, A. M., Cappellini, A., Pacifico, E., and others: Chromosome changes and their evolution in subjects with past exposure to benzene, Arch. Environ. Health **23**:385-391, 1971.

35. MacMahon, B., Alpert, M., and Salber, E. J.: Infant weight and parental smoking habits, Amer. J. Epidem. **82**:247-261, 1965.

36. Haddon, W., Jr., Nesbitt, R. E. L., and Garcia, R.: Smoking and pregnancy: carbon monoxide in blood during gestation and at term, Obstet. Gynec. **18**:262-267, 1961.

37. Division of Biology and Medicine, Prenatal x-ray and Children Neoplasia, U. S. Atomic Energy Commission Report, T. I. E., **12**:373, April 1, 1961.

38. Sigler, A. T.: Radiological health: father's radar exposure related to mongolism? Public Health Rep. **81**:225, 1966.

39. Medical Research Council, The Hazards to Man of Nuclear and Allied Radiation, A Second Report to the Medical Research Council, London, 1960, Her Majesty's Stationery Office.

40. Plummer, G.: Anomalies occurring in children exposed in utero to the atomic bomb in Hiroshima, Pediatrics **10**:687-692, 1952.

41. Yamazaki, J. N., Wright, S. W., and Wright, P. M.: Outcome of pregnancy in women exposed to the atomic bomb in Nagasaki, Amer. J. Dis. Child. **87**:448-463, 1954.

18
ECONOMIC POISONS

The term "economic poison" implies that a toxic agent, either desirable or actually needed in our daily life, is at the same time a hazard to health. In general, insecticides, fungicides, herbicides (weed and brush killers, defoliants), rodenticides, arachnicides (spider killers), and nematocides (worm killers) comprise this group. There are currently about 90,000 registered pesticide formulations that are based on 900 chemicals (Table 18-1).[1] Also included here are sprays for nonagricultural purposes, such as aerosols containing paints and cleaning compounds, cosmetics, drugs to be inhaled or applied to the skin, and sprays for many other purposes. Damage to health by these agents is determined mainly by the degree of their toxicity, the dose and duration of exposure, their concentration, and especially by a person's individual sensitivity and tolerance.

NONAGRICULTURAL USES

Individual spraying. It has been a common practice for a housewife to protect her child from flies and to avoid bacterial contamination by spraying in kitchen or bedroom with an insecticide. In her attempt to avoid one hazard to health she invites another—air pollution.

On the other hand, sprays that she uses on her hair or her windows with relatively low volume and low pressure pose little danger to persons around her although she herself might be subject to allergic reactions or even to low-grade systemic poisoning. Contact dermatitis and asthmatic attacks are often precipitated by sprays. For instance, in a person who contracted a severe dermatitis on the face, an arsenic-containing garden spray was identified as the culprit. The skin eruption appeared on only those parts of the face, forehead, and neck, unprotected by a scarf that she had been wearing around her hair at the time of the spraying. Similarly a painter's dermatitis was clearly demarcated by a sharp line on his forehead. His cap, which he always wore while using the sprays, had protected the skin under it (Fig. 18-1).

Large-scale spraying. Greater damage than in such individual incidents is brought about by large-scale spraying of buildings, greenhouses, and factories, particularly when many individuals are exposed over extended areas.

According to Hall[2] approximately 20% of all sprays and dusts are used in private homes and gardens and by public officials in buildings, parks, and streets. Commercial

Table 18-1. Tabulation of estimated 1970 production of pesticide chemicals in the United States

AMONG 34,500 REGISTERED PRODUCTS	
DDT products	59 million pounds
Mercury fungicides	105 million pounds
Aldrane toxaphane	89 million pounds
Parathion	50 million pounds
2,4,5-T	12 million pounds

establishments and industry employ less than 5% of the fumigants. In enclosed structures there is considerably less danger of widespread air contamination than in outdoor spraying of plantings on streets by city authorities, because the chemical is likely to drift far afield from the target area.

Medicinal spraying. Sprays are being used for medicinal purposes also, by means of atomizers for relief of skin diseases or for respiratory trouble, especially asthma, through inhalation. The most common propellants for this kind of treatment are the Freons, dichlorodifluoromethane (ordinary Freon) and dichlorotetrafluoroethane. One hundred and ten cases of sudden death have been reported in drug addicts as a result of sniffing vapors of airplane glue, solvents, and similar agents.[3] Victims of asthma have been found dead clutching an empty nebulizer in their hands. Until

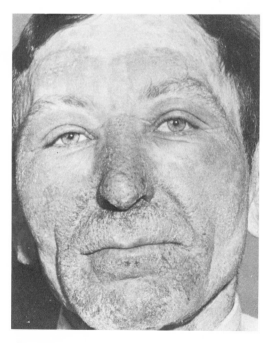

Fig. 18-1. Linseed oil dermatitis involving the face of a painter. The top of his forehead remained unaffected because it was protected by a cap worn while spray-painting.

recently it was believed that an overdose of the drug in the aerosol, not the propellant, was the culprit: the tight bond between the fluorine and the carbon atom of Freon was believed to render the propellant inert and perfectly harmless. Only recently has the propellant been identified as the most likely cause of death in such cases.[4] Because Freon is heavier than air it gravitates down through the small bronchi into the alveoli, where it displaces the air that is vitally needed, particularly in an asthmatic person. Furthermore, as shown in experiments on mice by Taylor and Harris[4] its toxic action may cause irregularities of the heart rate that can be fatal.

AGRICULTURAL USES

Eradication of such diseases as malaria or typhus would not have been possible had it not been for the use of insecticides.

Some of these agents, therefore, are indispensable regardless of their harmful side effects.

Mode of application

To eliminate a pest in agriculture, spraying, dusting, baiting, drenching, dipping, and painting are being employed. Pesticides are being added even to such consumer products as paints, household cleaning fluids, floor waxes, deodorizers, and shelf and drawer paper utilized in kitchen food storage areas. They vaporize through furnaces and ventilating equipment.

Some sprays are injected under the surface of the soil with or without a cover to reduce exchange with the atmosphere. Nonvolatile toxic fumigants reach the atmosphere by combining with dust that is blown into the air on windy days. In Long Island, for instance, schools had to be closed because the dust from potato fields carried arsenic and other insecticides[5] with it.

By far the most dangerous modes of pollution by a pesticide are spraying and dusting, especially spraying from a moving airplane. The dissemination of the poisonous agent is much more widespread when done in this manner than in crop spraying and in dusting from the ground. Ordinarily between 5% to 70% of sprays and 40% to 80% of dust applied from the air drift far afield from the target.[6] Dusts tend to drift farther than sprays.[7] A pesticide dust composed of particles 10 μ in diameter released at a height of 10 feet in a 3-mph wind drifted about 1 mile, whereas a 50 μ droplet of the same pesticide did not drift more than 200 feet. Only in forests is an airborne spray more likely to hit the intended target than in open areas. Tall growing crops with dense foliage like forests interfere with air movements. Weather conditions and topography of the land are the overriding factors influencing the drifting of a fumigant. A stable condition with little turbulence and little vertical motion, which is undesirable in a city atmosphere, is ideal for spraying a nonurban agricultural plot.

Kinds of pesticides

In the past, arsenic, lead, and cryolite (an aluminum fluoride [Na_3AlF_6] compound) have been prominent among insecticidal sprays. One of the most dangerous pesticides used in the 1930s was 1080, or sodium fluoroacetate, an organic fluoride compound. It was responsible for the death of thousands of wild life animals in their natural habitat. In recent years these agents have been partially replaced or supplemented* by two groups of chemicals—

---

*During 12 months in 1968 to 1969 about half a ton of lead arsenate was used by one city in Scotland to control worms and wasps on golf greens.[8]

Table 18-2. Symptoms of poisoning

	CHRONIC	ACUTE	FATAL DOSE MG/KG
DDT group			
DDT	Liver damage; brain disturbances	Tremor, convulsions	500
TDE (DDD)	Agranulocytosis, dermatitis, convulsions, coma, kidney damage	Lethargy, skin irritation	5000
Methoxychlor	Kidney damage	Skin irritation	7500
Aldrin toxaphane group			
Aldrin	Liver damage	Kidney damage, tremor, convulsions	3000
Chlordane	Liver damage	Convulsions, depression	
Dieldrin	Like DDT	Like DDT	
Heptachlor	Liver damage	Tremor, convulsions, kidney damage	1000 to 3000
Benzene hexachloride group			
Benzene hexachloride	Depression	Excitation, convulsions, depression	
Lindane	Liver damage	Dizziness, headache, vomiting, diarrhea, convulsions	150
Other chlorinated hydrocarbons			
p-Dichlorobenzene	Weakness, cataracts, anemia	Headache, nausea	

chlorinated hydrocarbons and the organo-phosphates (Table 18-2).

Chlorinated hydrocarbons

The chlorinated hydrocarbons include DDT, benzene hexachloride, lindane, diel-drin, endrin, aldrin, chlordane, isodrin, toxophene, and similar compounds designed to kill insects.

When insecticidal properties of DDT were discovered during World War II, the results of its initial use were so spectacular, particularly with reference to control of serious outbreaks of infectious diseases, that the Swiss chemist Carl Mueller, its discoverer, was awarded the Nobel Prize in 1948. It was not long before it became apparent that some pests had acquired resistance to DDT. Currently a total of 224 insects are resistant to one or more insecticides. Among these, 97 are of importance to public health or to the veterinarian; 127 attack field and forest crops or stored products.[9]

Some of these agents, especially DDT, have infiltrated practically everywhere—into the air we breathe, the water we drink, and the food we eat. They vaporize from storage containers, they reach the atmosphere from smokestacks, they are dumped into rivers and lakes, they evaporate from grocers' shelves.

Properties of DDT. DDT, dichlordi-phenyltrichlorethane and its breakdown products, TDE and DDE, are the most ubiquitous and most thoroughly studied chlorinated hydrocarbons, as well as some of the least expensive ones. The annual production of DDT in the United States reached 60 to 70 thousand tons (6×10^{10} grams) in 1969.[10] Its behavior is more or less typical of the whole group except that some of the other chlorinated hydrocarbons are more soluble in water and, therefore, of greater immediate toxicity in contrast to the characteristic long-term effect of DDT. Three properties render DDT one of the most dangerous pollutants[11]

1. It is extraordinarily stable; the half life of the residues ranges up to 20 years.[12]
2. Its high solubility in fat and low solubility in water enables it to penetrate into animal food products.
3. The high vapor pressure of DDT causes it to evaporate from soils and plants and to circulate widely in the atmosphere.

Distribution of DDT

In air. DDT has been discovered in migrating birds, fish, and seals in Antarctica, thousands of miles from the nearest point of use.[13] Insect populations high in unsprayed areas of California's Sierra Nevada Mountains were found infested with DDT. Its distribution, therefore, does not depend on water draining from agricultural land into the sea or on dumping of residues into sewers by manufacturers; most of the chemical moves via the air. When sprayed on a field, it evaporates and adheres to dust particles that carry it long distances until it is precipitated by rain or snow. It is estimated that more than 40 tons of DDT and related chemicals are thus deposited in England each year by rain.[9] Concentrations from 73 to 210 ppt have been reported in rainwater near regions where DDT has been used.[14]

In water. Water becomes saturated with as little as 1.2 ppb (parts per billion) DDT. The portion that does not dissolve quickly enters organisms living in water, particularly tiny invertebrate animals. Fish, which are extraordinarily sensitive to many pesticides, feed on these animals and further concentrate DDT in their bodies. Birds feed on fish and each link in the food chain presents an increasing build-up of DDT. After 7 days in water containing 10 ppb DDT, eastern oysters showed up to 151 ppm DDT.[15] In fatty tissue of gulls, concentrations as high as 3177 ppm were found.[9] Eventually DDT reaches humans when they consume fish, birds, other animals, and plants.

In the oceans. DDT residues circulate normally in the ocean at a depth up to 100 meters, from which they slowly descend to the lowest depths.[12]

In soil. Agricultural soils in the United States contain on an average 0.168 gm DDT/meter^2 (about 1.5 pounds per acre).[12] It remains in soil for a long time. Eight years after the introduction of 25 kg of DDT per hectare of soil, the Russian scientist Lazarev[16] still detected 44% in the soil. The mean lifetime of DDT in soil is about 5.3 years.[12] What little DDT is broken down to DDD and DDE is as persistent and indestructable as DDT itself. Carrots, potatoes, and leafy plants pick up DDT from the soil; but most other crops planted on DDT-containing ground do not accumulate the poison. Heavy rains remove only little DDT from soil with surface water. The major mechanism of removal of DDT and its residues from soil is evaporation.

In food. The widespread custom of spraying cows to control gadflies accounts for the presence of DDT in milk and butter. The usual range of DDT in these products is about 0.05 to 0.16 ppm. Tostanokskaya and co-workers[17] found 1.5 to 8 ppm DDT in fruit and berries, mainly in their rind or on their surface 3 weeks after they were sprayed with an oil emulsion of DDT. Fruit, vegetables, milk, and butter in the United States contain about 0.5 ppm DDT. Codliver oil from fish caught off the coasts of the Americas, Europe, and Asia contains DDT in concentrations that range from 1 to 300 ppm.[18]

On March 28, 1969, the United States government seized 35,000 pounds of Coho salmon, a pleasant tasting fish that had recently been introduced into the Great Lakes to the great delight of sportsmen. In its fatty tissue where DDT is resistent to breakdown by microbes, sunlight and water, up to 19 ppm of it was detected.

Biologic action of DDT. The effectiveness of DDT as an insecticide, as well as its long-term hazards, is the result of its strong affinity for fat. The fat of the skin of insects accounts for the easy penetration of DDT into their bodies. Although DDT can penetrate human skin, little absorption takes place in humans and animals in this way. Most DDT is taken up by the mammalian body through inhalation and ingestion of contaminated food.

In insects and other animals, DDT affects the central nervous system, causing convulsions and paralysis. In vertebrate animals it induces fatty degeneration of the heart muscle and of the liver. In fish, it blocks oxygen uptake at the gills and causes death by suffocation.

In experimental animals, especially in cats, DDT affects the liver, the cerebellum (the small brain), the spinal cord, and the adrenal glands. Sazonova[19] described the death of kittens suckled by cats that had ingested as little as 0.2 mg/kg DDT daily, a nontoxic dose.

Health effects of DDT in humans. Most people carry DDT in their fatty tissues in concentrations of 5 to 20 ppm.[9] Daily ingestion of DDT by the average American is estimated at 0.1 to 0.2 mg.[9]

Acute effect. In short-term experiments, Kalin and Hastings[20] exposed eight allergic individuals to inhalation of DDT dissolved in oil at concentrations of 10 (0.01 mg DDT per milliliter oil), 100, 1000, and 10,000 ppm. It was held 1 to 2 inches below the nostrils under carefully controlled double blind conditions. Within 2 to 10 minutes, blurred vision, headaches, perceptual abnormalities, and muscular weakness occurred. The degree of these symptoms was related to the dose of DDT. The muscular weakness was further confirmed objectively by electromyographic evidence, that is, measuring of the electric potential of muscles.

Long-term effect. Much of our knowledge concerning long-term effects of DDT has been obtained in workers employed in plants producing it. Here, damage to health can be pinpointed more readily than in other population groups. The early symptoms, described by Vashkov and associates[21] in 1955, are headaches, dizziness, loss of appetite, muscular debility, impairment of gait; in other words, an ill-defined disease similar to what occurs in many other kinds of chronic systemic poisoning.

In 1966 Krasnyuk[22] found a high incidence of liver and cardiovascular disease, as well as neurologic manifestations, in 261 workers at a DDT plant. She also noted a substantially decreased acidity of the stomach in these subjects. The National Cancer Institute includes DDT among 11 pesticidies with long-term cancer-producing effects as determined by animal experiments.

In a study on 24 prisoners who volunteered to take from 3.5 to 35.0 mg DDT per day by mouth for 21.5 months, Hayes and co-workers[23] noted a "high degree of safety." Some had accumulated 105 to 6119 ppm DDT in their fat tissue. Two individuals had to discontinue the test, one because of a myocardial infarct (clot in the heart muscle), the other because of hepatitis. Although studies of this kind suggest that DDT is innocuous to the general population, the limited number of 45 individuals observed for only a few years of their life-time among millions of people exposed to DDT does not necessarily prove DDT safe, particularly for individuals with a disturbed liver function.

DDT is now banned in many states in the United States and in some foreign countries, and in others its production is being restricted. Nevertheless, in 1970 about half as much DDT was manufactured as in 1963, the peak year. Whether further restriction will materially affect the incidence of insect-borne diseases such as malaria, typhus, and yellow fever and whether an adequate substitute can be developed that will be less harmful than DDT to environmental health is of considerable concern to governmental agencies and to the population at large.[24]

Among other chlorinated hydrocarbons the hazard of hexachlorophene, which is widely used in shampoos and aftershave lotions, has only recently come to the fore.[25]* It is absorbed through the skin in unpredictable amounts.

Five hundred ppm hexachlorophene in the diet of rats causes waterlogging of the white matter of the brain and paralysis after 2 weeks.[26] In humans, muscle twitching is often observed after treatment of burns with hexachlorophene.[27]

A baby washed five times daily with a 3% solution of hexachlorophene showed an average of 0.646 ppm hexachlorophene in his blood.[21] This is more than half the level that caused brain lesions in rats. The normal range in humans is 0.005 to 0.089 ppm.[28]

In March, 1972, more than 30 French babies died and a larger number of babies experienced a disease that began with a skin rash, loss of appetite, sleepiness, and increasing irritability followed by generalized muscular contractions. Talcum powder contaminated with 6% hexachlorophene was established as the cause. High levels of hexachlorophene were found in the blood and tissues; the abnormalities were indistinguishable from those produced by hexachlorophene in experimental animals.[†]

Case reports of poisoning by chlorinated hydrocarbons. In contrast to accidental poisoning with large doses through spillage, damage to health from long-term accumulation of DDT is either rarely recorded or the available reports are inadequately documented because the diagnosis is usually made in restrospect. Therefore, the following discussion includes data on cases in which the cause and effect relationship could not be completely "documented" by

---

*The effectiveness of hexachlorophene as a vaginal deodorant has been questioned because it does not attack the kind of bacteria that are chiefly responsible for the odor.[25]

†Hexachlorophene use limited to prescription products, editorial, Ann. Intern. Med. **77**:1-70, 1972.

the conventional criteria but for which sufficient circumstantial and clinical evidence is available to warrant suspicion that the disease is caused by the pollutant agents.

In 1965, a 21-month-old Negro girl who had always been in perfect health was brought to Harper Hospital, Detroit, with what appeared to be bruises on the skin, fever, and severe vomiting. During several months the parents had used DDT sprays, repeatedly, to kill flies. The last spraying had occurred on the day prior to the onset of the child's illness. A physician had treated the condition as "a cold." Laboratory findings revealed that the child's hemoglobin was approximately one tenth of the normal value, the red blood cells were slightly above 1 million (normal, 4 to 5 million). There was blood in the urine and the number of blood platelets had dropped to 59,000 (a normal person's blood contains 250 to 300 thousand). In spite of temporary improvement following a blood transfusion, death occurred 24 hours after admission to the hospital.

In Perth, Australia,[30] the same illness, hemorrhagic purpura, a bone marrow disease, followed a more protracted course. A 39-year-old housewife had been washing her dog with a 2% solution of benzene hexachloride, combined with lindane, once a week for 2 years.[29] She became fatigued, developed spontaneous bruises, anemia, and evidence of an aplastic (nonfunctioning) bone marrow. The disease persisted from May until August, when, in spite of multiple blood transfusions, her white blood count fell to about 800 (normal 6000 to 9000). She died in coma with high fever.

A case presumed to be caused by aldrin, another chlorinated hydrocarbon, was encountered by Dr. W. A. Gilpin of Detroit. A 15-year-old girl was seen on August 12, 1963, at his office in a highly emaciated state with a temperature of 99° F, considerable abdominal pain, nausea, and occasional rectal bleeding. Her illness began

in May 1959, a few days after large areas near her home in Bedford Township, southern Monroe County, had been dusted from the air with pellets of aldrin, one of the most toxic of all the chlorinated hydrocarbons. The condition became markedly aggravated in October 1961, immediately following a second spraying with aldrin. At that time birds, wildlife, and farm animals were found dead in the affected area. The soil contained 25 times the normal amount of aldrin.

By June 1963, 1 month after a third spraying she had lost considerable weight and was experiencing intermittent fever, pain, and nose bleeds. She was hospitalized in Toledo, where a battery of tests and examinations revealed a slightly enlarged liver. The bone marrow showed a noncancerous condition. At that time the urine still contained 0.25 ppm aldrin, more than twice the "normal" content. Four months later, however, cancer of the liver was diagnosed to which the child eventually succumbed. The relationship of this disease to the pesticide is not firmly established because of the absence of quantitative data concerning aldrin in blood, urine, and body tissues. Yet the marked aggravation of the disease immediately after the second spraying furnishes strong circumstantial evidence of the toxic action of aldrin. For this reason cases of this kind cannot be disregarded.

Another odd and unusual disease caused by a chlorinated hydrocarbon, so-called acquired toxic porphyria cutanea, was reported in the *Journal of the American Medical Association* in 1963. This skin disease is associated with excess formation of porphyrin (a pigment involved in the production of hemoglobin).[31] In 1954 the fungicide benzene hexachloride was introduced in Turkey for dressing grain in order to prevent growth of molds. During the years 1955 to 1959 some 3000 persons, 80% of whom were children, developed small blisters of the skin involving the whole body, loss of hair, scarring of the skin, and so-called hypertrichosis (excess hair growth) over the whole body. Because of a black discoloration of the skin and emaciation of the hands, the disease became known among peasants as "monkey disease." Enlargement of the liver and thyroid was common. The characteristic feature of this disease is the excretion of porphyrin in the urine, which gives it the color of port wine and renders it red-fluorescent with ultraviolet light.[32]

Organophosphates

The second group of pesticides, the organophosphates, includes such insecticides and such herbicides as parathion, malathion, azodrin, diazinon, TEPP, and phosdrin. These poisons are related to the nerve gas diisopropylfluorophosphate, which was developed in Nazi Germany during World War II. They attack a vulnerable part of the nervous system: Acetylcholine (an acetyl derivative of choline having blood pressure–lowering properties) is responsible for transmitting impulses from one nerve fiber to another and from nerves to muscles. The enzyme acetylcholinesterase (ACHE) breaks down this messenger chemical after it has completed its task. The organic phosphate pesticides and nerve gases disrupt this delicate mechanism by preventing the ACHE enzyme from breaking down acetylcholine. As a result, acetylcholine builds up in the body and the nerve impulses remain unchecked. Experimental animals succumb with muscular twitching and convulsions caused by excess stimulation of the nervous system.

Unlike the chlorinated hydrocarbons, the organophosphates produce no chronic effects in the ecosystems. Interestingly, some organophosphates, such as malathion, which are extremely poisonous to insects, have relatively little effect on mammals because of the carboxyesterase (an enzyme that destroys malathion) in the mammalian system.

The most important organophosphate pesticide in terms of its toxic action is parathion (0.0-diethyl-0-p-nitrophenyl thiophosphate). During the past few years it has caused serious illness as the result of spillage of the chemical during transport or storage. Three such epidemics occurred in 1967:

Near Blythe, California, almost pure parathion spilled from a truck on the surface of an interstate road.[33] The truck driver and six other people became ill but fortunately no lives were lost.

An accident in Tijuana, Mexico,[34] was more serious: sugar, contaminated by parathion during transport, was responsible for the illness of 300 persons and for the death of 17.

On November 25, 1967, in Colombia, some 600 persons were poisoned, 61% of whom were children younger than 15 years of age. On a truck en route from Bogota to Chiquinquira, one of the thirty bottles containing parathion had broken and had contaminated sacks of flour adjacent to the cargo. About 25% of the victims who had eaten bread baked with this flour experienced the mildest form of poisoning, namely abdominal pain, headache, blurred vision, tremor, dizziness, and general weakness. Some 10% to 25% sweated profusely, became irritable, and showed constricted pupils. A few manifested acute pulmonary edema with severe diarrhea, cyanosis (blue discoloration of the skin), and excessive excretion of saliva.

In another accident, two boys in Vancouver, B. C., were poisoned after using flannelette bed sheets that during their transport from Antwerp, Belgium, in the hold of the ship, had become contaminated by parathion. The blood pressure of one of the boys, 12 years of age, soared to 200/100. He became deeply comatose and developed respiratory failure. The pupils of his eyes were contracted, a characteristic feature of acetylcholinesterase poisoning.[35]

An almost fatal case[36] occurred in the

state of Washington, where parathion that had been spilled in a driveway had survived the winter's snow and rain and was ingested with mud by a 2-year-old boy playing on the ground. Although the soil contained 1% (8634 ppm) parathion, 11 ppm parathion was recovered in the child's feces. Paranitrophenol, a product of the hydrolysis of parathion, was excreted in the urine quite rapidly, clearing in about 30 hours after the ingestion.

Fortunately, in this kind of poisoning two drugs are available that provide prompt relief—injections of 0.6 mg atropine, a drug that counteracts the effect of organic phosphates upon nerve impulses, and PAM (pyridine-2-aldoxime methiodide) given intravenously in doses of 250 mg in normal saline solution.

Less dramatic than the acute phase of the disease is the chronic illness that affects agricultural workers engaged in picking, thinning, cultivating, and irrigating.[37] Parathion poisoning is often misdiagnosed as "food poisoning" or waterborne "gastroenteritis" when it occurs in large groups, as "heat stroke" when only a few persons are involved.

Involuntary twitching of the eyelids is an early diagnostic feature of the disease. In this case the skin rather than respiratory organs is believed to be the route by which parathion is absorbed. Contact of the skin with the sprayed vegetation, even as long as 12 to 33 days following spraying, induces poisoning. Moisture of the skin caused by perspiration in California's warm weather enhances absorption of parathion, whose concentration on leaves was found to be 8 ppm. Quinby and Lemmon[37] reported 11 such episodes of poisoning from contact with parathion residues involving more than 70 persons. Nevertheless, it appears that such accidents are rare both among workers and among those who are exposed to the pesticide under nonoccupational conditions. In 44 tobacco workers exposed to 0.05 to 4.65 ppm parathion, Guthrie and

associates[38] found no fall in the cholinesterase level of blood during the harvesting season except in one individual. These workers strictly adhered to the directives designed to prevent poisoning. Such data, although reassuring with regard to widespread damage to health, do not take into consideration that certain individuals in large population groups are likely to be intolerant to very low-grade exposure.

Little is known about the possible hazard of a popular pesticide called DDVP (0, 0-dimethyl-2,2-dichlorovinyl phosphate),[39] which is being marketed throughout the United States in some 300,000 retail outlets. This chemical impregnates a 10-inch plastic strip enclosed in a paper cage. Upon exposure of the strip to the air, the pesticide evaporates slowly over a period of about 3 months.

DDVP was sponsored by the U. S. Public Health Service in 1955 in their search for chemicals that would kill insects, particularly mosquitos aboard airplanes on international flights, to prevent and combat malaria and yellow fever.

Exposure to DDVP, which may reach a maximum concentration of 0.21 mg/meter^3 in the air, lowers the cholinesterase in the blood and affects the liver in a manner similar to that of the other organic phosphates. In plants and chick embryos, DDVP damages the chromosomes, an indication that it may eventually lead to birth defects and perhaps to cancer. However, not enough data are available at this time to arrive at final conclusions. Impregnation with DDVP of a plastic collar for the control of fleas in dogs has led repeatedly to contact dermatitis in humans handling the collar.[40]

Chlorinated biphenyls

Yusho disease. In 1968[41] about 1000 persons in southern Japan developed darkened skin, brownish pigmented nails, lips, and gums, a cheeselike discharge from the eyes, and severe acne. The patients experienced numbness and neuralgic pains and swelling in joints, especially in the heels, edema of the eyelids, transient visual and hearing disturbances, jaundice, and marked general weakness. On the soles and palms, scaling of the skin was associated with the brown discoloration.[42] Among 11 live and 2 stillborn babies, 10 exhibited the characteristic dark-brown skin at birth, 5 had dark-colored nails and gums, and 9 had discharge from the eyes. In many instances, the disease persisted for more than 3 years. Before people felt sick, 700,000 chickens had died of the same disease with edema in various parts of the body.[42a,43]

The illness was named "Yusho," or rice oil disease, because the patients had eaten food cooked with contaminated rice oil. The contaminant, Kanechlor 400, the main component of which is tetrachlorobiphenyl, had leaked from the pipe of a heat exchanger during manufacture of the oil. Some of the patients had consumed an average of 2 gm of polychlorinated biphenyl (PCB). The minimum dose at which symptoms appeared was about 0.5 gm. Material discharged from the eyes and the fat tissue of the skin contained 13.1 to 75.5 ppm Kanechlor. The placenta and the fatty tissue of the two stillborn babies also contained Kanechlor.

Properties and uses of polychlorinated biphenyl. Among the multitudes of chemical agents employed by industry, the PCBs play an extraordinary role as air pollutants that is comparable to that of DDT (Fig. 18-2).[44]

Whereas PCBs were first introduced in the United States in 1930, the first damage to human health was not detected until nearly four decades later. With increasing production over the years, by 1970 about 34,000 tons were being sold annually in the United States. Additional PCBs were being manufactured in Europe, Japan and U.S.S.R. In 1966, by an ingenious method, Jensen, a Swedish scientist, identified the chemical for the first time in a dead eagle found near Stockholm.[45]

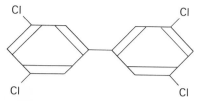

Fig. 18-2. Formula of chlorinated biphenyls.

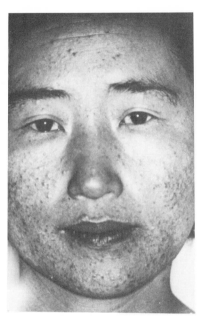

Fig. 18-3. A female patient with Yusho disease showing typical chloracne and brownish stain throughout the face. (Courtesy Dr. G. Umeda, Kitakyusyu Research Institute for Environmental Pollution in Japan.)

Polychlorinated biphenyls are noninflammable and have a high plasticizing ability. Because of their high dielectric constant they are used in transformers* (Fig. 18-3) and capacitors.† Furthermore they serve as hydraulic and heat transfer fluids, as plasti-

---

*A transformer consists of two coils insulated from each other. The two coils in an industrial transformer are submerged in insulating liquid such as PCB.

†An electrical device that consists of metal plates in an electrical insulating material, which may be paper or porcelain. In an industrial condenser or capacitor the insulating material can be a gas or a liquid such as oil or PCB.

Table 18-3. Incidents of PCB contamination of food

NUMBER	DATE	PLACE	FOOD INVOLVED	SOURCE	LEVEL OF PCB	COMMENT
1	July 1969	West Virginia	Milk	Spent transformer fluid used as vehicle for herbicides		Contaminated dairy cattle grazing areas were taken off production by state officials
2	April 1970	Ohio	Milk	Sealants in silos migrated to silage		Undetermined amount of milk destroyed
3	Aug. 1970	Florida-Georgia	Milk	Sealant in silos		11% PCB in silo coating
4	Dec. 1970	Three counties in New York	Chicken	Ground bakery goods, containing plastic wrappers, used as feed	Up to 26.8 ppm	140,450 chickens killed
5	July 1971	Throughout U.S.A.	Shredded Wheat	Packaging material contained 95% recycled paper in paperboard containers	Up to 5 ppm in food	PCB in paperboard ranged from 2 to 433 ppm
6	July 1971	East Coast Terminal, Wilmington, N. C.	Fish meal	Leakage from a heating system during pasteurization	14-30 ppm; one sample 350 ppm	One producer had to destroy 88,000 broilers
7	July 28, 1971	Illinois	Pasteurized meat meal	Heat treatment equipment		Contaminated product recalled
8	Aug. 1971	Minnesota, North and South Dakota	Turkeys	Not known	Up to 20 ppm (fat basis)	1 million turkeys withheld from market temporarily
9	Aug. 20, 1971	Oklahoma	Chickens	Not known		

cizers and solvents in adhesives, and as sealants.

Although chemically inert, they dissolve inorganic solvents; they adhere to smooth metal surfaces and to glass and thus prevent corrosion. They are used to coat electric wires. Mixed with asphalt, they form a protective coating for lumber, metal, and concrete. They render paints, varnishes, natural and synthetic rubber, and floor tile resistant to oxidation and to corrosive chemicals. They are added to printing ink and brake linings. In certain carbonless repro-

ducing paper, of the kind used in bank, library, and factory forms, PCBs were found at magnitudes of the order of 12 gm/kg paper.[43]

About 4000 tons enter the waterways principally through sewage, through leaching of lubricants, hydraulic, and heat-transfer fluids, and from dumps and landfills.[42] Between 1000 and 2000 tons per year escape into the atmosphere from plasticized materials. Concentrations of PCBs greater than the combined concentrations of organochloride pesticides DDT and DDE were found in nonmigratory bears within the Arctic circle.[42]

PCBs in food chain. In the food chain, PCB residues are found in fish, both the surface feeding varieties and those dwelling at great depths. In the Great Lakes region concentrations of PCB in Coho salmon have exceeded 5 ppm. In most species of North Atlantic fish, a range from 0.01 to 1.0 ppm is more typical. In heavily industrialized areas, PCB residues were found at magnitudes up to 100 times larger than DDT.[45]

Different kinds of fish vary in their susceptibility to PCBs. Bluegill and catfish succumb to concentrations of 20 to 50 ppb for several weeks; for trout, about 8 ppb and for shrimp, as little as 1 ppb[46] suffice. In cormorants and osprays (birds that feed on fish) concentrations between 300 and 1000 ppm are found.[47] Poultry feed has been contaminated by leaking heat exchangers.

To date no PCB poisoning in humans has been reported in the United States. However from July 1969 to August 1971 federal agencies have been taking action on "incidents," each of which could have had serious repercussions with regard to human health (Table 18-3).

Biologic action. In Sweden* the average intake of PCBs from all sources, mainly fish, has been estimated to be about 1 μg/kg of body weight per day.[45] Babies receive the highest doses per kilogram of body weight, largely from milk. In the United States, small residues in cereals have been traced to recycled packaging paper and to carbon paper.[48]

Polychlorinated biphenyls have a low solubility in water. Like DDT they degrade very slowly under natural conditions. The highly chlorinated PCBs seem to persist in the environment longer and are less toxic

than the more rapidly degradable low chlorine forms.

Storage of PCBs takes place in the body's fatty tissue. Of more than 600 samples of human fat tissue, 33% contained PCB residues of at least 1 ppm.[42] Some of their toxic effects have been attributed to trace amounts of dibenzofurans and other extremely toxic impurities.

PCBs inhibit growth of cultured cells, affect liver tissue, and interfere with the activity of a variety of enzymes.[49] In conjunction with DDT and organophosphate pesticides, they enhance the action of these toxic agents.

Damage to human health. Three categories form the potentials of damage by PCBs in humans:

1. Environmental contamination, mainly storage of PCBs in fish.
2. Industrial accidents, such as leakage or spillage of PCB-containing fluids, which contaminate food ingredients and animal feed.
3. Food packaging material containing PCB, which migrates into food.

There are four clinical phases of Yusho disease[50]:

1. *The latent type* occurs without significant physical signs or subjective symptoms in women who give birth to babies that display the typical manifestations of Yusho disease, especially when they are breastfed. In addition to the skin and eye manifestations, these children show a disturbance of growth.

2. *The visceral type* (affecting internal organs) does not exhibit any skin lesions. Instead, systemic symptoms such as general fatigue, nausea, vomiting, mild jaundice indicative of liver injury, coliclike attacks, diarrhea, and such respiratory manifestations as productive cough, chronic bronchitis, asthmatic attacks, and pneumonia are present. Sputum, blood, or material surgically removed from patients show an increase in triglycerides (fat) and pre(beta)lipoproteins (fat bound to pro-

---

*In January 1972, a Swedish law went into effect that prohibits use, import, manufacture, and sale of PCB.

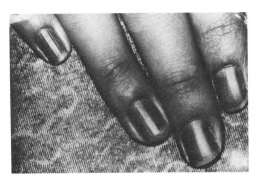

Fig. 18-4. Brownish discoloration of fingertips and nails in Yusho disease. (Courtesy Dr. G. Umeda, Kitakyusyu Research Institute for Environmental Pollution in Japan.)

tein). These cases are rarely diagnosed correctly by physicians.

3. *The manifest type* is characterized by acne eruption in the face (Fig. 18-4), by the dark-brown pigmentation of the skin, nails, and mucous membranes of the eye and mouth, and discharge from the eyes. Loss of hair, loss of sexual power, numbness in extremities, headaches, abdominal pain and vomiting, deformed nails, joints, and bones, and poorly developed teeth have been described.

4. *The delayed type* occurs 3 to 4 years after exposure to PCB. No explanation for these late occurrences has so far been given.

The disease may have aftereffects, such as permanent disturbances of the central nervous system, especially in young children who display the symptoms at birth. Changes in the heart and blood vessels and deformities of fingers, toes, ankles, wrists, and vertebrae, accompanied by pain, may linger on for long periods of time.

In early 1972 the Environmental Protection Agency issued waste disposal restrictions designed to keep PCB levels below 0.01 ppb in rivers and streams. They also prohibited the use of PCBs in materials for food containers and for application in food processing plants.

Phthalic acid esters

Phthalic acid esters are extensively used in industry, in homes, and in medical sciences. Approximately 1 billion pounds[51] were produced in 1972. Most phthalates are plasticizers. When incorporated into polyvinyl chloride (PVC) they impart flexibility and workability. They may account for as much as 40% of the final weight. Their esters are not chemically bonded to the matrix of PVC. They are interspersed between adjacent PVC chains. In spite of low solubility in water and low volatility they can escape out of the plastics into air and water where they become significant environmental pollutants.

Polyvinyl chlorides are used extensively for wall coverings, upholstery, and appliances. They are also valuable in the construction, housing, and transportation industries, particularly for the interior of automobiles. They are used in medical products such as blood bags for transfusions and in tubing in heart-lung and kidney machines. They also constitute ingredients for food packaging, pesticide sprays, and industrial oils. Cosmetics, perfumes, and insect repellents contain phthalates. The phthalic acid ester most commonly used is di-2-ethyl-hexyl phthalate (DEHP).

In the Charles and Merrimack rivers in Massachusetts phthalate concentrations range between 1 and 2 ppb.[52] In the Mississippi River in 1970, DEHP concentrations as high as 0.6 ppm were found.[51] Certain bacteria, fungi, and plants have the ability to synthesize phthalates, but the bulk of air and waterborne phthalate esters is probably derived from pesticides and volatilized PVCs.

Very little is known at this time concerning their degradability. In one experiment in a laboratory (where conditions may not be precisely the same as in the field) an "activated sludge" of microorganisms, such as those found in sewage treatment plants, eliminated within 48 hours more than 90% of the DEHP esters.[51]

Specimens of fish, crustaceans, and drinking water collected throughout North America[51] contain phthalates. They can therefore reach humans through the food chain.

The toxicity of phthalate esters to several fish species is relatively low.[51] In guppies however they increased the incidence of abortions; in zebra fish, survival of small fry was reduced. Because the poisoned zebra fish, following exposure to phthalates, expired in tetanic convulsions—an indication of low blood calcium—these esters are believed to affect the calcium metabolism.

When phthalic acid esters were injected into pregnant mice they increased the number of deaths in the newborn and caused abnormalities such as absence of tails and eyes, as well as leg and skeletal deformities in the offspring. Such effects of all eight phthalic acid esters occur in mice from relatively large doses (0.3 to 10.0 ml/kg of body weight).[51] The esters also reduced the ability of mice fibroblast cells to replicate when cultured in the test tube.

In humans, to date, except in large doses, no effect on life expectancy, food consumption, and body weight has been demonstrated. The so-called "subtle" effects from long-term uptake of phthalates in low concentrations or from special hazards to which individuals exposed to high concentrations might be subject require further investigation. Nutrient fluids in plastic bags, and blood used for transfusions in heart-lung and kidney machines, which circulate through the PVC tubing, contain phthalates. For instance, 50 to 75 ppm DEHP had migrated into blood that had been stored in PVC blood bags for 21 days at 4° C. Blood platelets used for transfusions in certain blood diseases showed levels up to 200 ppm.[53]

Whereas environmental phthalates have not been shown to pose an imminent threat to human health, certain risks are involved among individuals, for example, who receive multiple blood transfusions. Because of their wide distribution in the environment phthalates, even in low concentration, are likely to lead to untoward "subtle" effects upon human health.

Great progress has been made in the exploration of the biologic effects of the so-called economic poisons. However, the slow, inconspicuous development of illness as a result of their persistent uptake by the human organism, the vague symptoms, and the sparsity of clinical data concerned with long-term human exposure, precludes the recognition of their real significance in terms of the human life span and human health.

REFERENCES

1. Finkelstein, H.: Air pollution aspects of pesticides. Litton Systems, Inc., Bethesda, Maryland, September 1969, U. S. Department of Commerce, PB 188 091.
2. Hall, D. G.: Use of insecticides in the United States. Bull. Entom. Soc. Amer. 8:90-92, 1972.
3. Bass, M.: Sudden sniffing death, J.A.M.A. 212:2075-2079, 1970.
4. Taylor, G. J., and Harris, W. S.: Cardiac toxicity of aerosol propellants, J.A.M.A. 214: 81-85, 1970.
5. Carson, R.: AAAS report of air conservation commission, Publication No. 80, 1965, Washington, D. C.
6. Rollins, R. J.: California Department of Agriculture Bulletin 49, 1960, Sacramento, Calif.
7. Akesson, N. B., and Yates, W. E.: Problems relating to application of agriculture chemicals and resulting drift residues, Ann. Rev. Entom. 9:285, 1964.
8. Papworth, D. S., Taylor, J. K., Cutler, J. R., and others: Quantities of pesticides used by U. K. local authorities, Roy. Soc. Health J. 92:35-38, 1972.
9. Dahlston, D. L., Garcia, R., Laing, J. E., and others: Pesticides, New York, 1970, Scientists Instituted for Public Information.
10. U. S. Tariff Commission: Synthetic organic chemicals, U. S. production and sales 1969, Washington, D. C., 1970, U. S. Government Printing Office.
11. Kagan, Y. S., Fuedel-Ossipova, S. I., Khaikina, B. J., and others: On the problem of the harmful effect of DDT and its mechanism of action, Rückstands-Berichte 27:43-79, 1969.
12. Woodwell, G. W., Graig, P. P., and Johnson, H. A.: DDT in the biosphere: where does it go? Science 174:1101-1107, 1971.

13. Sladen, W. J. L., Menzie, C. M., and Reichel, W. L.: DDT residues in adelie penguins and a crabeater seal from Antarctica, Nature **210:** 670-673, 1968.
14. Tarrant, K. R., and Tatton, J. P. G.: Organochlorine pesticides in rainwater in the British Isles, Nature **219:**725-727, 1968.
15. Udall, S.: Testimony before U. S. Senate Subcommittee on Reorganization and Informational Organizations: Part I, Co-ordination of Activities Relating to the Use of Pesticides, Washington, D. C., May, 1963, U. S. Government Printing Office, p. 71-72.
16. Lazarev, N. V.: Problems of geohygiene and their connection with the task of investigating new insectifungicides and herbicides: In Hygiene, toxicology and clinical aspects of new insectofungicides, **22:**331, 1959.
17. Tostanokskaya, A. A., and Serebryanaya, S. G.: Methodical letters on the work of the sanitary inspector concerning control of DDT and hexachlorine application in agriculture. Coll.: Official Material Concerning Sanitation Control of the Application and Examination of Food Products, G.M.I., Ukr. S. S. R., 1960, p. 32.
18. The President's Science Advisory Committee Report: Uses of pesticides, White House, Washington, D. C., May, 1963, U. S. Government Printing Office.
19. Sazonova, N. A.: DDT toxic properties, Transactions of the Twentieth Session Plant Protection, Moscow, 1952, p. 37.
20. Kalin, E. W., and Hastings, A.: Cerebral disturbances from small amounts of DDT: a controlled study, Med. Ann. D. C. **35:**519-524, 1966.
21. Vashkov, V. I., Pogodina, L. I., and Sazonova, N. A.: DDT and its use, Moscow, 1955, Moscow Medik.
22. Krasnyuk, E. P.: State of health of workers engaged in DDT plants: In Hygiene toxicology and clinical aspects of insectofungicides. Moscow, 1959, p. 350.
23. Hayes, W. J., Jr., Dale, W. E., and Perkle, C. I.: Evidence of safety of long-term high oral doses of DDT for man, Arch. Environ. Health **22:**119-135, 1971.
24. Harrison, H. F., Loucks, O. L., Mitchell, J. W., and others: System studies of DDT transport, Science **170:**503-8, 1970.
25. Wade, N.: Hexachlorophene: FDA temporized on brain-damaging chemical, Science **174:**805-807, 1971.
26. Kimbrough, R. D., and Gaines, T. B.: Hexachlorophene effects on the rat brain: study of high doses by light and electron microscopy, Arch. Environ. Health **23:**114-118, 1971.
27. Larson, D. L., Abston, S., and Bachmann, R. C.: Hexachlorophene absorption from the burn wound. In Matter, P., Barclay, T. L., and Koníčková, Z., editors: Research in burns, Stuttgart, 1971, Hans Huber Publishers.
28. Curley, A., Kimborough, R. D., Finberg, L., and others: Dermal absorption of hexachlorophene in infants, Lancet **2:**296-297, 1971.
29. Woodliff, A. J., Connor, P. M., and Scopa, F.: Aplastic anemia associated with insecticides, Med. J. Aust. **1:**628-629, 1966.
30. Gilpin, W. A.: Personal communication, July, 1970.
31. Cam, C., and Nigogsyan, G.: Acquired toxic porphyria cutanea tarda due to hexachlorobenzene, J. A. M. A. **183:**88-91, 1963.
32. Quinby, G. E.: DDT and DDE content of complete prepared meals, Arch. Environ. Health **11:**641-647, 1965.
33. Warne, W.: Testimony before California Senate Fact Finding Committee on Agriculture, Sacramento, California, October 22-23, 1963.
34. Marquez Mayaudon, E., Fujigaki Lechuga, A., Moguel, A., and others: Problemas de contaminacion de alimentos con pesticides, Caso Tijuana, 1967, Salud Publica Mex. **10:**293-300, 1968.
35. Anderson, L. W., Warner, D. L., Parker, J. E., and others: Parathion poisoning from flannelette sheets, Canad. Med. Ass. J. **92:** 809-813, 1965.
36. Quinby, G. E., and Clappison, G. B.: Parathion poisoning: a near-fatal pediatric case treated with 2-PAM, Arch. Environ. Health **3:**538-542, 1961.
37. Quinby, G. E., and Lemmon, A. B.: Parathion residues as a cause of poisoning in crop workers, J.A.M.A. **166:**740-746, 1958.
38. Guthrie, F. E., Tappan, W. B., Jackson, M. D., and others: Cholinesterase levels of cigar-wrapper tobacco workers exposed to parathion, Arch. Environ. Health **25:**32-37, 1972.
39. Committee for Environmental Information: The price of Convenience, Environment **12:** 2-29, 1970.
40. Cronce, P. C., and Alden, H. S.: Flea collar dermatitis, J.A.M.A. **206:**1563, 1968.
41. Kuratsume, M., and others: Yusho, a poisoning caused by rice oil contaminated with polychlorinated biphenyls, HSHMA Health Rep. **86:**1083-91, 1971.
42. Goto, M., and Higuchi, K.: The symptomatology of yusho (chlorobiphenyls poisoning) in dermatology, Fukuoka Acta Med. **60:**409, 1969.
42a. Maugh, T. H.: Polychlorinated Biphenyls:

Still Prevalent, but Less of a Problem. Science, **173**:388, 1972.

43. Jensen, S.: The PCB story, Ambio **1**:123-134, 1972.

44. Hammond, A. L.: Chemical pollution: polychlorinated biphenyls, Science **175**:155-156, 1972.

45. Report of a new chemical hazard, New Scientist **32**:612, 1966.

46. Stallings, D. L., and Mayer, F. L., Jr.: Toxicities of PCB to fish and environmental residues, Environ. Health Persp. April, 1973. (To be published.)

47. Johnels, A. G.: PCB: occurrence in Swedish wildlife, Stockholm, Sweden, 1970, National Swedish Environmental Protection Board, Solna Research Secretariat, Proc. PCB Conference, pp. 29-42.

48. Edwards, R.: The polychlorbiphenyls: their occurrence and significance: a review, Chem. Industr. **47**:1340-48, 1971.

49. Berlin, M.: PCB: effects on mammals, Stockholm, Sweden, 1970, National Swedish Environment Protection Board, Solna Research Secretariat, Proc. PCB Conference, pp. 44-50.

50. Umeda, G.: Clinical aspects of PCB poisoning, Abstract of the Forty-fifth Congress of the Japanese Association of Industrial Health, Tokyo, April, 1972.

51. Marx, J. L.: Phthalic acid esters: biological impact uncertain, Science **173**:46-47, 1972.

52. Hites, R.: Transactions of the Conference sponsored by The National Institute of Environmental Health Sciences, in Environmental Health Perspectives, January 1973. (To be published.)

53. Autian, J.: Toxicity and health threats of phthalate esters: review of the literature, Oak Ridge, Tennessee, 1972, Oak Ridge National Laboratory.

19
HYDROCARBONS

DEFINITION

The term hydrocarbons comprises a wide variety of compounds whose molecules consist of atoms of hydrogen and carbon exclusively. They occur as gases, liquids, or solids. Hydrocarbons with 1 to 4 carbon atoms are gaseous at ordinary temperatures, whereas those with 5 or more carbon atoms are liquids or solids. Gasoline, for instance, consists of a mixture of liquid hydrocarbons. Hydrocarbons with more than 12 carbon atoms are generally not sufficiently abundant to reach atmospheric concentrations in the gas phase. They are however important as particulates.

There are three classes of hydrocarbons.

1. *Acyclic* hydrocarbons in which the carbon atoms are arranged in chains with or without branching chains but without rings (Fig. 19-1).

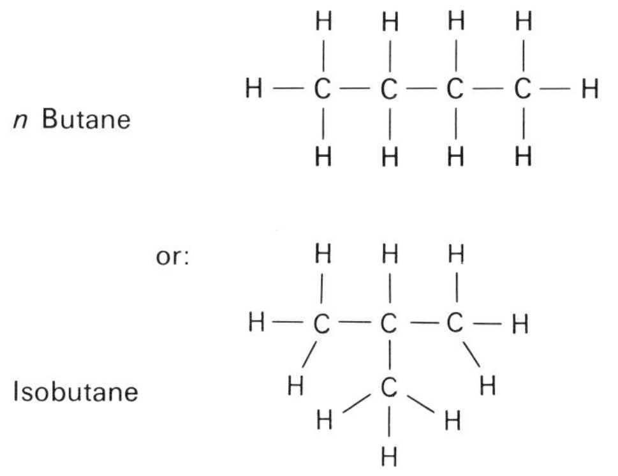

Benzene   Naphthalene

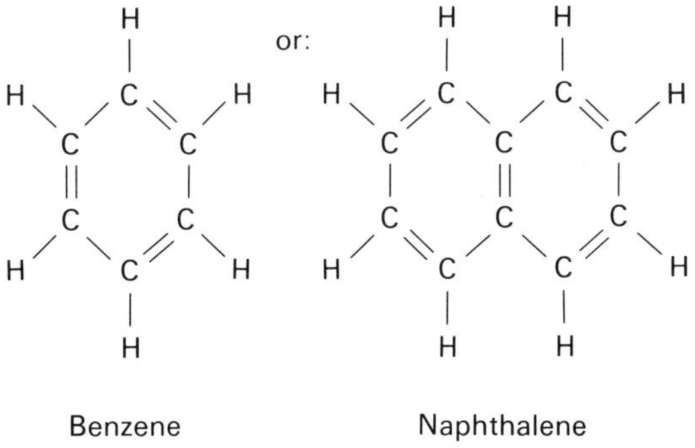

Fig. 19-2. Example of aromatic hydrocarbon.

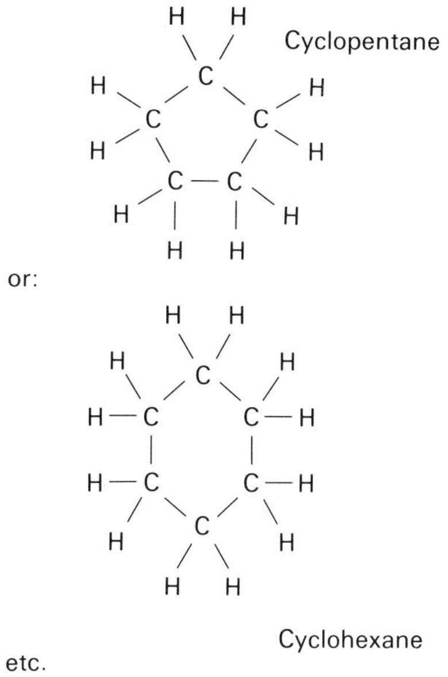

Fig. 19-3. Example of alicyclic hydrocarbon.

Fig. 19-1. Example of acyclic hydrocarbon.

2. *Aromatic* hydrocarbons in which the atoms are arranged in benzene rings, that is, in six-membered carbon rings with only one additional atom of either hydrogen or carbon attached to each atom in the ring (Fig. 19-2).

3. *Alicyclic or cycloaliphatic* hydrocarbons consist of saturated cyclic systems (Fig. 19-3).

The major role of hydrocarbons in air pollution is their participation in the production of secondary contaminants and of harmful reaction intermediates, ozone, nitrogen dioxide, and peroxyacetyl nitrate (PAN) as outlined in Chapter 7. The sunlight necessary for this action does not affect the hydrocarbons themselves.

SOURCES OF HYDROCARBONS

In air naturally. Hydrocarbons, particularly methane (CH_4),[1] are present naturally in the air. They originate from natural gas, coal, and petroleum fields and from natural fires. Methane, which is photochemically nonreactive, is generated in swampy and tropical areas. It is also found above the oceans in a concentration similar to that in ocean water. Other volatile hydrocarbons, such as terpenes and isoprenes, have been associated with vegetation throughout the world. The blue haze of the Appalachian Mountain region has been ascribed to formation of photochemical aerosols caused by these substances.

In nonurban air, methane levels range between 0.7 to 1.0 mg/meter³ (1 to 1.5 ppm). Other hydrocarbons, including various terpenes, are present in nonurban air at levels less than 0.1 ppm.

Man-made sources of hydrocarbons. In 1968, the United States Public Health Service estimated the nationwide emissions of hydrocarbons and of related organic compounds in urban areas at approximately 32 million tons.[2] Transportation accounted for 51.9%; industrial processes for 14.4%.

Approximately 63% of the total hydrocarbon emissions arise from urban areas. There

is a wide range in various regions of the country. In a survey of 22 metropolitan areas, the most formidable amounts were emitted in Los Angeles with 1,270,000 tons per year compared to 480,000 in Detroit and 95,000 in Pittsburgh.[3]

Moving sources. Transportation accounts for the bulk of local emissions, since hydrocarbon emanations are caused by inefficient combustion of volatile fuels. In gasoline engines, they are emitted from the engine exhaust, the crank case, the carburetor, and the fuel tank. Actually, hundreds of different hydrocarbons originate from this source.[4] Diesel engine exhaust contains substantially lower hydrocarbon levels and higher levels of aldehydes including formaldehyde than exhaust from gasoline engines. Formaldehyde is responsible for the distinctive odor of diesel exhaust.[5] Emission of hydrocarbon from the exhaust of gas turbines and aircraft jet engines is low.[6]

Table 19-1. Estimates of sources of hydrocarbon emissions (1968)

SOURCE	MILLION TONS		
Transportation	16.6		
Motor vehicles		15.6	
Gasoline			15.2
Diesel			0.4
Aircraft		0.3	
Railroads		0.3	
Vessels		0.1	
Nonhighway use, motor fuels		0.3	
Fuel combustion-stationary	0.7		
Coal		0.2	
Fuel oil		0.1	
Natural gas		Negligible	
Wood		0.4	
Industrial processes	4.6		
Solid waste disposal	1.6		
Miscellaneous	8.5		
Forest fires		2.2	
Structural fires		0.1	
Coal refuse		0.2	
Organic solvent evaporation		3.1	
Gasoline marketing		1.2	
Agricultural burning		1.7	
Total	32.0		

Stationary sources. Among stationary sources of hydrocarbons the production, processing, storage, and transfer of petroleum products, especially of gasoline and of organic solvents, are paramount. Leakage from oil fields and refineries, from gasoline storage tanks, and from gasoline loading facilities contribute to pollution. Other sources of hydrocarbon emissions are air-blowing of asphalt, blowdown systems, catalyst regenerators, processing vessels, flares, compressor pumps, and vacuum jets.

In addition, a wide variety of other industries that use organic solvents, namely chemical, drug, and pharmaceutical manufacturing plants emit hydrocarbons. Rubber and plastics, paints, varnishes, and lacquer undercoatings are composed to a large extent of organic solvents that evaporate during and after application of the coating. Dry cleaning of clothes, waste disposal by burning, particularly open burning of refuse, and inefficient incinerators are other contributors to hydrocarbon emissions.

HEALTH EFFECTS OF HYDROCARBONS

Although the gaseous hydrocarbons present in the atmosphere have very little, if any, direct effect on human health, the toxicity of their photochemical reaction products renders them hazardous. Formaldehyde and other aldehydes, ketones, and peroxyacetyl nitrates (PAN) contribute to eye irritation and to respiratory damage.[7]

1. Both the *aliphatic* and the *alicyclic* hydrocarbons have a slightly anesthetic and depressent effect on the central nervous system but only at concentrations 100 and 1000 times higher than those found in the atmosphere. Methane (CH_4), the most prevalent representative of the saturated aliphatic hydrocarbons, induces no ill-effect even at high concentrations in ambient air.

2. Vapors of *aromatic hydrocarbons*, which includes benzene, toluene, styrene, and xylene are more irritating to the mucous membranes than equivalent concentrations of the aliphatic and alicyclic hydrocarbons. They constitute serious occupational problems. Following long-term inhalation, abnormalities of the blood such as anemia, leucopenia (low white cells), and leukemia have been associated with exposure to aromatic hydrocarbons as, for instance, in chronic benzene poisoning.[8] No acute effects, however, have been reported at levels below 25 ppm.

3. *Oxygenated hydrocarbon derivatives.* Major interest in the air pollution literature centers about the role of two specific aldehydes, formaldehyde (CH_2O) and acrolein ($CH_2=CHCHO$). Their presence in the air can be detected by their irritant properties on eyes and respiratory mucous membranes. Indeed, the intensity of the odor, which they produce in diesel exhaust, parallels their concentration in the air.[9]

Formaldehydes act both as respiratory irritants to the eyes and nose and as allergenic agents. They give rise to lacrimation, sneezing, cough, dyspnea, sensation of suffocation, rapid pulse, headaches, weakness, and changes in the body temperature. Formaldehydes also induce allergic skin diseases.

Typical concentrations in Los Angeles in 1962 ranged from 0.02 to 0.19 ppm.[10] Eye irritation begins at levels of 0.01 to 1 ppm.[11] In the presence of solid and liquid aerosols, 1.8 to 3.3 μ (0.0018 to 0.0033 mm) in size, LaBelle[12] noted a synergistic effect on the death rate of mice and a high degree of pulmonary edema. Experimentally, after 18-hour exposures to formaldehyde vapor at 3.5 ppm[13] the alkaline phosphatase of the rat's liver increases and the ciliae in the bronchial tree become inactive. Exposure to 10 and 20 ppm causes breathing difficulties with shortness of breath, cough, burning of nose and throat, and extensive irritation in the trachea. Higher concentrations of 50 to 100 ppm cause serious pulmonary disturbances such as bronchopneumonia and pulmonary edema.[14] The threshold limit value for formaldehyde in industry is 5 ppm, but ambient air levels not higher than 0.1 ppm (.25 μg/meter³) are recommended.[2] Under the influence of sunlight, formaldehyde decomposes in the air into hydrogen and formyl radicals and into carbon monoxide.[15]

Dermatitis, a condition exemplified by poison ivy, is not infrequently caused by formaldehyde-impregnated fabrics. Whether or not atmospheric pollution levels can also induce such lesions on the exposed portions of the skin has not been established.

Acetaldehyde is believed to play an important role in the development of cardiovascular disease in smokers.[16]

The symptoms caused by vapors of acrolein resemble closely those caused by formaldehyde, but acrolein is considered more toxic to humans than formaldehyde. Asthmatic wheezing has been reported following inhalation of acrolein[14] at concentrations much lower than those at which formaldehyde causes pulmonary disease. Following exposure to 21.8 ppm (58,000 μg/meter³)[17] acrolein, pulmonary edema occurs immediately. However, the threshold for odor perception and eye irritation on volunteers is 0.3 ppm for acrolein as compared with 0.06 for formaldehyde according to observations by Russian workers.[18] Following inhalation of air containing 0.22 to 0.24 ppm acrolein, volunteers also experienced a decrease in the eye's sensitivity to light, indicative of an effect on the brain cortex.

In rats that inhaled from 0.06 to 0.57 ppm acrolein over a period of 24 days, loss of weight, changes in conditioned reflexes, decrease in cholinesterase activity of the blood, a fall of coproporphyrin excretion in the urine, and an increase in luminescent white blood cells were noted.[19]

Acetaldehyde (CH_3CHO), another aldehyde, formed from hydrocarbons and an important constituent of tobacco smoke (81 μg/40 ml per puff)[20] is practically nonirri-

tating to man at levels of 50 ppm. No untoward effects are known at concentrations that may be anticipated in the atmosphere.

REFERENCES

1. Migeotte, M. V.: Spectroscopic evidence of methane in the earth's atmosphere, Physiol. Rev. 73:519-520, 1948.
2. National Air Pollution Control Administration: Nationwide inventory of air pollution Emissions, 1968. Prepared by Division of Air Quality and Emissions Data, Bureau of Criteria and Standards, August 1970.
3. Ozolins, G., and Morita, C. B.: Sources and air pollutant emission patterns in major metropolitan areas. Presented at the sixty-second Annual Meeting of the Air Pollution Control Association, New York, June 1969.
4. Grant, E. P.: Auto emissions, Motor Vehicle Pollution Control Board Bull. 6:3, 1967.
5. Vogh, J. W.: Nature of odor components in diesel exhaust, J.A.P.C.A. 19:773-777, 1969.
6. Duprey, R. L.: Compilation of air pollutant emission factors, Durham, North Carolina, 1968, Public Health Service Publication Number 999-AP-42, National Center for Air Pollution Control.
7. Schuck, E. A., Stephens, E. R., and Middleton, J. T.: Eye irritation response at low concentrations of irritants, Arch. Environ, Health 13:570-575, 1966.
8. Gerarde, H.: Aromatic hydrocarbons. In Patty, F. A., editor: Industrial hygiene and toxicology, vol. 2, New York, 1963, Interscience Publishers.
9. Renzetti, N. A., and Bryan, R. J.: Atmospheric sampling for aldehydes and eye irritation in Los Angeles smog, 1960, J.A.P.C.A. 11:421-424, 427, 1961.
10. Technical Progress Report: Air Quality of Los Angeles County, vol 2, 1961, Los Angeles County Air Pollution Control District.
11. Air Quality Criteria for Hydrocarbons, National Air Pollution Control Administration, Washington, D. C., March 1970, U. S. Department of Health, Education, and Welfare.
12. LaBelle, C. W., Long, J. E., and Christofano, E. E.: Synergistic effects of aerosols, Arch. Industr. Health 11:297-304, 1955.
13. Murphy, S. D., Davis, H. V., and Zaratzian, V. L.: Biochemical effects in rats from irritating air contaminants, Toxic. Appl. Pharmacol. 6:520-528, 1964.
14. Fasset, D. W.: Aldehydes and acetyls. In Patty, F. A., editor: Industrial hygiene and toxicology, vol. 2, New York, 1963, Interscience Publishers.

15. Calvert, J. G., Kerr, J. A., Demerjian, K. L., and others: Photolysis of Formaldehyde by a hydrogen atom source in the lower atmosphere, Science **175:**751-752, 1972.

16. James, T. N., Bear, E. S., Lang, K. R., and others: Adrenergic mechanisms in the sinus node, Arch. Intern. Med. **125:**512-47, 1970.

17. Properties and Essential Information for Safe Handling and Use of Acrolein, Chemical Safety Data Sheet SD-85, Washington, D. C., 1961, Manufacturing Chemists Association.

18. Ryazanov, V. A.: Sensory physiology as basis for air quality standards: the approach used in the Soviet Union, Arch. Environ. Health **5:**480-494, 1962.

19. Gusev, M. I., Svechnikova, A. I., Dronov, I. S., and others: Determination of the daily average maximum permissible concentration of acrolein in the atmosphere, Gig. Sanit. **31:**8-13, 1966.

20. Newsome, J. R., Normal, V., and Keith, C. H.: Vapor phase analysis of tobacco smoke, Tobacco Science **9:**102-112, 1965.

20

POLLUTION BY RADIOACTIVE SUBSTANCES

Until the discovery of x-rays by Roentgen in 1895 exposure to ionizing radiation was the result exclusively of natural causes. In recent years, particularly since the advent of the atomic bomb and the harnessing of nuclear energy, human activities have contributed materially to atmospheric pollution by radioactive substances. This chapter will explore the possible damage to human health by radioactive pollutants.

TERMINOLOGY

It is a well-known fact that an atom consists of a nucleus with negatively charged electrons moving around it. The nucleus is comprised of protons, which are positively charged, and neutrons, which are electrically neutral. There are 103 known chemical elements arranged in alphabetical order. The Zth element in the periodic table has Z protons in the nucleus and, therefore, Z electrons, since the atom normally is electrically neutral. If A denotes the mass number, that is, the total number of nucleons (collective name for protons and neutrons), then the nucleus of a chemical element X is denoted by $_Z X^a$.

The atoms of a given element are not all exactly alike. The chemical properties of an element are determined solely by the number of electrons. Therefore, the number of protons in the nucleus of a specific element is fixed, but the number of neutrons may vary. Nuclei with different masses but the same number of protons are called isotopes of the element.

Not all atoms are stable. Some nuclei undergo changes through the process of radioactive decay in which particles are emitted and the nucleus changes into a different element. Radioactive material consists of unstable isotopes of various chemical elements such as carbon, hydrogen, iodine, strontium, uranium, and other elements called radioisotopes. Chemically, these unstable atoms behave like nonradioactive nuclei of the same atomic number.[1] Radioisotopes can be ingested with food, inhaled through the air, or administered medically. They are usually handled by the human body similarly to stable isotopes.

The resulting effects from ionizing radiation, which is emitted during the radioactive decay, depends on the amount of energy imparted by radiation per gram of a specific tissue as well as upon the type of ionizing radiation. The energy imparted by radiation per gram of tissue is called the "absorbed dose." Its unit is the rad (radiation absorbed dose) which is arbitrarily defined as 100 ergs (units of energy)/gm. The rate at which the dose is delivered, that is, the dose per unit time, is called the "dose rate." The roentgen (R) is the unit in which radiation exposure is measured. The curie (Ci) is the basic unit used to describe the activity of any radioactive isotope. One Ci represents approximately the rate of decay of one gram of radium, that is, the number of disintegrations per second from 1 gm of radium. The rem (roentgen equivalent mammal) is a unit of relative biologic dose or dose equivalent. In radiation biology, the rem describes the effectiveness with which a particular type of radiation produces a particular chemical or biologic effect.

KINDS OF RADIATION

Radionuclides in general give off three types of radiation: (1) alpha particles, which carry a positive charge, (2) beta particles with a negative or positive charge, and (3) electromagnetic gamma rays. The last mentioned have a short wave length; their effects are similar to those of x-rays.

Externally, alpha particles do not penetrate the skin. However they can produce serious damage when given off internally by items ingested or inhaled. Some beta rays can penetrate the protective layer of the skin but usually do not reach deep-seated organs when delivered externally. They can cause damage to the skin and may affect the eyes. Gamma rays are penetrating and can therefore be an external hazard.

Each radionuclide has a characteristic half-life (the time required to reduce the activity of a particular radioisotope to one half of its original value). For instance of 10,000,000 radon atoms, 5,000,000 will be left after 3.825 days (1 half-life), 2,500,000 after 7.650 days (2 half-lives), 1,250,000 after 11.475 days (3 half-lives) and so on. The half-lives of the known radionuclides range from a fraction of a second to thousands of years.[2]

SOURCES OF RADIOACTIVITY
Natural radiation

Radioactive gases, such as radon 222 and thoron 220, occur naturally both in the ground and in the atmosphere.

Radiation from soil. From the ground, radioactive gases are released by soil and rocks. Coal, for instance, contains radioactive material that escapes into the atmosphere when the fuel is burned.[3]

Solar radiation. In the atmosphere, radioactive agents are produced by cosmic radiation. Most natural radiation originates as solar particle beams produced by flares of the sun. During the first hour of the giant solar flare of February 23, 1956, radiation levels were estimated well in excess of 100 millirems (millirem = 1/1000 rem)[3] per hour at an altitude as low as 35,000 feet. Such occurrences constitute a hazard to commercial aviation, especially to supersonic transports. However, since the forecasting of solar flares has become possible, one can guard against them.

Radiation from stars. A third source of natural radiation is derived from the stars. Sizeable amounts are produced by neutrons and low energy protons; alpha particles are released in nuclear collisions of primary particles of high energy.

How much radiation from natural sources has affected and still is affecting human health is a moot question. For a crew of a supersonic transport plane with about 480 hours flying time per year at an average radiation level of 100 microrems (microrem = 1/1000 millirem) per hour, the resulting yearly dose would amount to 0.480 rem, which is slightly short of the official maximum permissible dose (MPD) of 0.5 rem for the public as determined by the International Commission on Radiologic Protection.[3] For the passengers of a supersonic plane, the dose per capita per year is about 0.36 millirem (Table 20-1).

Table 20-1. Population doses from radiation occurring in nature compared with man-made additions*

SOURCE OF RADIATION	DOSE EQUIVALENT (MILLIREMS PER YEAR)
Natural radiation	110
Medical x-rays	55
Fallout	10
Radiation workers	0.56
SST travel†	0.36

*Schaefer, H. J.: Radiation exposure in air travel, Science 173:780-783, 1971
†Assuming 77 million passenger hours at 33,000 feet.

Man-made radiation

Although natural radiation exceeds materially the amounts emitted from man-made sources, man has made essential contributions to radioactive contamination of the atmosphere, especially through harnessing nuclear energy. It should be emphasized however that under conditions of normal operations within existing regulations, there is no indication that either immediate or latent release of radiation causes damage to health.

The four possible sources of man-made radioactive contamination of the atmosphere are:

1. The production of nuclear fuel
2. The use of nuclear energy for propulsive power in ships, rockets, and aerospace vehicles
3. The use of radioisotopes in industry, agriculture, medicine, and scientific research
4. Testing of nuclear weapons

Each of these activities may under unfavorable circumstances release radioactive gases and dusts into the atmosphere,[4] but the health of employees rather than that of large populations is believed to be at risk.

Production of nuclear fuel

At power plants. The development of nuclear power plants promises to fill a great need in the rising production of electricity. Indeed, at the present time we are in the midst of an extraordinary increase in the size and numbers of such facilities.

After the fuels have been obtained and introduced into nuclear reactors, their operation releases radioactive waste into the confines of the reactor, from which it is a potential pollutant to the atmosphere. The waste originates with fission products that normally remain incorporated in the fuel (uranium). Waste is also produced by activation of extraneous products found mainly in coolants. A variety of radioactive gases are thus formed, particularly Iodine 131, Xenon 133 and 135, Krypton 85, Uranium 238, Thorium and Plutonium 239, Strontium 90, Cerium 144, Barium 140, and Zirconium 95 (Table 20-2). During the normal operation of a reactor, particularly if air cooling is utilized, Argon 41, an element normally present in the cooling air, is discharged into the atmosphere. Under certain conditions, inert dust contained in cooling air becomes radioactive and can escape into the environs. In general, however, air pollution is minimal for gas and water-cooled reactors and of negligible health significance, if normal operating procedures are followed.

At reprocessing plants. The most impor-

Table 20-2. The half-life of the most important fission products released from nuclear fuel*

		LONGER-LIVED (YEARS)			SHORTER-LIVED (DAYS)
^{3}H	(Tritium)	12.3	^{89}Sr	(Strontium 89)	51
^{85}Kr	(Krypton 85)	10.7	^{91}Y	(Yttrium 91)	57.5
^{90}Sr	(Strontium 90)	28	^{95}Zr	(Zirconium 95)	65
^{106}Ru	(Ruthenium 106)	1.0	^{95}Nb	(Niobium 95)	35
^{125}Sb	(Antimony 125)	2.0	^{131}I	(Iodine 131)	8.07
^{137}Cs	(Cesium 137)	30	^{133}Xe	(Xenon 133)	5.3
^{144}Ce	(Cerium 144)	0.78	^{140}Ba	(Barium 140)	12.8
^{147}Pm	(Promethium 147)	2.6			
^{151}Sm	(Samarium 151)	93			
^{155}Eu	(Europium 155)	1.7			

*Adapted from Radford, E. P.: Air pollution problems in nuclear power development. Presented at the American Medical Association Air Pollution Medical Research Conference, New Orleans, October 1970.

tant source of air pollution in the operation of a reactor fuel cycle is the chemical reprocessing of the spent reactor fuel. For economic management, nuclear reactor fuel must be recycled and reprocessed. In addition to Atomic Energy Commission plants such as that at Oak Ridge and Savannah River, three commercial reprocessing plants are currently in operation in the United States at West Valley, New York, at Morris, Illinois, and near Aiken, South Carolina.

During the process of separating unfissioned Uranium 238 and Plutonium 239 from the radioactive waste products, two significant radionuclides, Krypton 85 and Tritium (Hydrogen 3) are released. Krypton 85 is long-lasting (half-life, 10.76 years) and its quantity in the air is increasing. Tritium, the radionuclide of hydrogen present in water vapor has a half life of 12.26 years. It is extremely difficult to remove tritium from the liquid discharges of power and fuel reprocessing plants. However, it is not believed to concentrate in fish or in other links of the food chain.[6] Xenon 133 with a half-life of 5.3 days and Iodine 131 (half-life, 8 days) are also released from reprocessing plants and enter the atmosphere. Strict precautions have controlled to a large extent the health hazard of these agents.

Accidents. In the past, several accidents have occurred with nuclear reactors, which involved over 100 individuals.[4] On December 12, 1952, the reactor at Chalk River, Canada, emitted considerable radioactive material that spread over a large uninhabited area.[7] Another accident occurred at the National Reactor Testing Station in Idaho on January 3, 1961. Mainly because of the short half-life of Iodine 131 (Table 20-2), the contamination that extended about 100 miles southwest of the plant site was not considered hazardous.[8]

More significant was the environmental contamination in 1957 at Windscale, England.[2] Radioactivity spread over a large section of the country and airborne radioactive iodine was found on forage consumed by dairy cattle in a 200 square mile area. The milk from these cows had to be withheld from public consumption for 3 to 6 weeks.

Nuclear energy as a source of propulsive power. For some time past, nuclear energy has been in use for propulsion of submarines and surface vessels. The heat from the reactor transfers to liquid sodium and thence to water outside the reactor system. The steam drives standard steam turbines for propulsion.

Since radioactive contamination from propulsion of vehicles involves mobile sources (not stationary ones like an atomic power plant) it could conceivably constitute a danger for individuals residing distant from a reactor site as well as those in close proximity.

A relatively new potential source of atmospheric pollution is the use of nuclear energy for rocket propulsion and as a source of power for satellites. The first such device was placed in orbit in June 1962.[9] In our space satellite program Plutonium 238 and, more recently, Curium 244, both of which have a long half-life, are being employed as a source of power. Since they emit alpha rays, they do not present an external hazard during launching of the satellite and its reentry into the atmosphere. The hazard in their application is liable to occur should a satellite fail to go into orbit at the point of launching. In April 1964, an isotopic power device burned up over the Indian Ocean during reentry into the atmosphere, liberating traces of Plutonium 238. This material is still slowly descending toward the ground and is expected to produce atmospheric pollution.[10]

Radioisotopes in scientific research and medicine. A growing industry is the production of artificial radionuclides and compounds labeled with a specific radioactive atom, both in research establishments and in hospitals. They are employed for scanning of organs in order to determine the

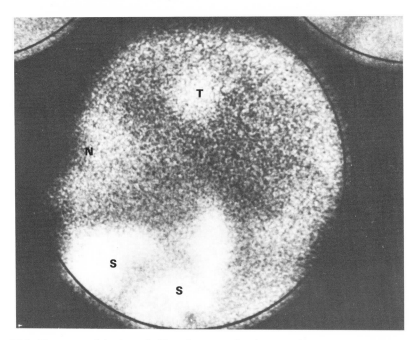

Fig. 20-1. Photoscan of brain with ^{99m}technetium, daughter product of molybdenum, obtained with a gamma camera, showing localization of brain density found to be a tumor, *T*. The light areas at bottom left represent normal localizations of the salivary glands, *S*; the area marked *N* represents normal nasal structures.

presence of certain disease processes in such organs (Fig. 20-1). Furthermore, radioisotopes are being used extensively in scientific research, mainly as tracers in industry, biology, and agriculture. These materials are discharged with the sewage into waterways. They can eventually reach both aquatic life and humans through their drinking water and the food chain. Radioactive material can also accumulate in the sludge of sewage. If the latter is used as a fertilizer, the radioactive material will be concentrated and remain attached to the fertilizer, thus contaminating both soil and plants.[11]

Most of these pollutants occur in the form of fine suspended particles. They are mainly beta-gamma emitters with a relatively short half-life. Furthermore, the doses of radioisotopes employed are small. Therefore, they are not considered sources of atmospheric pollution.[12] The radioiso-tope most commonly employed in medicine for external radiation is Cobalt 60 which is utilized for the treatment of malignant diseases. This radionuclide is probably the least potential pollutant.

Nuclear weapon testing. The principal potential source of radioactive pollution is the testing of nuclear weapons. During a nuclear detonation the fission products release an intensely hot fireball that cools as it rises and attracts dust particles from the ground into the fireball, which also become radioactive. As the fission products begin to cool, they form a nucleus for radioactive coating. Particles of the atomic cloud larger than 50 μ start falling back on the ground as soon as the cloud has reached its highest altitudes.[2] They are deposited within a few hundred miles downwind from the detonation. Most radioactive dust is suspended in the upper troposphere (30,000 to 50,000 feet). Dependent on the

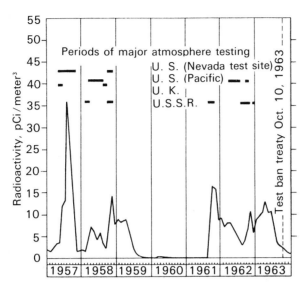

Fig. 20-2. Monthly mean concentrations of beta radioactivity as related to testing of nuclear weapons, 1957-1963. (From Miner, S.: Air pollution aspects of radioactive substances, Litton Industries, Inc., Bethesda, Maryland, 1969, U. S. Department of Commerce, PB 188-092.)

height of the detonation, on the energy yield of the bombs, on meteorologic conditions and the nature of the terrain, the products of instantaneous and delayed fallout are carried around the world several times. This fallout contains principally nuclear products with a short half-life, especially Iodine 131.

The lightest dust particles reach the stratosphere. It takes several years for the bulk of this radioactive material to be deposited on the ground. Since 1952, when the tests began on nuclear weapons with high explosive yields, fallout from the stratosphere has been more or less continuous (Fig. 20-2). Because of greater rainfall, the primary mechanism for removing radioactive material from the air, most nuclear fallout occurs in the temperate and polar regions of the earth rather than near the equator. Therefore, nuclear detonations at a U.S.S.R. test site in the arctic regions

produced a faster and less widely distributed fallout than those near the equator where the original United States testing was performed.

Nuclear testing has been followed by a marked increase in environmental pollution in northern Japan. In a survey conducted between 1962 to 1966, Takizawa and Sugai[13] reported an increase in the levels of Plutonium 239, Strontium 90, and Cesium 137, both in human tissue and in fish, shellfish, and seaweed.[13]

Underground testing in the Nevada test site produced relatively little air pollution. At high altitudes, however, detonations from nuclear fallout can damage jet engine turbines. Accumulation of radioactive dust interferes with the functioning of high temperature turbines.

The total radiation from nuclear testing has added about 10% to 15% to the normal natural radiation throughout the world.[14]

Fig. 20-2 shows the monthly concentration of beta radioactivity related to nuclear testing. The total explosive yields of all nuclear testing between 1945 and 1962 in the United States, United Kingdom, and Soviet Union was equivalent to 511 megatons of TNT.[15]

HEALTH EFFECTS
Distribution in the body

The doses of radiation from the release of a nuclide are dependent on the amount of the nuclide that is transferred from the point of release to the site from which the radiation reaches the human tissues. For certain nuclides this site may be outside of the body (external radiation), as for instance at the surface of soil where it was deposited. Other nuclides are absorbed into the body through dietary ingestion or through inhalation. They irradiate the body tissues from within. An example of an internal emitter of radiation is Potassium 40. Of the 140 gm of potassium, a vital element present in a "standard man," about 0.0165 gm is Potassium 40, a beta-gamma emitter that corresponds to about 0.1 μ Ci of Potassium 40.[2] Other nuclides irradiate tissues both from outside and inside the body.[1]

When inhaled, nuclides either remain in the lungs or are absorbed through the alveolar wall into the bloodstream and can be deposited in other organ tissues. A portion of inhaled radionuclides is expectorated and swallowed with saliva.

Biologic action of radionuclides

It is difficult to detect and relate long-term illness, such as an increase in the frequency of malignancies, or genetic damage to radiation. Therefore the estimates of such effects must be made principally by extrapolation from observations at much higher doses and dose rates. Critical factors in assessing damage to health are the kinds of radiation that are emitted, the half-life of the nuclides, how they are incorporated, how long they remain in the system, and the condition of the principal targets, the "critical organs."

Some of the radionuclides that can present significant health hazards to man are listed in Table 20-3:

1. Strontium 90 and Strontium 89, which principally irradiate the skeleton
2. Cesium 137, which concentrates in soft tissues and causes a generalized radiation
3. Carbon 14, which accumulates throughout the body and produces whole body radiation

Table 20-3. Examples of radionuclides causing damage to health

	KIND OF RADIATION	MAIN TARGET	HALF-LIFE	POSSIBLE EFFECT
Strontium 90	Beta	Skeleton	28 yrs.	Bone cancer (?)
Strontium 89	Beta	Skeleton	51 days	Bone cancer (?)
Cesium 137	Beta-gamma	Soft tissues Genital organs	27 yrs.	Gonadal tissue
Carbon 14	Beta-gamma	Whole body	5760 yrs.	—
Iodine 129	Beta-gamma	Thyroid	17 million yrs.	Cancer of thyroid (?)
Iodine 131	Beta-gamma	Thyroid	8 days	Cancer of thyroid
Plutonium 239	Alpha	Bones, liver, spleen	24,400 yrs.	Bone cancer
Krypton 85	Beta	—	10.7 yrs.	—
Tritium (H 3)	Beta	Whole body	12.3 yrs.	Gonads

4. Iodine 131, the target organ of which is the thyroid gland

Other short-lived fission products, which cause external irradiation on the body surface when they are deposited on the ground, are presented in Table 20-2.

Strontium 90, a bone seeker like calcium, is readily absorbed by plants through their roots and their leaves. Thus it reaches food derived from plant life. The amounts of ingested Strontium 90 can be sharply reduced by thoroughly washing vegetables and discarding the outer layers before consumption. Strontium 90 is also passed along to humans through the milk of animals that feed on the contaminated forage. When deposited in sufficient amounts in animals, Strontium 90 produced leukemia, bone cancer, and other skeletal diseases.[16] In humans these effects have not as yet been documented. In contrast to Strontium 89, with its short half-life of only 51 days, Strontium 90, which has a half-life of 28 years, is eliminated from the bones very slowly and can therefore damage the skeleton for a lifetime. Both are particularly hazardous in infants and children because of their presence in milk. Moreover, according to recent reports, Strontium 90 has a significant genetic effect[17] in research animals.

Cesium 137, a second radionuclide emitted from radioactive debris, is a major contributor to long-lived gamma ray activity. It irradiates the body externally and internally. This fact, as well as its long half-life of 27 years and its wide distribution throughout the human body, renders it a potential hazard. It is readily transferred through the food chain from cattle to milk and meat through which it enters the human diet.[18] Peaks in the average whole-body burden of Cesium 137 in man, following atmosphere nuclear testing, occurred in 1959 and 1964. They were 70 pc/gK (gram of potassium) and 120 pc/gK, respectively. The 1964 maximum peak was reached about 1½ years after the testing, a consequence of the prolonged duration of the worldwide fallout in the atmosphere and indicative of the transmission of Cesium 137 to man through the food chain. Since 1964, the body burden of Cesium 137 has declined rapidly following the moratorium on atmospheric nuclear testing.[2]

Carbon 14 has a long half-life of 5,760 years. It emits mainly weak beta rays. Its basic natural source is the cosmic rays. However, from 1955 to 1961 because of nuclear testing, Carbon 14 in carbon dioxide had increased by 30% in the northern hemisphere.[2] Since carbon is a basic element of all living matter, it is readily deposited throughout the body. It has a genetic as well as an immediate somatic potential (see Chapter 17).

It is estimated that 95% of Carbon 14 is precipitated into the ocean whence it can be incorporated in the food chain. The 5% remaining in the atmosphere constitutes a source of concern, particularly to the generations that follow the testing of an atmospheric weapon.

Tritium (H 3) (half-life 12.3 years) has been introduced into the environment as tritiated water or as tritiated water vapor. Tritium, like Carbon 14, can be present in any organic molecule. Therefore it is widely distributed throughout the body and constitutes a biologic hazard even when the body burden is very small. The duration of its storage in a given biologic system is influenced by the turnover of stable (nonradioactive) water. The uptake of tritium in plants from the soil occurs very rapidly. Tritium has been found in deer grazing near the Savannah River reprocessing plant. Their body hydrogen was uniformly labelled with tritium, eqivalent to water of 30 picocuries (pc, one trillionth curie) per milliliter. No data are available on humans residing near the plant who consume locally grown vegetables and water from surface springs.[5]

Iodine 131, although short-lived (its half-life is only 8 days), constitutes a hazard, particularly to children. Within a few days after it is deposited on the ground, milk produced by dairy cattle feeding on contaminated forage could possibly contain levels of Iodine 131 high enough to damage the thyroid gland in which it accumulates.[4] It is difficult to assess the harm of Iodine 131 in a particular area because its concentration varies from place to place and from time to time at the same site. Even after underground testing in Nevada, high levels of Iodine 131 were detected in the path of the fallout cloud.

Iodine 129 is a low-energy isotope with little penetrating power. Emitted from nuclear power plants, its half-life is 17 million years. Before 1945, little Iodine 129 was produced naturally by cosmic rays, and by fission of uranium in the earth's crust.[19] For every trillion iodine atoms, only about 5 were in the form of Iodine 129. A large increase in concentration between 1945 and 1959 was followed by a decline, probably because of installation of efficient effluent scrubbing equipment.[20]

A number of *short-lived* fission products with half-lives ranging from 14 to 369 days are deposited on the ground as a result of nuclear testing. They emit gamma rays that produce whole-body exposure and may be hazardous both to the health of the current generation and to that of their offspring.

Clinical features

Shortly after the discovery of x-rays, their ability to cause loss of hair, chronic ulcers of the skin and cancer was recognized. In the early part of the twentieth century, workers using radium in the luminous paint industry contracted bone cancer and aplastic anemia, a serious bone marrow disease. Use of radium as a nostrum for a variety of ailments such as arthritis and syphilis was responsible for additional fatalities. In 1949, a rise in the death rate caused by lung cancer in Joachimsthal, Czechoslovakia, was traced to high concentrations of radon and its daughter products

in metal mines. A similar situation[21] was reported in the United States uranium mining and milling industry[21] and in fluorospar mining.[22]

Acute exposure. Acute massive exposures are encountered mainly through accidents in workers in the nuclear industry or, in case of war, following a nuclear detonation. The effects of such events depends largely on the size of the dose that the body receives. Doses of 200 rems and above cause vomiting and nausea followed by a latent period of as much as 2 weeks. The symptoms that develop, known as radiation sickness, include loss of hair, sore throat, diarrhea, purpura (a disease characterized by reduction of blood platelets) hemorrhages of the skin and of other organs, manifestations indicative of damage to the blood-forming centers in the bone marrow and to the lymph glands.[23] Doses in the range of 350 to 450 rem may be lethal to man. The most radiosensitive tissues are the bone marrow, the lymphatic tissue and the lining of the intestinal tract.

Low-level exposure. Ionizing radiation, delivered for long periods of time, may cause a wide variety of effects. Changes in the texture and pigmentation of the skin and loss of hair are early signs; whereas such diseases as leukemia, cancer, and cataracts (opacities of the eye lens) may be delayed for 5 or more years. There is evidence that chronic radiation exposure can reduce the life expectancy and interfere with the body's immune mechanism.[2]

Leukemia. It is firmly established that early radiologists and patients exposed to radiation for therapeutic or diagnostic purposes as well as victims of the Hiroshima-Nagasaki bombing have developed leukemia. Patients treated with radioiodine in excess of 1 Ci showed a higher than normal incidence of leukemia. In the fetus, which is particularly vulnerable to the disease, doses from 2 and 10 rem have caused leukemia,[24]

Cancer. Various types of cancer are known to be caused by irradiation: skin cancer was reported among radiologists, within a decade after discovery of x-rays. Thyroid cancer is not uncommon among children who have received x-ray treatment in the neck region; lung cancer is not uncommon in miners occupationally exposed to radon and its daughter elements. Bone cancer occurred in radium dial painters and in other persons exposed to radium. The radionuclides, which may cause bone cancer (osteogenic sarcoma) are radioactive strontium, plutonium, thorium, and lead, agents that are ingested and metabolized in the bone. Lung cancer caused by radon and its daughter products has been reported in fluorospar miners.

*Cataracts.** Doses of x-rays and gamma rays at or above 600 roentgens[2] have been responsible for cataracts. Cataracts have been reported among Japanese survivors of the Hiroshima and Nagasaki atomic bomb disasters, among patients whose eyes were treated by x-ray and among physicians exposed to radiation from cyclotrons.[14]

Shortened life-span. During the early part of the century statistical evidence indicated that the life span of radiologists had been shortened although this development was not associated with radiation-induced fatal diseases such as leukemia.[25] This effect however was not observed among British radiologists. Furthermore, among 99,393 survivors of the Japanese bomb disasters who had been within 1200 meters of ground zero, mortality (excluding deaths from leukemia) between 1950 and 1960 was 15% higher than in a control group.[2] An acceleration of the aging process was documented further by experiments with animals.[26] Compliance with rigid protection techniques in recent times has reduced the threat of shortened life span among radiologists.

The genetic injury to populations by radiation is discussed in Chapter 17.

---

*Opacity of the eye lens with possible loss of vision.

Effects of bombing of Hiroshima and Nagasaki

Considerable knowledge about the health effect of radionuclides has been gleaned from the Hiroshima and Nagasaki atomic bomb explosions. Although the data on such massive single exposures does not necessarily apply to long-term exposures to radionuclides over extended periods, the two disasters serve as a pattern for assessing the overall effect of radiation.

Similar to irradiation by x-ray, the atomic bomb had an immediate and a delayed effect. Gastrointestinal injury, which in some cases was irreversible, occurred immediately.

Plummer[27] obtained a history of burns, loss of hair, fever, purpura (a disease characterized by tiny hemorrhages mainly on the skin), and gastrointestinal bleeding in 68 out of 250 pregnant women. Eleven were within 1200 meters of the hypocenter (the atmospheric center reflected on the ground) of the bomb's impact. The second peak of illness involving the bone marrow gave rise to anemia, hemorrhages, purpura, leukemia, and infections.[28]

Up to 1954, 10 years after the bomb disaster, 92 cases of leukemia among 216,176 survivors of the atomic bomb were recorded.[29] The first evidence of the disease appeared within 1 year following the bombing, but the peak did not occur until 6 to 7 years later. The blood showed a significant rise in basophile cells (white blood cells staining with basic dyes indicative of a toxic process) and the alkaline phosphatase activity in the white blood cells was markedly decreased. A higher than normal incidence of "radiation" cataracts was also noted in survivors who had been in the vicinity of the bomb explosion. In 1972, 22 cases of tumors of the salivary glands were reported, representing five times the "normal" incidence that had occurred between 1957 and 1970 among atomic bomb survivors in Hiroshima-Nagasaki. These patients had been exposed to a dose of radiation that ranged from 89 to 606 rad.[30]

The prolonged latent period following exposure, which precedes the development of symptoms, adds further to the complexity of identifying the source of illness in a patient whose health may be deteriorating as the result of radioactive pollution. Most illness caused by radioactivity is not only incurable but it is also likely, under certain conditions, to be transmitted to future generations.

The discovery of x-rays and of nuclear energy has led to remarkable scientific advances that are responsible for saving numerous lives. Many phases of this great achievement have been accomplished with relatively little environmental damage compared with that derived from natural radioactive emission. Protective measures have reduced the incidence of diseases caused by radiation and will undoubtedly lead to further control of this ever-present, vexing problem.

REFERENCES

1. Report of the United Nations Scientific Committee on the Effects of Atomic Radiation. General Assembly, Official Records, twenty-fourth session, Supplement No. 13 (A/7613), New York, 1969, United Nations.
2. Arena, V.: Ionizing radiation in life, St. Louis, 1971, The C. V. Mosby Co.
3. Schaefer, H. J.: Radiation protection: recommendations of the International Commission on Radiological Protection (ICRP) Publication No. 9, New York, 1966, Pergamon Press.
4. Smats, H. B.: A review of nuclear reactor incidents. In Reactor safety and hazards evaluation techniques, vol. 1, Proceedings of a Symposium, Vienna, 1962, pp. 89-110.
5. Radford, E. P.: Air pollution problems in nuclear power development. Presented at The American Medical Association Air Pollution Medical Research Conference, New Orleans, October, 1970.
6. Environmental Quality: The first annual report of the Council on Environmental Quality. Transmitted to Congress, August 1970, Washington, D. C., U. S. Government Printing Office.
7. Lewis, W. B.: The accident to the NRX reactor on December 12, 1952, AECL. 232, Chalk River, Ontario, 1953, Atomic Energy of Canada Ltd.
8. Horan, J. R., and Gammill, W. P.: The health physics aspect of the SL-1 accident, Health Phys. 9:177-186, 1963.
9. Stern, A. C.: Air pollution, New York, 1968, Academic Press, Inc.
10. Report of the United Nations Scientific Committee on the Effects of Atomic Radiation, New York, 1966, United Nations.
11. Proceedings of the Second United Nations International Conference of the Peaceful Uses of Atomic Energy, New York, 1958, United Nations.
12. Jammet, H. P.: Radioactive pollution of the atmosphere, Monograph Series 46, Air Pollution, 1961, World Health Organization.
13. Takizawa, Y., and Sugai, R.: Plutonium 239, Strontium 90 and Cesium 137: concentrations in human organs of the Japanese, Arch. Environ. Health 23:445-450, 1971.
14. Miner, S.: Air pollution aspects of radioactive substances. Bethesda, Maryland, September 1969, U. S. Department of Commerce, National Bureau of Standards, PB 188 092, Litton Industries, Inc.
15. Federal Radiation Council Report, No. 4: Estimates and evaluation of fallout in the United States from nuclear weapons testing conducted through 1962, Washington, D. C., May 1963, U. S. Government Printing Office.
16. Air Conservation: Report of the Air Conservation Commission of the American Association for the Advancement of Science, Publication Number 80, Washington, D. C. 1965.
17. Luning, K. G., Frolen, H., Nelson, A., and others: Genetic effects of Strontium 90 injected into male mice, Nature 197:304-305, 1963.
18. Garner, R. J.: An assessment of quantities of fission products likely to be found in milk in the event of aerial contamination of agricultural land, Nature 186:1063, 1960.
19. Kohman, T. P., and Edwards, R. R.: Iodine as a chemical and ecological tracer: progress report to Environmental Science Branch, Division of Biology and Medicine, U. S. Atomic Energy Commission, November 30, 1966.
20. Novick, S.: Seventeen million years, Environment 13:42-47, 1971.
21. Wagoner, J. K., Archer, V. E., Lundin, F. E., Jr., and others: Radiation as the cause of lung cancer among uranium miners, New Eng. J. Med. 273:181-188, 1965.

22. Cooper, C. W.: Uranium mining and lung cancer, J. Occup. Med. **10**:82, 1968.

23. Wald, N., Thoma, G. E., Jr., Brown, G., Jr., and others: Hematologic manifestations of radiation exposure in man. Progr. Hemat. **3**:1, 1962.

24. Chadwick, D. R., and Abrahams, S. P.: Biological effects of radiation, Arch. Environ. Health **9**:643-648, 1964.

25. Warren, S.: Longevity and causes of death from irradiation of physicians, J.A.M.A. **162**:464, 1956.

26. Mole, R. H.: Shortening of life by chronic irradiation: the experimental facts, Nature **179**:456, 1957.

27. Plummer, G.: Anomalies occurring in children exposed in utero to the atomic bomb in Hiroshima, Pediatrics **10**:687-692, 1952.

28. Cronkite, E. P., Bond, V. P., Chapman, W. H., and others: Biological effect of atomic bomb gamma radiation, Science **122**:148-150, 1965.

29. Maloney, W. C.: Leukemia in survivors of atomic bombings, New Eng. J. Med. **253**:88-90, 1955.

30. Belsky, J. L., Tachikawa, K., Cihak, R. W., and others: Salivary gland tumors in atomic bomb survivors Hiroshima-Nagasaki, 1957-1970, J.A.M.A. **219**:864-868, 1972.

21
SMOKING

In 1953 in the *Journal of the American Medical Association*[1] I described a disease caused by smoking, which I termed "smoker's respiratory syndrome." The 23 patients whose cases were reported had been complaining of constant irritation in the throat, expectoration of mucus, cough, wheezing localized in the upper air passages, and shortness of breath, particularly in the morning. Their unusual susceptibility to upper respiratory infections caused them to miss work frequently. Subsequently, several hundred additional cases were encountered most of whom improved promptly once they had discontinued smoking. The number of cigarettes that they smoked during the course of one day did not necessarily determine the severity of the disease. In some persons, smoking as few as five cigarettes a day had caused as much trouble as in others who smoked as many as thirty, an indication that factors other than smoking entered the picture, perhaps exposure to additional air pollutants, perhaps an inherited or acquired resistance to the smoke, or varying smoking practices.

In many respects, the condition resembled what was noted in previous years in patients residing near the Bay City-Midland area (Chapter 15). The smoker's syndrome, however, could be much more clearly defined than that caused by pollution in an industrial region because most smokers made a dramatic recovery as soon as they stopped smoking.

This disease, which often leads to emphysema, is perhaps the most common of all disabilities caused by smoking and, at the same time, probably the most neglected. Examination of the patients invariably reveals a chronically inflamed throat and slight asthmalike wheezing localized in the upper bronchial tree, not severe enough to disquiet either the patients or their physicians.

Smoking elicits other more serious disabilities, particularly chronic emphysema and lung cancer. It affects the blood vessels, the heart, the stomach, and the adrenal glands.[2]

INGREDIENTS OF SMOKE

Such a variety of effects must be anticipated when one realizes that tobacco smoke is a composite of numerous pollutants inhaled in rather high concentrations. Whereas *carbon monoxide* in persons employed in fume-laden garages, tunnels, and behind automobiles reaches levels of 100 ppm, concentrations of cigarette smoke may rise as high as 42,000 ppm.[3] Fortunately, the smoker does not breathe in such heavily polluted air nor is the inhalation of carbon monoxide–laden air as consistent as in the above-mentioned workers. In a poorly ventilated room laden with tobacco smoke, however, concentrations of carbon monoxide can easily reach several hundred parts per million, thus exposing smokers and nonsmokers alike to its toxic fumes.

Similarly, *nitrogen dioxide,* which in the Los Angeles area has reached a maximum concentration of 3 ppm, is found in smoke at the level of 250 ppm. Smoking one cigar in a home raises the particle count from 10 to 100 times, depending on particle size.[4]

Numerous other chemicals make up the *particulate matter* in tobacco smoke. In condensed form, these millions or even billions of particulates form a brown sticky mass, the cigarette "tar." At least ten hydrocarbons found in cigarette tar have pro-duced cancer in animals, particularly benzo[a]pyrene.

Inexpensive cigars, for the manufacture of which reconstituted tobacco sheets are used, contain a variety of inorganic particles such as clays, quartz, glass fibers, and fibers of aluminum silicate (Fig. 21-1).[5] On heating to about 700° C, the temperature of a burning cigar, they break up into finer particles, mainly crystobalite.[5]

Nicotine is another powerful poison of which about 0.5 to 2 mg are found in a

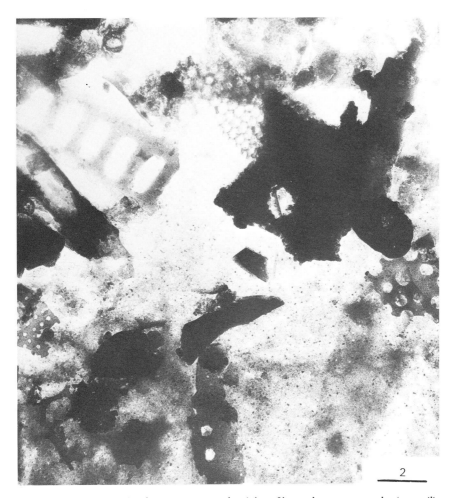

Fig. 21-1. Photomicrograph of inorganic particles (glass fiber, glass, quartz, aluminum silicates, and others) that are present in tobacco smoke. (Courtesy Selikoff, K. J., and Langer, A. M.: Inorganic particles in cigars and cigar smoke, Science **174:**585-586, 1971. Copyright 1971 by the American Association for the Advancement of Science.)

cigarette. Nicotine is marketed as a powerful insecticide under the name of Black Leaf 40.

Phenols, which are also present in tobacco, tend to destroy the protective action of the cilia, the small hairlike projections that line the respiratory tract. Although phenols themselves are not carcinogenic, they potentiate the carcinogenic action of benzo[a]pyrene.

Acetaldehyde, a strong irritant that inhibits the ciliary action and damages the lining of the upper respiratory tract, is found in the vapor phase of tobacco smoke in relatively high concentrations (81 μg/40 ml puff).[6]

Metals. Among other chemicals in cigarrettes are cadmium (30 μg per pack) of which 70% passes into the smoke,[7] lead (20 to 60 μg per pack),[8] and fluoride (48.8 μg per pack).[9] They enter the tobacco plant through the roots and leaves from soil and air, respectively, either as the result of sprays or of otherwise polluted air. The average smoker absorbs 10 mg more lead per day than a nonsmoker.[10] Necropsy studies revealed that accumulation of cadmium in the organ tissues of smokers is related to the number of packs of cigarettes smoked per year.[10a]

Some toxic agents in cigarette smoke have no counterpart in ordinary air pollution. Hydrogen cyanide, for instance, impairs the action of respiratory enzymes. Long-term exposure to this agent at 10 ppm is considered dangerous. The concentration in cigarette smoke is almost 1600 ppm.[2]

HEALTH EFFECTS

A significant amount of tobacco smoke is absorbed in the nasal cavity in experimental animals.[11] In humans, smoking taxes the defense mechanism of the lungs as indicated by the presence of pigmented macrophages (scavanger cells) in the lungs of smokers. These cells are related to the number of cigarettes smoked per day. No pigmented macrophages were found in the alveoli of nonsmokers.[12]

It has already been shown that smoking enhances a person's susceptibility to the toxic effect of many atmospheric contaminants such as carbon monoxide, sulfur dioxide, cadmium, asbestos, and teflon fumes, when this plastic is heated above 400 C. In coal miners, cigarette smoking contributes materially to the development of emphysema.[13]

Cancer

Lung cancer and chronic emphysema are the most serious respiratory diseases that can be attributed to smoking. In the last 30 years, deaths from lung cancer in the United States have increased strikingly over deaths from cancer in other organs.[14] Whereas in 1940 only 371 deaths from lung cancer were reported in the United States, in 1968 the number rose to 55,300. The annual consumption of cigarettes per person above 15 years of age living in the United States, which amounted to 1828 in 1940, increased to 4,003 in 1967.[2]

In distinction to air pollution, the smoke from a cigarette, pipe, or cigar is inhaled directly through the mouth, throat, and bronchi. Thus, it by-passes the filtration mechanism of the nose, which normally removes about 75% of particulate matter from the air.[2] In cancer of the mouth, throat, and larynx, tobacco plays a major role. Pipe smoking, particularly, has been linked with cancer of the lip. Cessation of smoking in persons whose cancer has been removed successfully reduces the risk of new cancerous growth.[15] Cancer of the urinary bladder, of the pancreas, and of the kidney have also shown an association with smoking,[16] although other sources may have been contributing factors.

Emphysema

That emphysema and chronic bronchitis can result from smoking has been documented by numerous statistical studies. One of the most convincing surveys on over a million men and women by Hammond[17] revealed a death rate from bronchitis and

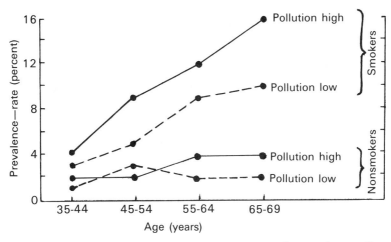

Fig. 21-2. Age trends in respiratory disease in relation to smoking and air pollution. (From Lambert, P. M.: Smoking, air pollution, and bronchitis in Britain, Lancet 1:853-857, 1970.)

emphysema in men aged 45 to 64, 6 times as high in smokers as in nonsmokers. Above age 75, the mortality rate was four times higher. Unlike lung cancer, which is fatal after a relatively short period, emphysema caused by smoking tends to linger on for decades. A British study of 9975 men and women age 35 to 69 showed that the incidence of chronic bronchitis rises with increasing levels of air pollution in both smokers and nonsmokers. As pollution increases there is a widening gap between smokers and nonsmokers, as shown in Fig. 21-2.[18]

By incubating in test tubes, lymphocytes (the round white blood cells) from eight allergic persons exposed to cigarette smoke Savel[19] demonstrated the development of allergy to tobacco smoke. In conjunction with the known irritating property of some of the ingredients of tobacco, smoking thus further unbalances the equilibrium in allergic patients.

Cardiovascular disease

Coronary thrombosis and myocardial infarction (blood clots in the blood vessels of the heart, and its musculature) are more prevalent in smokers than in nonsmokers.[20] In Hammond's study the death rate from coronary heart disease for men and women 45

to 54 years of age was 2.8 times as high for men who smoke a package or more of cigarettes a day as in nonsmokers. In women, this proportion was slightly lower. Johnson[21] noted 50% more abnormal electrocardiograms in smokers than in nonsmokers. Although smoking is not the only risk factor in the development of coronary heart disease, carbon monoxide and nicotine present in tobacco smoke are dominant causes: nicotine increases the demand of the heart for oxygen, and carbon monoxide decreases the ability of the blood to furnish the needed oxygen.[16]

Thromboangiitis obliterans, or Buerger's disease, has been identified with tobacco for many years.[22] In this disease, narrowed capillary blood vessels hamper the blood flow into the extremities, a process that leads eventually to gangrene of fingers and toes.

Other effects

Smoking also affects the endocrine glands. Nicotine increases the amount of adrenal hormones on the average of 47% in a person who smokes cigarettes for 30 minutes.[23] Cigarette smoking is also connected with higher death rates from peptic ulcer, especially stomach ulcer. It reduces the effectiveness of the standard ulcer treatment and slows down healing of the ulcer.[16] Smoking two unfiltered cigarettes decreases the electrooculogram readings (the electric potential of the eyes) significantly.[24]

In a survey on 12,992 births, MacMahon and associates[25] showed that the birth weight of children decreases significantly with the amount of maternal smoking. The father's smoking did not affect the infant's weight. Carbon monoxide concentrations in blood of pregnant women are significantly higher in smokers than in nonsmokers.[26]

The above data indicate that smoking damages a wide variety of organs in addition to the lungs.

REFERENCES

1. Waldbott, G. L.: Smoker's respiratory syndrome: a clinical entity, J.A.M.A. **151**:1398-1400, 1953.
2. Diehl, H. S.: Tobacco and your health: the smoking controversy, New York, 1969, McGraw-Hill Book Co.
3. Abelson, P. H.: A damaging source of air pollution, Science **158**:1527, 1967.
4. Lefeve, N. M., and Inculet, I. I.: Particulates in domestic premises. Part I, Ambient levels and control air filtration, Arch. Environ. Health **32**:230-238, 1971.
5. Langer, A. M., Macklar, A. D., Rubin, I., and others: Inorganic particles in cigar and cigar smoke, Science **174**:585-587, 1971.
6. Newsome, J. R., Normal, V., and Keith, C. H.: Vapor phase analysis of tobacco smoke, Tobacco Sci. **9**:102-111, 1965.
7. Nandi, M., Gick, H., Slone, D., and others: Cadmium content of cigarettes, Lancet **2**:1329-1330, 1969.
8. Schroeder, H. A., Balassa, J. J., Gibson, F. S., and others: Abnormal trace metals in man: lead, J. Chron. Dis. **14**:408-425, 1961.
9. Oelschlager, W.: Personal communication, Universität Hohenheim, Stuttgart/Hohenheim, April, 1970.
10. Ullman, W. W.: Lead in the Connecticut environment, Conn. Med. **35**:360-362, 1971.
10a. Lewis, G. P., Jusko, W. J., Coughlin, L. L., and others: Contribution of cigarette smoking to cadmium accumulation in man, Lancet **1**:291-292, 1972.
11. Dalhamn, T., Rosengren, A., and Rylander, R.: Nasal absorption of organic matter in animal experiments. Part I, experimental technique and tobacco smoke absorption, Arch. Environ. Health **22**:554-556, 1971.
12. McLaughlin, R. R., and Tueller, E. E.: Anatomic and histologic changes of early emphysema, Chest **59**:592-599, 1971.
13. Naeye, R. L., Mahon, J. K., and Dellinger, W. S.: Effects of smoking on lung structures of Appalachian coal workers, Arch. Environ. Health **22**:190-193, 1971.
14. Wynder, E. L.: The epidemiology of cancer of the bronchus: facts and suppositions, Arch. Otolaryng. Rhinol. Laryngol. **76**:228-37, 1967.
15. Moore, C.: Cigarette smoking and cancer of the mouth, pharynx and larynx, J.A.M.A. **218**:553-558, 1971.
16. Facts: Smoking and health, National Clearinghouse for Smoking and Health, HSM Number 72-7508, Rockville, Maryland, Revised September 1971, U. S. Department of Health, Education, and Welfare, Public Health Service.
17. Hammond, E. C.: Smoking in relation to the death rates of 1 million men and women, Monograph 19, National Cancer Institute, January 1966, pp. 127-204.
18. Lambert, P. M., and Reid, D. D.: Smoking, air pollution, and bronchitis in Britain, Lancet **1**:853-857, 1970.
19. Savel, H.: Clinical hypersensitivity to cigarette smoke, Arch. Environ. Health **21**:146-148, 1970.
20. Doyle, J. T., Dawler, T. R., Kannel, W. B., and others: The relationship of cigarette smoking to coronary heart disease, J.A.M.A. **190**:108-112, 1964.
21. Johnson, H. J.: A study of 2400 electrograms of apparently healthy males, J.A.M.A. **114**:561, 1940.
22. Harkavy, J.: Tobacco allergy and cardiovascular disease: a review, Ann. Allerg. **26**:447-459, 1968.
23. Kershbaum, A., Pappajohn, D. J., Bellet, S., and others: Effect of smoking and nicotine on adrenocortical secretion, J.A.M.A. **203**:275-278, 1968.
24. Schmidt, B.: The effects of cigarette smoking on the EOG, Klin. Mbl. Augenheilk. **156**:523-31, 1970.
25. MacMahon, B., Alpert, M., and Salber, E. J.: Infant weight and parental smoking habits, Amer. J. Epidem. **82**:247-261, 1965.
26. Haddon, W., Jr., Nesbitt, R. E. L., and Garcia, R.: Smoking and pregnancy: carbon monoxide in blood during gestation and at term, Obstet. Gynec. **18**:262-267, 1961.

22
WATER POLLUTION

Since time immemorial man has used water for disposal of his wastes. In the year 4000 B.C. the palace of Knossos in Crete featured an elaborate drainage system that emptied into the Mediterranean Sea. Rome channeled its sewage into the Tiber river by means of aqueducts built to last for many centuries. During the Middle Ages, waste disposal systems in large European cities such as Paris and London served simultaneously as a dump and as a source of water supply with the result that epidemics of typhoid fever, cholera, and dysentery were rampant. Our own century has seen rivers, lakes, and oceans become the outlet for sewage and many other pollutants, particularly industrial wastes and detergents.

Two major pollutants, inorganic phosphates and nitrates, are playing the principal role in water pollution since, to date, our current water treatment procedures are not effective in removing them from sewage. Many other chemicals that contaminate the atmosphere are likewise present in water (Table 22-1). Damage to health arises directly through imbibing polluted water or indirectly through ingesting food, particularly fish, poisoned through the food chain.

The scope of water pollution comprises the following areas:

1. Waterborne viruses and bacteria
2. Waste heat
3. Radioactivity
4. Salinity and acidity
5. Eutrophication
6. Industrial pollutants

MICROORGANISMS

Throughout the early part of the twentieth century, such waterborne infections as typhoid fever and infectious enteritis were major causes of death.

An illness that can occasionally be spread through drinking water is infectious hepatitis, a virus disease associated with fever and jaundice. It often leads to permanent liver damage. In the presence of organic material, the viruses are unusually resistant to disinfection or to water treatment.

At the present time these diseases occur only sporadically. They are being controlled by strict sanitary engineering. Only during floods, earthquakes, and other great disasters is there a threat of waterborne epidemics.

Nevertheless a 1970 surveillance of 969 water systems in the United States covering 182 million persons showed that 90% of our water supply systems do not meet the criteria set up by the government for freedom from contamination.[1] The smallest communities, especially those with water supplies derived from springs and surface waters, had the poorest record. Of 22 communities with a population greater than 100,000, only 36% satisfied the surveillance criteria.

Table 22-1. Limits for contaminants in drinking water*

CONSTITUENTS	RECOMMENDED	MANDATORY
Alkyl benzene sulfonate	0.5 mg/liter	—
Arsenic	0.01 mg/liter	0.05 mg/liter
Barium	—	1.0 mg/liter
Boron	1.0 mg/liter	5.0 mg/liter
Cadmium	—	0.01 mg/liter
Chloride	250 mg/liter	—
Chromium (hexavalent)	—	0.05 mg/liter
Coliform organisms	—	0.01 ml
Cyanide	0.01 mg/liter	0.20 mg/liter
Fluoride	0.8—1.7 mg/liter†	1.4—2.4 mg/liter†
Gross beta activity	—	1000 pCi/liter
Iron	0.3 mg/liter	—
Lead	—	0.05 mg/liter
Manganese	0.05 mg/liter	—
Nitrate	45 mg/liter	—
Radium 226	3 pc/liter	—
Selenium	—	0.01 mg/liter
Strontium 90	10 pc/liter	—
Sulfate	250 mg/liter	—
TDS	500 mg/liter	—
Zinc	5 mg/liter	—

*Compiled from Community Water Supply Study, Analysis of National Survey Findings, July 1970, U. S. Department of Health, Education, and Welfare, Public Health Service, Environmental Health Service, Bureau of Water Hygiene.

†Established according to annual average temperatures.

WASTE HEAT

The temperature of water has a direct influence upon the toxicity of many pollutant chemicals and upon growth of microorganisms and viruses. Electricity generating plants dissipate considerable heat in the condensation of circulating water. Absorption of this heat is particularly troublesome when waste water is emitted into small rivers where it damages aquatic life. The use of large cooling towers has not solved this problem; when the cooling water returns to the river only a quarter to two thirds of the heat has been dissipated by evaporative cooling.[2] A temperature increase in river water to 12° F (6.7° C) within 1 mile of the cooling tower reduces plankton life for a distance of 10 to 12 miles downriver.[3] Removal of brush and shade trees along streams in rural areas was shown by Brown and Krygier[4] to cause a rise in annual maximum temperatures of streams from 57° to 85° F (14° to 30° C).

RADIOACTIVITY

In the vicinity of mining and milling activities, where radionuclides are used in industry, research, and commerce and where atomic bombs are being tested, radioactive materials have been released into waters. In late 1963, measurements at 128 stations in the United States revealed a rise of Strontium 90 levels in rivers from a low of less than 1 picocurie per liter (pc/liter) in 1960 to almost 4 pc/liter late in 1963.[5]* In 1965, following cessation of testing of atomic bombs, the level returned to about 1 pc/liter. Downstream from two uranium milling sites, the Colorado River showed a

---

*Drinking water standards permit a maximum concentration of 10 pc/liter.

significant rise in beta radioactivity with the greatest magnitude in the algae and successively less in mud and drinking water. Excessive concentrations of radioactive materials were noted at a distance of about 50 miles.[6] Although such levels do not constitute an immediate hazard to human health, continued accumulation of radionuclides in the bottom sediments and their concentration in the food chain, particularly in fish, may conceivably reach hazardous levels.

The waters of the Gulf of Mexico are constantly being contaminated by uranium from North American rivers at an estimated annual increase of 0.3 μg/liter.[7] In fifteen rivers flowing into the Gulf, uranium contrations ranged between 0.9 to 2.7 ppm. Uranium in the rivers is derived from their flow through uranium-bearing strata, the ore of which contains between 0.1% to 0.5%. In the Colorado River Basin, uranium waste piles leaked approximately 4,000 gm of Radium 226.[8] Although Uranium 238 itself is not taken up by vegetation, its radioactive decay products, namely Radium 226, Lead 210, and Plutonium 238, are readily absorbed by plants and thus constitute a potential hazard to humans.

SALINITY AND ACIDITY

Salinity of water refers to its total content of dissolved minerals. Soluble salts are either extracted from plants or enter the water naturally through springs that flow over rocks and through soil. Man-made sources of salinity include irrigation, domestic, and industrial effluents, drainage from mines, and oil wells.

A hardness above 100 ppm is troublesome to domestic users. Salts that exceed a few hundred parts per million affect the taste of water. Larger amounts may have long-term effects on people, especially on those afflicted with heart and kidney disease.

During recent years scientists have become concerned about the increasing acidity of rainwater and its effect on rivers and lakes.[9] Ordinarily rainwater is slightly acid with a pH of 5.7. The degree of acidity is regulated by carbon dioxide gas present in the atmosphere.[10] Recent studies have revealed much stronger acidity in rain and snow with pH values between 3 and 5.[9] This rise is attributed to increasing amounts of sulfuric and nitric acids, which are derived from sulfur dioxide and nitrogen oxides emitted into the atmosphere by combustion.

In Scandinavia,[11] where pH values in rainwater as low as 2.8 have been recorded,[9] sulfur is believed to drift in from industrialized regions of England and of the Ruhr Valley. In the United States, measurements in the range of 3.52 to 4.29 have been recorded in the Finger Lakes region of New York and in New Hampshire, particularly during winter months when greater local combustion of fossil fuels takes place.[12]

The effect of this newly observed phenomenon on the ecosystem is difficult to forsee. Sampling stations in Scandinavia have shown a trend toward a rising acidity in almost all lakes and rivers between 1965 to 1970.[13] Although other pollutants dumped into the aquatic ecosystems must be taken into account as a contributing factor, "unpolluted" rivers showed increases in acidity by 1.4 times during the same 5 years. In southern Norway salmon eggs no longer develop and salmon runs have been eliminated, presumably as the result of increase in the water's acidity. Swedish ecologists have felt that the acid rainfall has also affected the forest growth in their country.

EUTROPHICATION

The process of fertilizing waters with mineralized nutrients, mainly phosphates and nitrates, is termed eutrophication. It leads to excess growth of algae and rooted water plants. Respiration of these plants and their decay consumes oxygen that is vital to fish and other aquatic life. Thus, eutrophication renders water less desirable for domestic, industrial, and recreational uses as well as for fish and wildlife.

Sites

Impounded waters such as small lakes, slowly flowing rivers, or dammed reservoirs are predilective sites for eutrophication; the coastal areas of large lakes and rivers, especially the portion below the point of waste discharge from large cities, are highly susceptible to overfertilization. A favorite site is the estuary where a river enters the sea. Here, the interaction of river flow, tides, and coastal currents combine to settle sediment that had been held in suspension down river for long distances. As the river slows down upon its entrance into the estuary, the suspended material is deposited in mud and sand. It attracts algae and plankton, which thrive in salt and brackish marsh.

The planktonic blue-green algae that accumulate along the shores of slow-moving waters produce ill-smelling and decaying scum that is toxic to domestic and wild life. The identity of the principal toxin released by decaying algae has not been determined, in spite of considerable research.

Oysters, clams, crabs, and terrapins as well as a wide variety of water birds, feed on the nutrient material. River estuaries are also excellent nursery grounds for coastal fishes. Much of the harvest of seafood in the United States is composed of species that pass through or whose existence depends on, this entrance zone enroute to spawning grounds.

Phosphates

In hard carbonate lakes, the concentration of total phosphorus in the surface waters in summer ranges usually between 0.02 to 0.1 ppm.[2] In alkaline lakes, whose hardness is above 240 ppm of calcium carbonate, phosphate concentrations are particularly high. They give rise to extensive growth of blue-green algal blooms.

The high phosphorus concentrations of sewage is largely attributable to the use of detergents. Phosphates are added to detergents for a threefold purpose: (1) in combination with calcium and other dissolved minerals, they soften wash water; (2) they maintain a desirable level of alkalinity in water; and (3) they act as a "surfactant" and loosen dirt in clothing. Liquid detergents contain 20% to 30% polyphosphates; in some locations, as much as half of the phosphorus in sewage effluents is derived from detergents. Nitrates, however, leach through the soil and, therefore, reach the drainage waters more readily than phosphorus.

Nitrogen compounds

Nitrates. The nitrates are taken up by plants almost as rapidly as they appear in water. Vegetables and drinking water constitute our major source of nitrates. In addition nitrates are used as food additives in the meat-curing process. Ordinarily nitrate-nitrogen concentrations in lakes and other impounded waters tend to be below 0.1 ppm.[14] In well water, health agencies have established a limit of 10 ppm, but this concentration is frequently exceeded.[15]

Nitrates accumulate in water through *natural* run-off and through seepage from the soil, particularly if it is porous and if the water table is underlain by solid rock formation. In streams draining from farm lands, nitrate levels are higher than in drainage water from forests. Rain also provides an appreciable amount of nitrogen. Furthermore, wild animals, water fowl, and fish fertilize water with their excrement, which is high in nitrogen.

The major man-made sources of nitrates are sewage and wastes from domestic animals, from ships and boats, garbage, drainage from land fertilized with agricultural chemicals, industrial wastes, and remnants of manufactured chemical products. Shallow wells are susceptible to contamination by nitrates caused by seepage from septic tanks, from manure that has been spread on porous soil, and from run-off and seepage from cattle feed lots.

In the quantities normally occurring in water and food, nitrates are rapidly excreted by the human organism and are not toxic. If imbibed in sufficient quantities, they form the starting point for a chain of reactions resulting in toxic substances. In the digestive tract of humans and animals, the nitrates are reduced to nitrites by some of the common intestinal bacteria, particularly the coli bacillus. The nitrites are by far the most dangerous compounds.

Occasionally in cattle, nitrates cause enteritis (inflammation of the bowels) and diarrhea before they are converted into nitrites. Under certain conditions, further conversion takes place from nitrites to the harmless ammonium form and subsequently, to amino acids and proteins. When this conversion procedes with sufficient rapidity, ingested nitrates may have little apparent effect.[16]

Nitrites. Nitrites, formed in the bowels, are responsible for two important changes in the human body: they transform the oxygen-carrying oxyhemoglobin of the blood to methemoglobin. Thus, they interfere with release of oxygen to the cells of the body. This inhibition of cell breathing induces a bluish discoloration of the skin, a condition known as cyanosis. Nitrate-nitrogen levels in water above 8 to 9 ppm can precipitate this illness. The Public Health Service recommends restriction of the daily intake of nitrites in man to 0.4 mg/kg body weight.[17]

The other effect of nitrites is their capacity to dilate capillary blood vessels, which induces stagnation of the circulating blood and increases the oxygen hunger of the organism.

The diagnosis of nitrite intoxication is usually difficult, particularly in adults. Increase in the heart and respiration rates, shortness of breath, excess production of saliva, weakness, subnormal temperature, and a progressively bluish-dark discoloration of the skin characterize the illness.

Some victims manifest listlessness, diarrhea, and frequent urination.

Infants too young to consume solid foods are particularly subject to nitrite cyanosis and to methemoglobinemia caused by nitrates in drinking water. The U. S. Public Health Service considers more than 45 ppm nitrates in water unsafe for infant feeding. Boiling of water and the concomitant evaporation causes the concentration of nitrates in the remaining water to rise and thereby increases their tendency to induce cyanosis. In adults, the major discomfort from nitrates is diarrhea.

Carlson and Shapiro[18] reported the case of a 56-year-old Minnesota farmer with a kidney disease who began home dialysis (treatment with the artificial kidney for the purpose of dialyzing harmful metabolic products out of the system). The patient developed nausea, vomiting, sleepiness, weakness, and low blood pressure. After he had terminated the dialysis in February 1969, the vomiting and mental confusion persisted; he remained cyanosed (blue); his arterial blood appeared to be black. Upon discovering that the nitrate-nitrogen content of his well water was as high as 94 ppm, it became apparent that nitrates from the water used in the kidney machine had been transferred to the bloodstream and thence into the bowels. Carlson and Shapiro considered it likely that the nitrates, which were reduced by intestinal microorganisms to nitrites, were subsequently reabsorbed into the bloodstream. The patient's condition was aggravated by the fact that he had a low red blood count of the kind usually associated with chronic kidney failure, which further reduced the oxygen transport into the body tissues. This patient recovered promptly upon receiving intravenous injections of a solution of methylene blue, the antidote for nitrite poisoning.

Other nitrogen compounds. Nitrilotriacetic acid (NTA) has been recommended and used in the United States and in Sweden as a substitute for phosphates. About

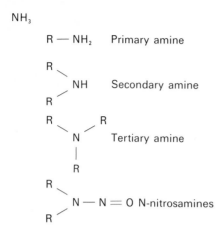

Fig. 22-1. Formula for nitrosamines.

90% of NTA is converted to nitrite and nitrate. Thus, the substitute for phosphates in detergents is another agent causing eutrophication.[19] Furthermore NTA accumulates in bones. Although its toxicity is relatively low, it is a chelating agent and can dissolve and mobilize heavy metals such as mercury from lake sediment, which reach the human organism. NTA, a tertiary amine (Fig. 22-1), breaks down to secondary amines particularly to iminodiacetic acid and then to primary amines. During this process, secondary amines combine with nitrites in acid conditions to form the carcinogenic nitrosamines[20] (See Chapter 16).

WATER POLLUTION BY INDUSTRIAL PRODUCTS

The number of chemical substances in water derived from industry is legion. We have already pointed to the chemicals present in agricultural soils, mainly fertilizers and spray residues that reach the water through run-off or seepage through soil. Other modes of contamination such as the pollution of lakes by airborne mercury, by windblown dust near chemical factories, or from airborne volatile pesticides have also been discussed.

The three principal modes of contamination by chemicals are:

1. Discharge of wash water and industrial wastes
2. Dumping of trash and debris into bodies of water
3. Oil spills

Waste discharge

The direct dumping of chemicals into rivers and seas has been practiced by certain industries for many years. As long ago as 1950, an Oregon farmer's family, beef cattle, and farmland sustained serious injury as the result of a Vancouver, Washington, aluminum company having dumped 1000 to 7000 pounds of fluoride waste each month into the Columbia River.[21]

According to the 1958 statistics, 84% of all water used by United States industry during the course of that year was discharged into waterways by four major industries producing paper, chemicals, primary metals (in contrast to metals reprocessed from scrap), and petroleum.[22] They accounted for 91% of all brackish water. Only one-fourth of all wastes discharged by the four industries received any sort of treatment prior to discharge.[22] Most of the above-mentioned industries are concentrated at seashores or on large rivers, namely the paper industry in the Pacific Northwest and in the southeastern states of Alabama and Mississippi; chemical plants in the Gulf and middle Atlantic states; the petroleum industries in New Jersey, Louisiana, Texas, and California. The wastes are derived directly from the manufacturing process; in many instances, they constitute the contaminated wash water from air pollution control devices. Use of wet collectors enhances the total quantity of liquid waste that must be discharged into water courses.

Some industries conduct their wastes into artificially produced lagoons where they are treated and subsequently metered into rivers or lakes.[23] Effluent water from such an artificial lagoon at a southwest Florida fertilizer facility (Fig. 22-2) contained up to 21,500 ppm phosphates and 5150 ppm fluo-

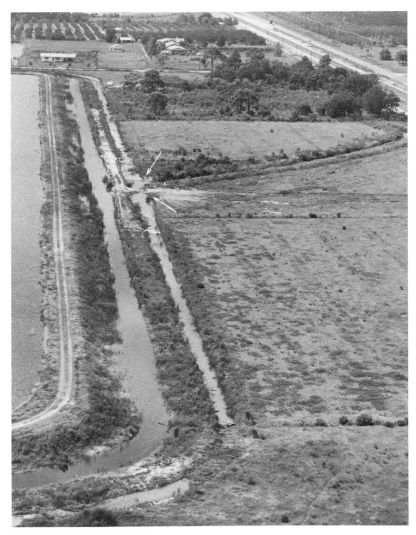

Fig. 22-2. Aerial photograph of a wall break (arrows) in an artificial southwest Florida lagoon. The effluent was highly acid (pH 1.6 to 1.8). Water from a phosphate fertilizer plant contained high concentrations of fluoride and phosphates. (Photograph by Tim Murphy.)

ride.[24] The high acidity of the water (pH 1.6 to 1.8) rendered it especially harmful to the environment. In summer, when the water levels of these lagoons recede, dust containing the chemical wastes is blown from their edges into the air and is dispersed by the wind.

Even more serious damage occurs when there is a break in the retention dam of such dikes as, for instance, in the December 3, 1971, dam break near Arcadia, Florida.[25] About three billion gallons of sludge, at some places three feet high, were released from the two-hundred acre pond into the Peace River. It killed an estimated 1,956,-000[26] fish as well as a complete crop harvest near the seafood center of Charlotte Harbor. Five secondary state roads, as well as pasture lands in the area, were covered by the sludge. Bird life, alligators, water insects, and reptiles were adversely affected by the spill. Damage to human health is bound to ensue because of consumption of contaminated produce, or because of direct intake of fluoride. Less severe breaks had occurred in the 10 years prior to this episode.[25]

Some of the most publicized water pollution episodes in recent years are mercury contamination of the Great Lakes caused by discharge from manufacturing of chlorine and other chemicals, nickel contamination of rivers from the automobile industry, cadmium and cobalt pollution released from metal smelting. Chemical water pollutants associated with petroleum by-products are oil, cement, white lime, and caustic soda. In Texas, hydrocyanic acid and lactonitrile have killed gulf-coast fishes and invertebrates within 24 hours at levels below 0.3 ppm.[22] In Florida, because of an increasing number of superphosphate plants on the Peace River, the fluoride content, at ten different locations from Bartow to Fort Ogden 1957 through 1961 ranged between 0.5 to 46 ppm.[27]

In a relatively uncontaminated area at Narragansett Bay, Rhode Island, an extremely thin layer of coherent film ranging from 100 to 150 μm contained surface-active substances such as fatty acids and fatty alcohols. In this film, lead, iron, nickel, copper, fatty acids, hydrocarbons, and chlorinated hydrocarbons were found in concentrations 1.5 to 50 times higher than in the water 20 cm below the surface. These agents are believed to reach the water surface through atmospheric transport, through rivers, sewage, and industrial effluents, dumping, and spills. Since they are readily accessible to bacteria, plankton, and other microorganisms these pollutants initially at the surface will enter the food chain and eventually become concentrated in higher animals.[28]

Angino and co-workers[29] of the Kansas Geologic Survey found 2 to 8 ppb arsenic in the Kansas River, which approaches the

Table 22-2. Water supplies tested for toxic ingredients*

	NUMBER OF SYSTEMS EXCEEDING CONSTITUENT LIMIT	PERCENT OF ALL WATER SUPPLIES STUDIED
Arsenic	2	1
Barium	1	1
Cadmium	3	1
Chromium (hexavalent)	4	1
Colibacillus	120	12
Fluoride	24	2
Lead	14	1
Selenium	5	1

*Compiled from Community Water Supply Study, Analysis of National Survey Findings, July 1970, U. S. Department of Health, Education and Welfare, Public Health Service, Environmental Health Service, Bureau of Water Hygiene.

Public Health Service limit of 10 ppb. It is believed to originate from detergents that contain arsenic levels as high as 72 ppm.

Among the 969 water systems tested for toxic ingredients in 1970, the numbers listed in Table 22-2 exceed the mandatory limits.

These are but a few instances of gross chemical pollution from industrial wastes.

Application of pesticides to agricultural land constitutes another significant source of water pollution. The extent of contamination usually corresponds closely to the amount applied. The water-soluble pesticides are detectable in samples of tap water, whereas the less soluble agents (for instance, DDT) accumulate in the bottom of rivers and lakes (see Chapter 18).

Dumping of trash and debris

Tires, tin cans, market baskets, useless lumber, paper, and plastic boxes are often discharged into rivers and lakes. Near Washington, D. C., about 150 tons of debris are being retrieved from the Potomac River every 6 months.[3] Little, if any, information is available on the possible increase in viral and bacterial contamination resulting from dumping such material into waters.

The National Institute of Public Health of the Netherlands in Utrecht[23] analyzed 80 samples from drums containing chemical wastes, which had been "caught" by Dutch fishermen during their fishing operations in the North Sea. Other drums have been washed ashore along the Dutch coast. These drums contained very toxic agents including endosulfan and derivatives, trichlorotoluidines, dichlorotoluidines, dichloronitrobenzenes, and other products.

An example of poisoning of aquatic life caused by dumping wherein thousands of fish, frogs, snakes, tadpoles, and worms died, occurred in a little waterway called Crooked Creek south of the Missouri town of Troy.[8] A pest control operator had disposed of some excess material. He pulled his truck off the main road and dumped the chemical on the ground in a shady spot, 100 yards from the creek into which it seeped. The cargo contained chlordane, malathion mixed with xylen, a preparation to control termites.

Oil spills

Pollution of coastal waters has become a threat to marine life as a result of oil spills either through accidents of oil-carrying freighters or through eruptions of oil during off-shore drilling operations.

On January 28, 1969, for instance, an off-shore oil well in California's Santa Barbara Channel erupted when operators tried to replace a drilling rig.[30] The oil, which escaped at the rate of 1500 barrels an hour for 11 days blackened 40 miles of southern California's beaches and formed an oil slick of 400 square miles in the Pacific Ocean. The noxious fumes were found 1000 feet above sea level.[30]

On February 13, 1970, the Greek tanker Delian Apollon, while attempting to maneuver into a Florida oil port during a dense fog, ran aground in Tampa Bay. Before tugs could get the tanker off the sandbar, some 10,000 gallons of heavy oil had spilled into the Bay through the ship's ruptured hull. In the notorious Torrey Canyon shipwreck of 1967, in the English Channel, about 100,000 tons of crude oil were lost.

During a 3-year period, 1964 to 1967, 91 tankers were stranded in various parts of the world and 238 vessels were involved in collisions with tankers and other vessels. In 39 cases cargo spillage or leakage occurred.[31] The yearly spill of petroleum from tankers and other commercial vessels into the ocean is estimated to amount to 3½ million tons.[32]

Scientists[33] at the Woods Hole Massachusetts Oceanographic Institution pointed out that disappearance of visible evidence of an oil spill on the surface of the sea does not coincide with the disappearance of biologic damage. Crude oil and oil products are not readily biodegraded (broken down to simple substances) by bacteria. They settle unaltered to the bottom of the ocean and are retained in the mud for many months. Particularly, the more toxic aromatic hydrocarbons that are not being detoxified by bacteria remain in the sediments.

Moreover, oil-laden sediments can move with bottom current and contaminate unpolluted areas off shore long after the initial accident. Thus the sea bottom in wide areas near an oil spill remains toxic to animals for long periods following the initial spill.

Furthermore oil (just as the fat of fish and shellfish) concentrates other fat-soluble poisons such as many insecticides and chemical intermediates.[34] When this material is taken up by plankton and algae it is likely to reach edible seafood and, eventually, constitute danger to human health.

The numerous modes of water contamination are apt to induce illness either by direct consumption of contaminated water or through the food chain. Short of an epidemic of illness of catastrophic proportion, it is rarely possible for a physician or for the patient himself to recognize its source.

REFERENCES

1. Community Water Supply Study: Analysis of national survey findings, July 1970, U. S. Department of Health, Education and Welfare, Public Health Service Environmental Health Service, Bureau of Water Hygiene.
2. Water quality. In Restoring the quality of our environment, Report of the Environmental Pollution Panel, President's Science Advisory Committee, Appendix X7, The White House, November 1965, p. 71.
3. Wolman, M. G.: The nation's rivers, Science **174**:905-918, 1971.
4. Brown, G. W., and Krygier, J. T.: Effect of clear cutting on stream temperature, Water Resour. Res. **6**:1133-39, 1970.
5. Water pollution surveillance system, annual compilation of data 1962-1963. Public Health Service, Publ. No. 663, 1963, p. 5.
6. Morgan, J. M., Jr.: A stream survey in the uranium mining and milling area of the Colorado Plateau, Colorado and Gunnison Rivers. Baltimore, 1959, Johns Hopkins University.
7. Spalding, R. F., and Sackett, W. M.: Uranium in run-off from the Gulf of Mexico, distributive province: anomalous concentrations, Science **170**:629-631, 1971.
8. Novick, S.: Radioactive mining wastes, Environment **8**:10-15, 1966.
9. Likens, G. E., Bormann, F. H., and Johnson, N. M.: Acid rain, Environment **14**:33-40, 1972.
10. Barrett, E., and Brodin, G.: The acidity of Scandinavian precipitation, Tellus **7**:251-257, 1955.
11. Engström, A.: Air pollution across national boundaries: the impact on the environment of sulfur in air and precipitation. Report of the Swedish Preparatory Committee for the U. N. Conference on Human Environment. Stockholm, 1971, Kungl. Boktryckeriet P. A. Norstedt et Söner, p. 96.
12. Pearson, F. J. Jr., and Fisher, D. W.: Chemical composition of atmospheric precipitation in the northeastern United States, Geol. Surv. Supply Paper 1535-P, 1971, pp. 23.
13. Odén, S., and Ahl, T.: The acidification of Scandinavian lakes and rivers, Ymer, Årsbok, 1970, pp. 103-122.
14. Moyle, J. B.: Aquatic Blooms. In Restoring the quality of our environment. Report of the Environmental Pollution Panel, President's Science Advisory Committee, Appendix Y9, November 1965, The White House, p. 178.
15. Wolff, I. A., and Wasserman, A. E.: Nitrates, nitrites, and nitrosamines, Science **177**:15-19, 1972.
16. Hanway, J. J., Herrick, J. B., Willrich, T. L., and others: The nitrate problem, Ames, Iowa, August 1963, Iowa State University of Science and Tech. Cooperative Extension Service on Agriculture and Home Economics, Special Report Number 34.
17. Orgerson, J. D., Martin, J. D., Caraway, C. T., and others: Methemoglobinemia from eating meat with high nitrite content, Public Health Rep. **72**:189-193, 1957.
18. Carlson, D. J., and Shapiro, F. L.: Methemoglobinemia from well water: a complication of hemodialysis, Ann. Intern. Med. **73**:757-759, 1970.
19. Thomson, F. E., anl Duthie, J. R.: The biodegradability and treatability of NTA, J. Water Pollut. Contr. Fed. **40**:306, 1968.
20. Lijinsky, W., and Epstein, S. S.: Nitrosamines as environmental carcinogens, Nature **225**: 21, 1970.
21. Oregon rancher asks $200,000 of aluminum co., The Seattle Times, December 16, 1952.
22. Pimentel, D.: Effects of pollutants on living organisms other than man. In Restoring the Quality of Our Environment, Report of the Environmental Pollution Panel, President's Science Advisory Committee, Appendix Y10, November 1965, The White House.
23. Greve, P. A.: Chemical wastes in the sea: new forms of marine pollution, Science **173**:1021-1022, 1971.
24. Cross, F. L., and Ross, R. W.: Fluoride emissions from phosphate processing plants, Fluoride **2**:97-105, 1969.
25. Spill seen costing $1 million in crabs, Fort Myers News-Press, December 9, 1971, p. 1.
26. Peace River given over to buzzards. Fort Myers News-Press, December 12, 1971, p. 1.
27. Memorandum: Lamar Johnson, Consulting Engineer to Peace River Valley Water Conservation and Drainage District, Bartow, Florida, November, 1961.
28. Duce, R. A., Quinn, J. G., Olney, C. E., and others: Enrichment of heavy metals and organic compounds in the surface microlayer of Narragansett Bay, Rhode Island, Science **176**:161-163, 1972.
29. Angino, E. E., Magnuson, L. M., Waugh, T. C., and others: Arsenic in detergents: possible danger and pollution hazard, Science **168**:389-390, 1970.
30. Environmental tragedy in oil, Time, Feb. 14, 1969, pp. 23-24.

31. Gerber, W.: Coastal conservation, Editorial Research Rep. **1:**141-149, 1970.
32. Blumer, M.: Scientific aspects of the oil spills problem. Paper presented at the Oil Spills Conference Committee on Challenges of Modern Society, N.A.T.O., Brussels, 1970.
33. Blumer, M., Sanders, H. L., Grassle, J. F., and others: A small oil spill, Environment **13:**2-12, 1971. (Contribution number 2630 of the Woods Hole Oceanographic Institution.)
34. Hartung, R., and Klinger, G. W.: Concentration of DDT by sedimented polluting oils, Environ. Sci. Technol. **4:**407, 1970.

23
FIRES

Individual fires as well as mass fires are important sources of atmospheric pollution. As already indicated, during any kind of combustion a vast variety of agents is emitted into the air as gases, smoke, and particulates in combination with heat, the dominating factor. The composition of the combustion products, the wind velocities,* the concentrations of the materials being burned, and the location of a fire determine its role as an air pollutant.

The U. S. Armed Forces have made extensive studies,[1] particularly of the results of the great fires in Japan and Germany during World War II, which were produced by incendiary bombs, and of the major fires that occurred naturally in the United States and elsewhere during the past century. Heat was the foremost cause of serious damage to human health. The other source of high mortality was the wide variety of gases and dusts evolved by fires. Damage to the lungs and other organs developed immediately upon exposure to the fire; subsequently the delayed effects became apparent.

HEAT

In a burning structure, particularly on the upwind side, the temperatures are likely

to be in excess of 1090° C (2000° F). Free-standing fuel as, for instance, fallen timbers piled with rubble burns faster and hotter than enclosed material because oxygen has free access to it. Fuel not readily exposed to oxygen reaches its highest temperature more slowly and burns longer. Temperatures above 2000° F occur only for short periods over small sites at very specific locations. They are not nearly as damaging as the lower temperatures that are encountered over extended areas for prolonged periods of time.

Transfer of heat. Heat is transferred to a human being by means of hot air, by direct contact with hot objects (conduction), and by radiation from hot surfaces and gases.[2] Radiant heat is largely dependent on the distance from the original fire. The U. S. Forest Service has recorded radiation intensities of 0.2 calories per cm per second at distances of 90 feet from burning fuel.[3] Heat radiation rises quickly to its peak with the fire and falls off promptly as the fire dies.

Conductive heat in burning and smoldering debris will prolong a fire and ignite new areas, particularly when free-standing timber collapses.

Health effect of heat. According to Buettner[4] the pain threshold of the skin ranges between 42° and 46° C (108° and 115° F). Burns will occur whenever the skin exceeds 54° C (129° F). In experiments on goats and dogs, Moritz and associates[5] observed se-

---

*Wind speeds in the 1906 San Francisco fire varied from 20 miles per hour (mph) to a low of 5 mph and then back up to 26 mph. In the great Chicago fire, wind velocities from 4 to 7 mph were reported.

vere pulmonary edema that was not related to inhalation of hot air but to circulatory failure incidental to systemic hyperthermia (overheating of the body). High temperatures are usually associated with intolerable pain.[6]

KINDS OF POLLUTANTS

Carbon monoxide. Among the numerous air pollutants released during combustion, carbon monoxide is the most abundant one. The magnitude of its emission depends on the chemical composition of the fuel, the amount of oxygen present, and the temperature in and around the combustion zone.[7,8] In the immediate area of burning material, extremely high levels of carbon monoxide are found. However, they endure for short periods only and their concentration decreases rapidly with increasing distances from the fire. In open fires, the highest carbon monoxide level recorded at horizontal distances of 9 feet or greater, has been 0.08%. In enclosed fires, concentrations of carbon monoxide are higher and persist longer.

Oxygen. The other dangerous feature of a fire is the low oxygen levels in the air. Under certain conditions, they can reach near zero for short periods. Low atmospheric oxygen starves the blood and tissues of oxygen and can thus lead to death.

Inspired air normally contains 20.9% oxygen, whereas the oxygen content of expired air is 15.4%. The difference is caused by combustion of oxygen in body tissues. Insufficient oxygen in the air, as may happen in a fire, causes so-called anoxia and hypoxia (absence or low oxygen supply) of the blood. There are three typical stages:

During the *first* stage, breathing becomes rapid. In the *second* stage, respiration grows irregular and convulsive. The patient may lose consciousness. The skin, especially the face, turns into a gray color as opposed to the blue coloring that is characteristic of asphyxia (strangulation). In the *third* stage, collapse and convulsions occur in the extremities; the respiration becomes shallow; face, neck, and body become rigid and arched backward. The pulse is slow and respiration stops.[9] Persons inhaling less than 10% oxygen fall into a stupor; their bodies became weak and they become somewhat euphoric (a feeling of well-being).[10] A good test for a low oxygen content of the air is the behavior of a lighted candle: when the atmospheric oxygen falls below 17.5% (normal 20.9%), the light is extinguished.

Carbon dioxide. Carbon dioxide is not considered a toxic gas ordinarily. As little as 2% in the inspired air stimulates respiration; at 3% the ventilation of the lungs is doubled.[11] At 4.5% to 5% carbon dioxide, breathing becomes extremely labored and nausea occurs. When air contains 8.5% carbon dioxide, the blood pressure is no longer obtainable, breathing becomes difficult, and the lungs become congested. A concentration of 7% to 10% carbon dioxide in the air is fatal in a short period.[12] Since carbon dioxide is usually associated with the absence of oxygen and the presence of car-

Table 23-1. Concentrations of chemicals in the flue gases in ppm by volume of dry gas, corrected to 12% carbon dioxide*

COMPONENT	PPM
Nitric oxide, NO	53.0—115
Sulfur dioxide, SO_2	55.7—195
Chloride, Cl	214—1250
Cyanide, CN	0.02—0.10
Fluoride, F	2.6—34.2
Phosphate, PO_4	0.36—6.3
Organic acids as CH_3COOH	35.1—178
Aldehydes and ketones as CH_2O	1.25—12.6
Phosgene, $COCl_2$	0.5
Chlorine, Cl_2	0.2

*Compiled from Carotti, A. A., and Kaiser, E. R.: Concentrations of twenty gaseous chemical species in the flue gas of a municipal incinerator, J. Air Pollut. Contr. Ass. **22:**248-253, 1972.

bon monoxide, it is difficult to establish clearly the effects of either gas.

Other gases. Which additional gases are emitted from a given fire is a complex question, because the number of chemicals and other materials present in a burning structure is legion. They include chlorine, hydrogen chloride, carbonyl chloride ($COCl_2$), hydrogen cyanate (HCN), ammonia (NH_3), hydrogen sulfide (H_2S), and nitrogen oxides.[1] During the burning of a large rubber warehouse, for instance, large quantities of hydrogen sulfide and sulfur dioxide are freed; a woolen mill, during burning, emits hydrogen cyanide and a plant producing chlorinated products generates chlorine gases.

Smoke, another major atmospheric pol-

Table 23-2. Illness caused by combustion of plastics

NAME	SOFTENS WHEN HEATED TO	DECOMPOSITION PRODUCTS	SYMPTOMS
Acrylic plastic $\left(-CH_2-CH-\atop \quad\quad OAc\right)_n$ or $\left(CH_2-\underset{\;}{\overset{CH_3}{\underset{OAc}{C}}}-\right)_n$	121° C (250° F)	Hydrochloric acid Carbon monoxide	Irritability Headache Anorexia Somnolence Hypotension
Polyethylene $-(CH_2-CH_2)_n$	100° to 127° C (212° to 260° F)	Paraffin hydrocarbons	
Polystyrene $-(CH-CH_2)_n$	250° to 350° C (482° to 662° F)	Styrene Styrene	Headache Fatigue Nausea Vomiting Drowsiness
Polyurethane $-(\overset{O}{\overset{\|}{C}}-O-R-O-\overset{O}{\overset{\|}{C}}-NH-R_1-NH)_n$	150° to 250° C	Diisocyanates Glycols, polyols, amines, carbon monoxide, carbon dioxide	Asthma Nasal and eye irritation Hives
Polyvinyl chloride $-(CH_2-CH)_n \atop \quad\quad\; Cl$	300° C (572° F)	Hydrochloric acid Carbon monoxide, carbon dioxide	Pulmonary irritants Headaches, drowsiness
Polyvinyl acetate $-(CH_2-CH)_n \atop \quad\quad\;\; OAc$	250° C (482° F)	Vapors of acetic acid	
Polyvinyl alcohol $-(CH_2-CH)_n \atop \quad\quad\;\; OH$	200° C (392° F)	At temp. below 170° C narcotic ethers are formed	Drowsiness
Polyvinyl methyl ether $-(CH_2-CH)_n \atop \quad\quad\;\;\; OCH_3$	195° to 320° C (382° to 608° F)	Monomers, alcohol Alcohols	

lutant released by fire, irritates the eyes and produces pharyngitis and tracheitis. During combustion of refuse plastics a wide variety of poisonous chemicals is released into the atmosphere. Table 23-2 presents a tabulation of the major plastics, their decomposition products, and the symptoms that they induce.

It is evident from the foregoing discussion that aside from damage to lungs by heat, a variety of toxic gases, especially carbon monoxide and lack of oxygen, are the foremost sources of illness and death.

REFERENCES

1. Pryor, A. J., and Yuill, C. H.: Mass fire life hazard, Defense Document Center, September 1966, Defense Supply Agency, AD 642 790.
2. Buettner, K., and Richey, E. O.: Effects of extreme heat on man. Part IV, mechanism of heat transfer in an open gasoline fire, Project No. 21-26-002, July 1951, USAF School of Aviation Medicine.
3. Countrymen, C. M.: Mass fires and fire behavior, USFS PSW—19, 1964.
4. Buettner, K.: Effects of extreme heat on man, Part III, Surface temperature, pain, and heat conductivity of living skin in experiments with radiant heat, USAF School of Aviation Medicine, Project No. 21-26-002, 1951.
5. Moritz, A. R., Henriques, F. C., Henriques, F. C., Jr., and others: Studies of thermal injury. Part IV. Arch. Path. 43:22, 1947.
6. Webb, P.: Aerodynamics heating. Mechanical Engineering 82:60-62, 1960.
7. Easton, W. H.: Smoke and fire gases, Industr. Med. 11:3, 1942.
8. Easton, W. H.: Irritating vapors produced by burning cellulosic materials. J. Industr. Hyg. Toxicol. 27:211-216, 1945.
9. Sollman, T.: Systemic action of gases: A manual of pharmacology, ed. 7, Philadelphia, 1948, W. B. Saunders Co., pp. 693-711.
10. Kraines, S. H.: The correlation of oxygen deprivation with intelligence, constitution and blood pressure, Amer. J. Psychiat. 93:1435-1446, 1937.
11. Viessman, W.: Air conditioning for protective shelters, Heating, Piping and Air Conditioning, December 1954.
12. Yuill, C. H., and Bieberdorf, F. W.: An investigation of the hazards of combustion products in building fires. Report Project 3-1273-3 SwRI, Contract No. PH86-62-208, San Antonio, Texas, October 1963, U. S. Public Health Service.

24
PROPHYLAXIS AND TREATMENT

Of all the illnesses in which prevention can accomplish more than treatment, disease caused by air pollution is paramount. Indeed, once a person has developed emphysema, crippling arthritis, hypertension, liver or kidney damage from long-term exposure to a pollutant, relatively few therapeutic measures are effective.

In reviewing prophylactic measures to combat airborne disease I shall consider the role of the physician, of the patient, of industry, and of government.

THE PHYSICIAN

During the last three decades, a new medical discipline pertaining to the study of environmental diseases has developed. Unfortunately, this area of medicine has not as yet made very much impact upon the medical practitioners who are not engaged in this particular specialty.

Recognition of disease caused by air pollution

Such minor ailments as intermittent sore throats, cough, dizzy spells, stomach upsets, or merely general weakness (for which the usual routine laboratory procedures have failed to give a clue to the diagnosis) do not necessarily represent evidence of a low-grade infection, an endocrine disorder, a vitamin deficiency, or a psychosomatic ailment; such manifestations can be the early signs of a slowly progressive illness caused by air pollutants.

Neither is the other cardinal feature of airborne illness sufficiently appreciated, namely that ingestion of contaminated food and water might be of equal if not greater significance than inhalation of contaminated air.

Lack of diagnostic tools

Diagnostic tools to establish the effects of air pollutants are not readily available to the average physician. Expansion of laboratory facilities is needed in order to make them readily accessible to practicing physicians and to community hospitals so that they will have the means to establish proof of adverse health effects by pollutants. Only a few physicians, when they encounter a chronic unexplained disease, habitually analyze urine, blood, body tissues, food, drinking water, and ambient air for pollutants that prevail in the area of the patient's residence. Most laboratories that carry out such assays are attached to industrial establishments and to scientific institutions to which the practicing physician has no ready access. Poisoning centers have been established in recent years in large United States communities. However, they deal mainly with acute intoxication, not with the chronic, slowly developing disease the cause of which is difficult to pinpoint.

Documentation of health hazards

As pointed out repeatedly, the slow insidious onset of most environmental diseases,

Table 24-1. Manifestations of the principal pollutants (at large doses)

MANIFESTATION	POLLUTANT
Aging (premature)	Ozone; PAN; other oxidants, radiation
Alopecia (loss of hair)	Lead, arsenic, radiation
Anemia	Lead, molybdenum, vanadium
Asthma	
Allergic	Fungi, pollen; TDI, cobalt, epoxy resins,
Nonallergic	respiratory pollutants
Ataxia	Manganese, mercury, lead
Bone disease	Strontium, fluorides
Brain involvement	Boron, carbon monoxide, lead, mercury, zinc
Bronchitis	Irritating gases
Cancer	
Abdomen	Nickel carbonate
Bones	Strontium
Gallbladder	Nitrosamines
Lungs	Asbestos, beryllium, nickel carbonate
	benzo[a]pyrene
Nose, sinuses	Selenium, nickel carbonate, chromium, strontium
Skin	Arsenic
Testicles	Cadmium
Coronary heart disease	Carbon monoxide, cadmium, hydrogen
	sulfide
Cyanosis	Nitrites, carbon monoxide
Dental caries	Selenium
Dermatitis	Nickel, chromium, arsenic, formaldehyde,
	organophosphates
Emphysema	Most respiratory pollutants
Eye irritation	Ozone, PAN, formaldehyde, nitrogen
	oxides, acrolein, ammonia
Fever	Manganese, zinc, boron, other metals
Fibrosis (scarring) of lungs	Quartz, silica, selenium, cobalt, iron
Gastroenteritis	Lead, mercury, fluorides, arsenic, zinc,
	selenium
Hypertension, arteriosclerosis	Cadmium, barium, organophosphates,
	carbon monoxide
Headaches	Lead, fluoride, carbon monoxide
Kidney disease	Lead, mercury, selenium, cadmium
Leukemia	Atomic explosions, radionuclides
Liver disease	Molybdenum, selenium, chlorinated
	hydrocarbons
Melanosis (dark skin)	Arsenic
Mesothelioma	Asbestos
Myalgia (muscle weakness	
and pain)	Fluorides, lead
Mutagenic agents	Chlorinated hydrocarbons, lead,
	arsenic, cadmium, radionuclides,
	mercury
Nasal irritation (septum)	Nickel, chromium, arsenic, selenium
Visual reduction	Ozone, selenium, fluoride

Table 24-2. Laboratory features in diseases caused by major pollutants

POLLUTANTS	BLOOD	URINE	OTHERS
Arsenic	Arsenic ↑ *		Hair, urine (As ↑)
Asbestos			Sputum, ferruginous bodies
Barium	Potassium ↓ *	Potassium ↑	
Beryllium	Uric acid ↑		Sputum, Schauman bodies
Cadmium	Alkaline phosphatase ↑	Microglobulin ↑ sulfur ↑ Glucose in urine	Nails (Cd ↑)
Carbon monoxide	Carboxyhemoglobin ↑		
Cobalt	Cobalt ↑		
DDT (chlorinated hydrocarbons)			Fat (DDT ↑)
Fluorides	Alkaline phosphatase ↑ Fluorides ↑	Fluorides ↑	Hair, bones (F ↑)
Hydrogen sulfide	Sulfhemoglobin		
Lead	Red blood cells (stippled) Delta aminolevulinic acid ↓	Coproporphyrin III ↑, lead ↑ Delta aminolevulinic acid ↑	X-rays of bones, abdomen
Manganese	Lymphocytes ↑		Hair (Mn ↑)
Mercury	Mercury ↑ uric acid ↑		
Nitrites	Methemoglobin ↑		
Organophosphates	Cholinesterase ↓	Nitrophenol ↑	
Pulmonary irritants			Chest x-ray
Selenium		Selenium ↑	
Vanadium	Cholesterol ↓ serotonin ↑		

* ↑ = increase; ↓ = decrease.

the vague symptoms of chronic poisoning, and the frequent absence of specific diagnostic criteria often preclude adequate documentation of the diagnosis of chronic poisoning. Therefore medical editors hesitate to publish data on chronic illness caused by air pollution, short of a major disaster that involves the health of a large segment of the population such as the Minamata mercury epidemic or the Itai Itai disease caused by cadmium in Japan. On the other hand, proof of the diagnosis by means of epidemiologic statistics is equally as difficult to establish because of the many variables encountered in chronic illness, especially in the composition of polluted air and in individual susceptibility of afflicted persons. Experimental studies in animals rarely take into account that human exposure to a pollutant can last throughout life,

that interaction of many pollutants can modify the clinical picture to such an extent that the characteristic features are unrecognizable, and that nutritional and prevailing environmental conditions cannot be duplicated in the animal experiment. Furthermore, susceptibility to disease in animals differs from that in humans.

I have repeatedly encountered patients with chronic diseases as a result of environmental causes who had been consulting outstanding physicians and leading medical centers for years before the diagnosis of intoxication as the result of a specific air pollutant was finally established. Even when the medical practitioner is informed concerning airborne illness, economic, political, and emotional factors weigh heavily in the interpretation of the clinical data with which he is confronted.

Table 24-3. Clinical characteristics of certain pollutants

POLLUTANT	CHARACTERISTIC
Arsenic	Dark skin, loss of hair
Asbestos	Ferruginous bodies
Barium	Thyroid disease
Boron	Brain damage
Cadmium	Hypertension, emphysema, osteoporosis
Carbon monoxide	Carboxyhemoglobin
Chromium*	Nasal irritation
Cobalt*	Thyroid disease, asthma
Fluoride	Skin (maculae), dental fluorosis
Iron*	Siderosis
Lead	Anemia, gastrointestinal symptoms
Hydrogen sulfide	Rotten egg odor
Manganese*	Ataxia, tremor
Mercury	Tremor
Nickel carbonate	Nasal irritation
Nitrites	Cyanosis
Ozone	Eye irritation
Quartz	Silicosis
Selenium*	Odor of garlic, tooth decay
Tellurium	Garliclike odor
Titanium	Yellow discoloration of skin
Vanadium	Respiratory symptoms
Zinc*	Fever

*Trace quantities of these elements are essential for life.

Some of the features that serve in the diagnosis of diseases caused by air pollution are outlined in Tables 24-1 to 24-3.

Denial of the existence of illness caused by air pollution

Textbooks and treatises concerned with certain pollutants often emphasize that no adverse effects on humans have ever been reported. In a strictly scientific sense this is perhaps true for certain pollutants but the conclusion that, therefore, no damage to health has occurred is unwarranted. A common trend among some scientists has been to disregard the possibility of damage to human health. For instance, in an article on lead intoxication of horses near a British Columbia lead smelter, damage to the animals is thoroughly aired, but ill-effect to humans is casually dismissed without adequate investigation.[1]

In a review of health effects by atmospheric pollutants one of the nation's most respected industrial toxicologists[2] attributes to fluorides only "beneficial" action on humans. He fails even to consider the possibility that they might be harmful at levels present in the atmosphere. Similarly, the effect of DDT and other pesticides on human health is being minimized in a large array of scientific publications. Another study regards arsenic and its compounds as relatively harmless poisons.[3]

The difficulties encountered in convincing the scientific community of environmental poisoning are described by Dr. Harriet Hardy,[4] who deserves much credit for the recognition and control of beryllium poisoning. Referring to the effects of this metal Dr. Hardy states:

Initially, much time elapsed because of poor communication between different investigators and between various countries. Next, suspicion centered upon a number of other toxic substances associated with beryllium especially fluorine. Then, different forms of the disease and similar problems in widely varying industries failed to be related. An emotional, and sometimes irrational, response by industry and the problems of trade secrets delayed progress. A number of animal experiments led to misleading conclusions. Governmental agencies mistakenly exonerated beryllium at a crucial time. Finally, with full recognition of the hazard, the solution came from relatively simple measures of industrial hygiene.[4]

These experiences point up the need for coordinated efforts by the leaders of the medical profession and call for an unemotional, straight-forward, and realistic approach to the subject. Communication between the environmental specialist and the practicing physician is one of the foremost requirements for further progress.

THE AFFLICTED PERSON
Avoidance of exposure

A person whose health is threatened by pollution is relatively limited in carrying out prophylactic measures. True, certain activities associated with pollution, such as idling of the motor of a bus or taxicab in a parking area can be discontinued. Habitual burning of refuse and leaves can be abandoned. Spraying with insecticides can be limited to the requirements necessary to prevent disease. Exercise in polluted air, that is, jogging or bicycling on a busy highway can be avoided. More difficult for some is to discontinue smoking, one of the greatest threats to health both in a polluted and nonpolluted region.

Change of residence

To persons residing close to a polluting factory or a busy highway the problem is more complex. The only effective way for them to avoid undue exposure to pollutants is a change in location. Owners of farms near an industrial plant cannot readily sell their land once the threat to health associated with the pollution becomes known, because of the concommitant depreciation of real estate values. Even temporary absence from their homes should be encouraged, since intermittent exposure to certain pollutants can mitigate illness caused by them (Chapter 6).

Consumption of contaminated food

In surveying the health of individuals in several polluted areas, I have encountered greater damage among residents who consumed produce grown in their own garden plot or small farm than among those who purchased their food from other sources. It is well established that most leafy vegetables and root plants contain higher levels of lead, fluoride, and cadmium when grown in an industrial area than they do when grown at a distance.

THE GOVERNMENT

Accomplishments. Governmental agencies on the international, national, state, and local levels have made great strides in recent years in the control of atmospheric pollution. Two outstanding examples of the effectiveness of governmental action is the reduction of sulfur dioxide and particulate emissions in London, England, as the result of the 1956 and 1968 Clean Air Acts, which prohibits burning of soft coal and encourages oil combustion for heating. It is said that London is enjoying 50% more sunshine now than prior to the passing of these acts. More than fifty types of birds that have been absent for years have returned to the parks of central London.[5]

An example of a significant breakthrough in environmental research (carried out in cooperation with the Los Angeles county and California state air pollution control agencies) is the discovery in 1950 of the chemical reaction of hydrocarbons and nitrogen oxides emitted from motor vehicles, which yields ozone and other toxic agents in the presence of sunlight, that is, the California smog.[6] The State of California has set the pace for effective pollution control. The output of pollutants in Los Angeles county has been reduced by legislative measures from an expected level of 26,000 tons to 14,000.[9] Other remedial legislation is the banning of mercury-containing fungicides for dressing grain in Sweden (1968), the prohibition by the city of New York, February 26, 1972,[8] of the spraying of asbestos fire-proofing, and the restriction of the use of certain pesticides in several states of the United States in 1972.

The U. S. Environmental Protection Agency. On July 9, 1970, the Environmental Protection Agency was formed. It is a strong, independent federal regulatory agency charged with responsibility to mount and integrate attacks on environmental problems. This agency is believed to be less plagued by conflicts than some of the other arms of government entrusted with the protection of the public. The Atomic Energy Commission, for instance, is charged with protecting the environment from radiation hazards, while at the same time it must promote nuclear power. The

U. S. Department of Agriculture, whose duty it is to control the use and the abuse of agricultural chemicals, must at the same time aggrandize farm yields.

One of EPA's first achievements was the establishment of standards for six pollutants—sulfur oxides, primary particulate matter, carbon monoxide, photochemical oxidants, nitrogen oxides, and hydrocarbons. Such standards are vital to legislatures in their efforts to institute measures to protect the nation's health.

Since contamination of food by certain atmospheric poisons is of equal if not greater significance than inhaled air in the causation of ill-effect, standards based solely on air quality cannot by themselves be considered adequate criteria for assessing health effects. Poisons in soil, vegetation, food, and water must all be taken into consideration in determining possible damage to human health.

The EPA has developed a system of year around monitoring of ambient air for its content of pollutants in a wide network throughout the country. There are three National Environmental Research Centers, each a complex of laboratories and associated facilities with continuing research teams. They are the Western Environmental Research Laboratory at Corvallis, Oregon, the EPA Center at Research Triangle Park in Durham, North Carolina, and the Cincinnati Center.[9]

Air quality data obtained from such studies furnish useful guidelines concerning overall distribution of pollutants both in urban and rural communities throughout the country. Valuable as these data are, they must be interpreted with discretion. Attention should be given to the residential areas in the environs of factories and superhighways, since the values obtained in such areas deviate considerably from the averages. Furthermore, sudden short-term outbursts of pollutants in a contaminated area are not reflected by charting the daily averages. The level of pollutants in ambient air does not parallel the magnitude of chemicals deposited over months and years on the soil, their entry into edible vegetation, their uptake by cattle from soil and forage.

The EPA has sponsored a wide variety of research projects. One of its joint research ventures with industry is the letting of contracts for "Clean Car" incentives to stimulate the private development of the "clean car" and the development of an experimental "clean" motor vehicle engine.

With respect to control of water pollution the agency has taken action to prohibit discharges of mercury and other industrial waste into lakes, rivers, and streams. New treatment of effluents and sewage for removal of phosphates from water, the use of pure oxygen instead of ordinary air in secondary treatment of sewage, the utilization of sewage for industrial purposes, and other projects have been developed largely with the financial support and advice of EPA.

By the end of 1971, EPA had closed 5,000 of the 15,000 open dumps across the nation. In 14 months they converted 800 of these sites into sanitary landfills.[9] Efforts are underway to separate waste material into commodities for recycling and to convert sanitary landfills into parks or golf courses.

The Community Health and Environmental Surveillance Studies (CHESS) compare the health of those who breathe polluted air with that of persons residing where the air is less polluted. Studies are underway on more than 38,000 volunteers whose health is being monitored. They involve the effect of pollution on respiratory diseases, on school absenteeism, on frequency of asthmatic episodes, on the death rate, on heart attacks, and so on. The findings are being distributed to industry, to scientific and educational organizations, and to agencies training workers for pollution control.

Systematic assays of human organs for suspected airborne toxic agents have not, as yet, been adequately carried out. Results of such assays could be related to the history and environment of the diseased person, to the residence, habits, occupation, nutrition, smoking, and other factors. They might thus contribute materially to recognition and prevention of damage to populations.

The Environmental Protection Agency sponsors fellowships and makes grants to universities for training future experts in environmental management.

Other subjects that deserve careful consideration by governments are the selection of sites for factories, the zoning of areas near polluting industries, particularly with respect to erection of dwellings, agricultural development, and forestry.

All these programs have enhanced our knowledge of air pollution as well as its control. Their effectiveness, however, must necessarily be gauged by the extent to which they avoid interference with industrial progress and economic development.

INDUSTRY

A vexing problem. Pollution has plagued industries for centuries. However, until the last two decades industry had been slow in introducing effective preventive measures.

Some corporations have attempted to solve their problem by buying up the land close to their factories in order to avoid damage to humans. Some have heightened their smokestacks, which reduces damage to the immediate environs. These measures have only limited value, since they fail to take into account the dispersion of pollutants into more distant regions. Others have installed pollution control devices at tremendous cost, but they have proved to be relatively little effective after they are installed.

Table 24-4. Tools for reducing industrial air pollution

METHODS	MODE OF OPERATION	SUITABLE FOR
Solid particles		
Mechanical cyclonic collectors	Whirling around in a funnel followed by gravitation into a funnel	Coarse particles; ore crushing; trapping flyash
Electrostatic precipitators	Gas-stream passes across electrically charged plates; particles are drawn to plates, then discharged into a storage hamper	Small particles (size: $> 1/10\ \mu$) Power plants, incinerators, smelters, paper mills
Wet scrubbers	Washing out contaminants	Removal of SO_2, H_2S, HCl; crushing and grinding plants
Fabric filters (bag-houses)	Principle of vacuum cleaner	Cement plants, iron foundries, steel furnaces
Gaseous		
Gas absorption	Use of a liquid to remove soluble gases that react chemically with the liquid	Fumes from plating and galvanizing tanks
Gas adsorption	Gaseous molecules adhere to surface of solids (carbon)	Dry cleaning; dye operations in textile mills
Gas combustion	A gas flame burns up the contaminant	Stack gases of refineries; paint oven fumes

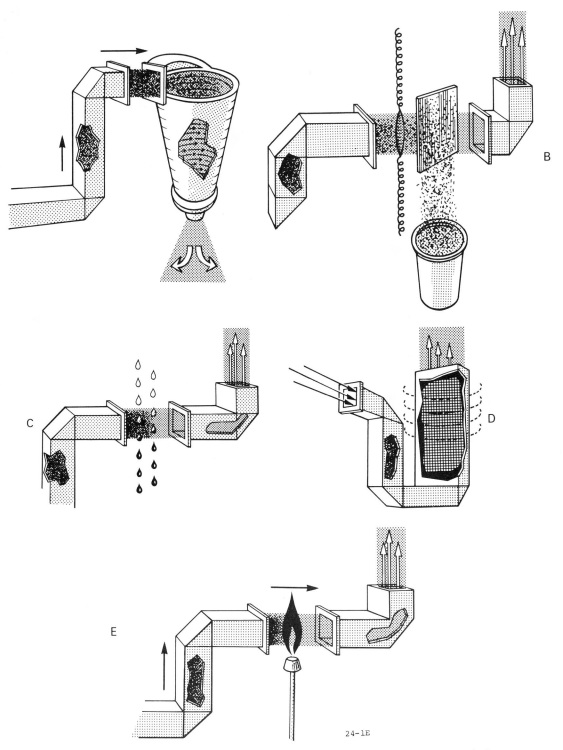

Fig. 24-1. Principles of removal of pollutants from stationary sources. **A,** Mechanical dust collectors. **B,** Electrostatic precipitators. **C,** Wet scrubbers. **D,** Fabric filters. **E,** Combustion removal of gases through flame.

Industry has established research centers throughout the United States, mainly in order to determine the action of air pollutants and to safeguard the health of its employees. Research at these institutions has led to significant advances in our knowledge, but clinical data on individuals or populations whose health is threatened by pollution are sparse.

Control of emissions. Measures for the control of pollution concern both stationary and moving sources.

Control of emissions from smokestacks. The major devices designed to control emissions of smoke are outlined in Table 24-4. The kind of antipollution equipment must be chosen according to the types of industrial operations, their size, and the chemical and physical properties of the contaminating agents. Whether the pollutants are gases or particulates must also be taken into account (Fig. 24-1).

Two serious problems have handicapped the control of emissions from factories, namely the fact that storage bins of raw, unfinished materials constitute a constant source of contamination inside and outside of a factory. This is true particularly in the fertilizer and cement industries where dust emissions are very difficult to control. Pollution control through wet scrubbers necessitates disposal of the dirty wash water. If conducted into rivers and lakes, the air pollution remedy becomes a water pollution problem.

Control of emissions from moving sources. A vast body of research is being conducted to reduce the output of air pollutants from automobiles, trucks, ships, and trains. The automobile industry is engaged in improving existing facilities and in searching for new sources of power such as the external combustion engine, gas turbines, and electric power. The chemical industry has been studying new fuels.

Emission from motor vehicles consists mainly of hydrocarbons, the unburned portion of fuel, of nitrogen oxides which are instrumental in formation of photochemical smog, of carbon monoxide and particulate solid matter, mainly lead particles. They are emitted from the crank case, the ex-

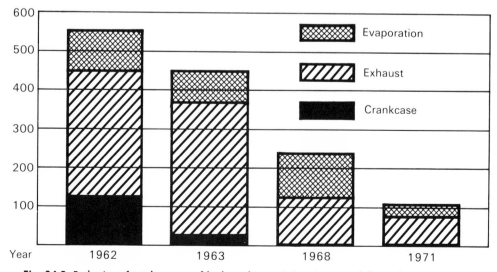

Hydrocarbons (grams per car per day)

Fig. 24-2. Reduction of total amount of hydrocarbon emissions in automobiles in the U. S. A.

haust pipe, and through evaporation of unburned fuel from the fuel tank and carburetor of an automobile.

The ideal solution to the problem would require the elimination of carbon monoxide as well as unburned and partially burned hydrocarbons and nitrogen oxides, by complete combustion of hydrocarbons and carbon monoxide to carbon dioxide and water vapor and simultaneous removal of nitrogen oxides.

Crankcase. Devices to recirculate unburned hydrocarbons in the crankcase have reduced their output by 20% according to data released by automobile manufacturers (Fig. 24-2).

Exhaust pipes. Emission of gases from exhaust pipes is being counteracted by installation of an afterburner that creates further burning by means of a regulated jet of air before the gases are released (Fig. 24-2). Other methods now in use involve a redesign of the engine with extensive modification of the combustion chamber, the fuel induction system, the ignition distributor, and other engine components.

Fuel tank, carburetors. Unburned hydrocarbons that evaporate from the fuel tank and the carburetors are being conducted into storage areas such as the engine crankcase or through a canister of activated charcoal granules where they are stored and burned when the engine is restarted.

Some of the other tasks to which industry is addressing itself concern the control of water pollution, recycling and re-use of trash, and replacement of harmful chemicals by less toxic ones.

TREATMENT

With respect to treatment of diseases caused by air pollution, only a few principles and major guidelines can be included here. As discussed in Chapter 5, the toxic agent might affect the activity of enzymes, it might combine with cell constituents and it might elicit secondary action because of its presence in the human organism. Each of these factors must be taken into account in establishing therapeutic measures. Treatment seeks to aid the system in its defense, by eliminating, detoxifying, or neutralizing the toxic agents and to counter their undesirable effect in the body.

Measures customarily employed in the treatment of acute poisoning such as the use of cathartics and emetics (vomiting-inducing drugs) are of relatively little value in chronic poisoning. They are of course often very beneficial in acute episodes of intoxication following ingestion of food contaminated by atmospheric poisons.

The overall management depends largely on the specific action of each pollutant. Antagonists for certain agents have already been named. For instance, sulfur will counteract cadmium; ammonia fumes neutralize sulfur oxides; calcium, aluminum, or magnesium compounds tend to combine with fluorides and render them less absorbable. Selenium and sulfur serve as antidotes for arsenic. Agents that counter oxidation such as vitamin E, and para-aminobenzoic acid (PABA) tend to lessen damage caused by the oxydizing action of ozone.

Poisoning from metals can be effectively ameliorated by the use of chelating agents such as calcium, EDTA, and levodopa.

Atropine combats the effect of acetyl cholinesterase deficiency in poisoning from organophosphate pesticides (Chapter 18). Oxygen is a valuable agent for carbon monoxide and hydrogen sulfide poisoning. Blood pressure reducing agents might benefit cases of chronic cadmium poisoning. For some toxic atmospheric pollutants such as silica, beryllium, asbestos, or the chlorinated hydrocarbons no effective antidotes are known. Therefore for such conditions as well as for respiratory diseases caused by most other respiratory pollutants physicians must rely upon purely symptomatic medication.

Drugs such as theophylline and epinephrine relax bronchospasm. Antihistaminics control the formation of mucus. Expectorants promote its elimination from the bronchial tree. Antibiotics counter secondary infection, which often supervenes following exposure to respiratory pollutants. Steroids (cortisone preparations) aid in the treatment of pulmonary fibrosis and granulomatous lesions of the lungs.

The early recognition and treatment of lung cancer has made considerable strides in recent years; prompt surgery combined with anticancer medication has led to complete cures. Allowance should be made for the fact that individuals show great variations in their response to toxic agents and that the human organism is not a statistical entity but is highly individualized. Nor can the findings in animal experiments, desirable as they are, be applied to the human organism without reservation.

REFERENCES

1. Schmitt, N., Brown, G., Devlin, E. L., and others: Lead poisoning in horses, Arch. Environ. Health **23**:185-197, 1971.
2. Stokinger, H. E.: The spectre of today's environmental pollution—U.S.A. brand: new perspectives from an old scout, Amer. Industr. Hyg. Ass. J. **30**:195-217, 1969.
3. Frost, D. V.: Arsenicals in biology: retrospect and prospect, Fed. Proc. **26**:194, 1967.
4. Hardy, H. L.: Beryllium poisoning: lessons in control of man-made disease, New Eng. J. Med. **273**:1188-1199, 1965.
5. Stewart, A. B.: Co-operation in prevention of air and water pollution, Roy. Soc. Health J. **92**:3-5, 38, 1972.
6. Haagen-Smitt, A. J.: Carbon monoxide levels in city driving, Arch. Environ. Health **12**:548-551, 1966.
7. Chass, R. L.: Profile of Air Pollution Control, Los Angeles, California, 1971, County of Los Angeles Air Pollution Control District.
8. Spraying of asbestos prohibited, Local Law 49 in Air Pollution Control Code of the City of New York. Sec. 1403.2-9.11 New York City Department of Air Resources, August 25, 1971.
9. Environmental Protection—1971. Washington, D. C., 1971, 0-450-479 United States Environmental Protection Agency, U. S. Government Printing Office.

APPENDIX

Threshold limit values of major contaminants adopted by the American Conference of Governmental Industrial Hygienists

Concentrations for a 7- or 8-hour work day and 40-hour work week

Acrolein	0.1 ppm	Molybdenum (soluble compounds)	5 mg/meter³
Aldrin	0.25 mg/meter³	Nickel, metal, and soluble compounds	1 mg/meter³
Arsenic and compounds (as As)	0.5 mg/meter³	Nitrogen dioxide	5 ppm
Arsine	0.05 ppm	Ozone	0.1 ppm
Barium (soluble compounds)	0.5 mg/meter³	Phosgene (carbonyl chloride)	0.1 ppm
Beryllium	0.002 mg/meter³	Phosphorus (yellow)	0.1 mg/meter³
Boron oxide	10 mg/meter³	Selenium compounds (as Se)	0.2 mg/meter³
Cadmium (metal dusts and soluble salts)	0.2 mg/meter³	Silicon	10 mg/meter³
Carbon dioxide	5,000 ppm	Sodium fluoroacetate (1080)	0.05 mg/meter³
Carbon monoxide	50 ppm	Sulfur dioxide	5 ppm
Chlorine	1 ppm	Sulfuric acid	1 mg/meter³
Chromic acid chromates (as CrO_3)	0.1 mg/meter³	2, 4, 5 T	10 mg/meter³
Cobalt	0.1 mg/meter³	TEDP	0.2 mg/meter³
DDT	1 mg/meter³	Tellurium	0.1 mg/meter³
Fluoride	2.5 mg/meter³	TEPP	0.05 mg/meter³
Fluorine	1 ppm	Tetraethyl lead (as Pb)	0.100 mg/meter³
Formaldehyde	2 ppm	Vanadium (V_2O_5 fume) as V	0.05 mg/meter³
Hydrogen chloride	5 ppm	Vinyl acetate	10 ppm
Hydrogen fluoride	3 ppm	Zirconium compounds (as Zr)	5 mg/meter³
Hydrogen sulfide	10 ppm		
Iron salts, soluble, as Fe	1 mg/meter³		
Lead	0.15 mg/meter³		
Lead arsenate	0.15 mg/meter³		
Lindane	0.5 mg/meter³		
Manganese and compounds	5 mg/meter³		
Mercury (alkyl compounds)	0.01 mg/meter³		
Mercury (nonalkyl)	0.05 mg/meter³		

GLOSSARY

acne skin disease involving mainly the face; consists of multiple individual papules—"pimples" filled with either a cheeselike mass or pus

acrolein toxic colorless liquid aldehyde with an acrid odor

adenocarcinoma malignant tumor with cells arranged like glands

adenoma benign tumor with a glandlike structure

aerosol solid particles or liquid droplets smaller than 100 μ in diameter, suspended in a gas

airway resistance resistance to the flow of air in the passage to the lungs

aldehyde organic compounds containing the group R-CHO; intermediate in state of oxidation between primary alcohols and carboxylic acids

allergenic allergy-inducing agent

alveolus (pl. alveoli) small, saclike dilation at the terminal end of the airway

antibody serum globulin synthesized by lymphoid tissue in response to an antigenic stimulus

antigen high molecular weight substance, usually protein; forms a specific antibody

atelectasis the collapse of all or part of a lung

atherosclerosis diseased arteries containing fatty substances

autosomes ordinary chromosomes in contrast to sex chromosomes

benzo[a]pyrene polycyclic aromatic hydrocarbon liable to produce cancer

bronchiectasis chronic dilation of a bronchial passage

bronchiole one of the fine subdivisions of the bronchial tree

bronchus (pl. bronchi) one of the large air passages in the lungs

carcinogen substance capable of causing living tissue to become cancerous

carcinoma cancer; malignant growth made up of cells derived from epithelial tissue

cardiovascular pertaining to the heart and blood vessels

cerebral cortex outer portion of brain

cholinesterase any one of several enzymes that hydrolize choline esters; occurring most frequently in nerve tissue and the blood

cilium (pl. cilia) small, hairlike process attached to a free surface of a cell

cyanosis bluish discoloration of the skin caused by excessively reduced hemoglobin.

dehydrogenase any one of various enzymes that accelerate removal of hydrogen from metabolites and its transfer to other substances, thus playing an important role in biologic oxidation-reduction

dermatitis

   contact allergic skin disease involving mainly the epidermis (uppermost layer of skin) caused by direct contact of the causative agent

   atopic involves mainly the second layer of the skin, caused by antigenic agents distributed through the bloodstream (food, pollen, and so on)

dyspnea labored breathing

edema accumulation of abnormally large amounts of fluid in the spaces between the cells of the body

effluent liquid discharged as a waste

emphysema, pulmonary overdistension of air spaces resulting in destruction of alveoli and loss of functioning lung tissue

epithelium sheet of cells arranged in one or more layers, covering the surface of the body and lining hollow organs

fetus unborn child

fibrosis development of fibrous (scar) tissue

gastric pertaining to the stomach

gastrointestinal pertaining to stomach and intestines

histamine substance that produces dilatation of capillaries

hydrocarbon compound containing only hydrogen and carbon

hyperplasia increase in number of cells with retention of normal function and cellular structure

hypertension high blood pressure

interstitial situated in the space between cells

larynx the voice box; situated at the upper end of the trachea

lipid fat

lymph fluid coming from body tissues; flows in the lymphatic vessels and eventually into bloodstream

lymph node accumulation of lymphatic tissue situated throughout the body

macrophage large phagocytic cell found in connective tissue, especially in areas of inflammation

mesothelioma tumor at the lining of a body cavity

motion, Brownian rapid random motion of small particles caused by bombardment by surrounding molecules, which are in thermal motion

mucus (adj. mucous) clear viscid secretion of a mucous membrane

mutagen agent inducing genetic mutations

nasopharynx part of the pharynx (throat) above the level of the soft palate

node circumscribed swelling

olefin class of unsaturated aliphatic hydrocarbons of the general formula C_nH_{2n}

phagocyte cell that ingests microorganisms and other small particles

pharynx upper expanded portion of the alimentary canal lying between mouth and nasal cavities

placenta organ inside pregnant uterus, which carries blood to and from fetus

pneumoconiosis fibrous reaction in the lungs caused by retention of certain inhaled dusts in the lungs

pneumonitis inflammation of the lung

radioautograph (autoradiogram) radiographic portrayal of an object or organism made by the inherent radioactivity of the object or organism

rale abnormal respiratory sound heard in the chest

sclerosis development of fibrous tissue

silicosis type of pneumoconiosis caused by inhalation of silica dust

spore a reproductive element of many lower organisms

stoma (pl. stomata) a small opening in the epidermis of a plant

synergism combined action of two or more agents

systemic relating to the whole body rather than to its individual parts

teratogen producing physical defects in developing embryo

trachea windpipe extending from the larynx to the two mainstream bronchi

urticaria hives; allergic skin disease that somewhat resembles mosquito bites

AUTHOR INDEX

A

Aaronson, T., 142
Abbasi, A. H., 144
Abe, M., 88
Abelson, P. H., 250
Abernethy, R. F., 110, 172, 174, 199
Abrahams, S. P., 211, 246
Abramowicz, M., 124
Abston, S., 222
Ackley, A. B., 184, 185
Addington, W. W., 196
Adelson, L., 127
Agate, J. N., 152
Ahl, T., 257
Ahlmark, A., 99
Akashi, S., 102
Akesson, N. B., 219
Akio, K., 203
Alaire, Y., 81, 83
Alden, H. S., 225
Algeri, E. J., 210
Allen, E. R., 82, 84
Allensworth, D. C., 124
Allison, A. C., 101
Alpert, M., 214, 254
Altshuller, A. P., 84
Ambrose, M. E., 170
Amdur, M. L., 176
Amdur, M. O., 8, 57, 81-84, 95, 103, 117
Anderson, D. O., 81
Anderson, L. W., 224
Anderson, R. F., 124
Anderson, R. P., 176
Anderson, W. A. D., 165
Andreeva, E. C., 88
Angino, E. E., 203, 262
Ansari, A., 102
Aranyi, C., 88
Archer, V. E., 246
Arena, V., 239, 241, 242, 244-247
Armstrong, W. D., 153
Aronson, A. L., 49
Ascher, M. S., 182
Ashenberg, N. J., 57
Aston, B. C., 103
Astrup, P., 124, 126

Athanassiadis, Y. C., 116, 117, 172, 174
Attala, R., 138
Autian, J., 230
Ayers, S. M., 68

B

Bachmann, R. C., 222
Bacon, J. F., 158
Bader, M. E., 199
Bader, R. A., 199
Baetjer, A. M., 201
Balassa, J. J., 133, 134, 161, 162, 173, 175, 200, 201, 252
Balazova, G., 159
Banford, F. N., 131
Bannon, J. H., 93
Bansal, B. C., 8, 154
Barach, A. L., 84
Bardelli, P., 49
Barnako, D., 132
Barrett, E., 257
Barry, P. S. I., 135
Bass, M., 218
Bates, D. V., 90, 91
Battigelli, M. C., 31, 69, 83
Battistini, V., 136
Baumslag, N., 202
Bazell, R. J., 49, 133
Bear, E. S., 236
Beard, R. R., 124
Beath, O. A., 169, 170
Beck, H., 86
Becker, R. O., 135
Beckman, H., 194
Beeckmaus, J. M., 117
Beland, J., 89
Bell, G. H., 152
Bellet, S., 253
Belsky, J. L., 247
Bercovici, B., 154
Berg, B. A., 173
Berg, E. W., 135
Bergmann, M., 111
Berlin, E., 132, 133
Berlin, M., 145, 228
Berman, E., 132

284

SUBJECT INDEX